Paediatrics
For UKMLA and Medical Exams

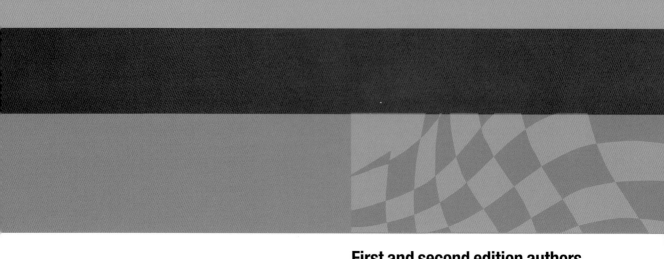

First and second edition authors

Christine Budd

Mark Gardiner

David Pang

Tim Newson

Third edition author

Shyam Bhakthavalsala

Fourth edition authors

Rajat Kapoor

Katy Barnes

Fifth edition authors

Anna Rodgers

Jessica Salkind

6th Edition
CRASH COURSE

SERIES EDITOR

Philip Xiu

MA (Cantab), MB BChir, MRCP, MRCGP, MScClinEd, FHEA, MAcadMEd, RCPathME
Honorary Senior Lecturer
Leeds University School of Medicine
PCN Educational Lead
Medical Examiner
Leeds Teaching Hospital Trust
Leeds, UK

FACULTY ADVISOR

Gerry O'Hare

MBBS, MRCPCH, FRCEM
Consultant Paediatrician
Leeds Children's Hospital
Leeds, UK

Paediatrics
For UKMLA and Medical Exams

Alyce Hayes

MBChB, BSc (Hons), MRCPCH, PGCertMedEd
Paediatric Registrar
Leeds Children's Hospital
Leeds, UK

Andrei Pobischan

MBChB, MRCPCH, BSc, MSc, PGCert Health research
NIHR Paediatric Academic Clinical Fellow
Leeds Children's Hospital
Leeds, UK

ELSEVIER

First edition 1999

Second edition 2005

Third edition 2008

Fourth edition 2013

Fifth edition 2019

Sixth edition 2025

Notices

ISBN: 978-0-4431-1537-0

Content Strategist: Trinity Hutton
Content Project Manager: Ayan Dhar
Design: Miles Hitchen
Marketing Manager: Deborah Watkins

Printed in India by Thomson Press (Ltd)

Last digit is the print number: 9 8 7 6 5 4 3 2 1

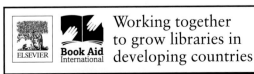

Series editor's foreword

With great honour and pride, we present the latest edition of the *Crash Course* series. This series has traversed a journey of nearly a quarter-century, stemming from the vision of Dr. Dan Horton-Szar, and his legacy continues to walk with us on this pathway of knowledge.

The series has been popular with students worldwide, selling over **1 million copies** and being translated into more than **8 languages**, reinforcing our commitment to global learning.

We remain extremely grateful for your unwavering trust. The series has once again been refreshed and fully upgraded in accordance with the rapidly changing medical guidelines, ensuring the content is comprehensive, accurate and fully up-to-date.

This latest series continues our tradition of integrating clinical practice with basic medical sciences, tailored meticulously for today's medical undergraduate curriculum. A central highlight of this instalment is our emphasis on high-yield exam content designed specifically for the UKMLA curriculum.

The addition of the **Rapid UKMLA Index** at the beginning of the book enhances this offering, serving as a valuable aid to students to track their exam preparation efficiently. We have also revised all self-assessment questions to align with the single best answer format in line with the latest UKMLA examination style. We have also added ***High-Yield Association Tables***. These are essential tools designed to aid students in recognizing clinical patterns and acing vignette-style exam questions. By condensing complex medical scenarios into digestible, manageable insights, these tables ensure efficient learning. They connect symptoms, diagnosis and treatment, bolstering understanding and confidence in tackling the rigorous UKMLA exams. This comprehensive approach makes these tables an indispensable asset in your exam preparations.

Utilizing student feedback, we have strived to maintain the core principles of this series: delivering precise and readable text that brings together depth and clarity. The authors are experienced junior doctors who successfully navigated these exams recently, ensuring practical and tested guidance. A team of expert faculty advisors from across the United Kingdom ensures the content's accuracy, making it resilient and reliable.

As we turn a new chapter with the latest edition, we honour the past, cherish the present, and embrace the promise of the future. We wish you every success in your journey of learning and growth and hope that this series adds value to your life, both as students and as future medical professionals.

Philip Xiu

Prefaces

Authors

Paediatrics is a far-reaching speciality encompassing numerous subspecialties within it. Looking after children and young people is extremely rewarding but the scope of practice is vast, and as such, a good breadth of knowledge is essential. Our hope and aim with this book is to condense information into clear summaries that can be easily absorbed during revision. Useful and pertinent information has been highlighted in boxes to add to your insight into clinical practice, gain extra points in exams and become competent doctors.

This book has been updated with the UKMLA in mind and has a wealth of new content included. Not only that, but this book also reflects recent changes in knowledge and practice within the field, for example, the COVID-19-induced PIMS-TS illness. This edition also reflects the multipronged assessment modalities used in medical schools, and as such there are numerous single best answer (SBA) questions, short answer questions (SAQs) and OSCE stations included to test your understanding and retention.

We hope that you enjoy studying with this book and that this may inspire some of you to consider an exciting career in paediatrics. Paediatrics is a challenging but constantly absorbing and interesting speciality that we would wholeheartedly recommend! We wish you all the best for your studies and future careers.

Alyce Hayes and Andrei Pobischan

Faculty advisor

I'm thrilled to be writing the preface to this, the sixth edition of *Crash Course Paediatrics*. This has afforded me an opportunity not only to work with an incredibly talented team, from the authors to Dr. Xiu and the Elsevier team, but also to explore, refine, and crucially explain child health – paediatrics - which is, unquestionably, simultaneously the widest ranging, the most challenging and the most rewarding discipline in medicine.

Crash Course Paediatrics, sixth edition, not only nails the key points, with an engaging layout, integrated tables and illustrations, but it is also full of explanations and gems that I find valuable every day; the self-assessment sections are fantastic at highlighting key areas and questions that you will encounter not only on the wards and clinics but also in formal assessments.

This crucially not only streamlines learning but also endows more time to spend with your paediatric patients - the (very) best bit!

Crash Course Paediatrics, sixth edition, is essential for students of every age. I hope you find it as rewarding reading as we have had writing and collating a brilliant text that will see you thrive through undergraduate into postgraduate child health!

Gerry O'Hare

Acknowledgement

We would like to thank our fantastic faculty advisor, Dr. Gerry O'Hare, for all his guidance and support during the writing process. His breadth of knowledge and up-to-date pearls of wisdom have been paramount in producing the sixth edition of this text. We would also like to extend our thanks to the series editor, Dr. Phil Xiu, and the whole team at Elsevier for their help and input during this project. In addition, thank you to our family and friends for supporting us in this endeavour.

Alyce Hayes and Andrei Pobischan

Series editor's acknowledgement

We would like to express our sincere gratitude to those who have provided their support and expertise in preparing this sixth edition of the *Crash Course* series. Our junior doctor contributors' participation in crafting the manuscript has been indispensable. Their first-hand experience and current medical knowledge have infused realism and practicality into our content.

Our faculty editors deserve a special note of thanks. They have extensively validated the correctness of the information, ensuring that the content is not just accurate but also contemporaneous, credible, and aligns with the latest medical standards.

We extend our heartfelt thanks to our publisher, Elsevier. Their staff have demonstrated an unwavering commitment to quality, maintaining the high standards set since the first edition. Their insights have routinely enriched the content and process alike.

Our Commissioning Editor, Jeremy Bowes, deserves a special mention for his consistent support and guiding hand throughout the development process. His directions and advice have bettered this edition and spurred us on our quest for excellence.

We are greatly indebted to Alex Mortimer for her wisdom, practical insights and valuable guidance. A big thank you to our Content Strategists, Trinity Hutton and Cloe Holland-Borosh, who need special acknowledgement for meticulously outlining the direction and scope of the content. They've managed to mix details with a strategic plan, keeping our readers in mind.

Lastly, much gratitude is owed to our Content Product Managers, Taranpreet Kaur, Ayan Dhar, Shivani Pal and Tapajyoti Chaudhuri, who have juggled the numerous day-to-day tasks with utmost dedication and perseverance. Despite the ever-approaching deadlines, they have shown remarkable patience and steadfast determination, ensuring that each step of the book's development was accomplished seamlessly.

In conclusion, we sincerely thank each of these wonderful people for their outstanding contributions and support, without which this work wouldn't have been achieved. Their passion, commitment and collaborative effort have helped us bring this edition together.

Philip Xiu

Rapid UKMLA Index

Table 2 UKMLA Presentations and Where to Find Them

Contents

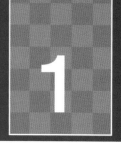

1

While most adult patients will comply with history and examination, it often takes skilled communication to perform these critical aspects of assessment in paediatrics. Building rapport with the child or young person, as well as their caregivers, is vital. Your approach should be age appropriate and flexible. The only way to gain these skills is by clinical experience, so make the most of your paediatric placements, taking opportunities to interact directly with babies, children and adolescents wherever possible.

When summarizing the clinical history and examination, think about how you would investigate and manage the case. It is good to practise this skill as a student, as it will be expected of you once you become a foundation doctor.

PAEDIATRIC HISTORY TAKING

Introduce yourself and establish who is in the room, taking time to develop rapport. While taking a history directly from the parent/carer can be tempting, especially where a child is shy or anxious, it is much better to take your account, at least partly from a child who can speak, wherever possible. This is particularly important where child protection concerns have been raised.

COMMUNICATION

It is vital to establish who everybody is and not make assumptions about how people are related (it is highly embarrassing to incorrectly assume an older mother is a grandmother or a two-dad family as a father and uncle!). A helpful approach can be to ask a verbal child, 'who have you brought with you today?' and confirm precise relationships with the adult(s).

ETHICS

The initial clerking is the appropriate time to establish parental responsibility, which is vital if consent for investigations or treatment is needed or if there are any child protection concerns. See Chapter 19 for more information on parental responsibility.

Presenting complaint

As with any history, begin with open questions to establish the reason for the presentation. Explore the nature of any symptoms, the onset, duration and precipitating factors. In addition, explore associated symptoms. If the child has a possible infection, find out if anyone is currently unwell at home, whether they have travelled abroad or eaten anything unusual. It is helpful to establish which symptoms worry the child and their parents most. Do not dismiss parental anxiety: a parent who tells you, 'my child is not himself/herself,' may have picked up on something you missed.

Medical history

Explore any previous diagnoses, hospital admissions and previous treatment. Many children will have no prior conditions, but some children, for example, those who were born very prematurely or with congenital syndromes, may have a list of medical history as long as many adult patients you have seen. It can be helpful to read previous discharge letters or clinic correspondence, especially if the child is under the care of a specialist centre.

Drug history

If known, take a complete history of current and previous medications, including doses, frequencies, route of administration and indication. It is essential to explore compliance with treatment – lack of compliance may be a safeguarding concern. Document carefully any drug allergies, including whether the child has taken that drug and the nature of the allergic reaction. Inquire about whether the child is up to date with their immunizations, and if not, explore the reasoning behind this. It may be that they are open to having catch-up immunizations which can be arranged via their general practitioner.

Birth history

In an older child, you only need to briefly establish any key events around birth (e.g., prematurity or congenital conditions). For neonates and infants, the birth history is critical (see the 'Neonatal history' section).

Developmental history

Ask about the age at which key developmental milestones were reached, including any concerns about vision or hearing. It is sometimes helpful to use phrases such as, 'is he/she able to keep

Example (autosomal dominant inheritance)

Fig. 1.1 How to draw a family tree.

up with their peers in PE?' or 'does he/she have the same skills as their friends at school?' See Chapter 17 for more details.

Family history

Ask about medical and mental health problems within the family. In paediatrics, drawing a family tree can be very useful in diagnosing heritable conditions and establishing the social history (see Fig. 1.1). Ask specifically about parental consanguinity, which can increase the likelihood of autosomal recessive conditions (e.g., metabolic conditions).

Social history

You must establish whom the child lives with, contact with parents/other caregivers they do not live with, and any social care involvement.

COMMUNICATION

Always ask about other services involved, particularly whether the family has any current or historical involvement with social care. You can preface the question by explaining, 'this is a routine question we ask all paediatric patients'.

Other important things to ask about include the following:
- parental occupations
- any difficulty at home (e.g., divorce, recent bereavements and domestic violence)
- pets at home and exposure to other possible allergens

- parent/carer smoking, alcohol or drug use. These questions should also be asked of an adolescent patient (see the 'Adolescent history' section).

RED FLAG

A thorough social history will allow you to identify children at risk of abuse. The 'toxic trio' are three factors identified together as high risk for child abuse:
- domestic violence
- parental mental health problems
- substance misuse

ADOLESCENT HISTORY

The key consideration when taking a history from an adolescent is always to offer to speak to the young person alone. This is important for two reasons. First, young people should be supported to take responsibility for their health, including interacting with the doctor or healthcare professionals. Second, and very importantly, there are many essential things that a young person may not be comfortable saying in front of their parents.

COMMUNICATION

An excellent way to speak to the adolescent alone is simply to say, 'we routinely speak to all young people of your age on their own and also with their parents/carers, are you happy for us to do that now?' and ensure you find a place somewhere for their parents to sit which is well out of earshot.

ETHICS

Confidentiality can be complex when working with adolescents, especially if they disclose a potential safeguarding risk. It is essential to be upfront with the young person by explaining that there may be situations where you would have to share what they have told you with another healthcare professional, and potentially their parents, but this is not common. You would always discuss it with them before doing so.

Adolescents generally appreciate honesty, so be upfront and acknowledge that some topics might be difficult to talk about. If you seem embarrassed, they are likely to be too.

The Home, Education/Employment, Eating, Activities, Drugs, Sexuality, Suicidal ideation and Safety (HEEADSSS) framework has been developed to explore different aspects of a young person's life.

- Home: find out where they live, whom they live with and whether there are any difficulties at home.
- Education/employment: find out about school/college and explore their plans/ambitions. Discuss friendship groups and any problems such as bullying.
- Eating: it is helpful to explore eating habits to detect any eating disorders which commonly start in adolescence. See Chapter 18 for more information.
- Activities: find out what they do in their free time, exploring hobbies and interests. This is an opportunity to discuss social media use, including potential risks like cyberbullying, 'sexting' and meeting up with people they have spoken to online.
- Drugs: explore smoking, alcohol and drug use and whether they have felt any peer pressure to use substances. You may want to explore how they are paying for any substances used.
- Sexuality: you may need to preface this by acknowledging that some young people find these issues embarrassing to talk about. Explore any relationships, whether they are having sex, using any forms of protection, and whether there are any issues around consent. Explore their feelings and whether they have felt pressured or unsafe during sexual activities.
- Suicide/low mood: ask about sources of stress and whether they feel down or anxious. If they do, you should specifically ask about self-harm and thoughts or plans of ending their own life. Evidence shows that asking about suicide does not make it more likely.
- Safety: you may have covered this already, but make sure you have established potential sources of danger at home, school, online or other arenas. Specific safeguarding risks include joining gangs, radicalization, child trafficking and grooming.

You will need to use your judgement: often, many of these areas need only to be briefly covered. If you feel unsure or things warrant further discussion, seek senior paediatric advice and help from your local child protection team.

COMMUNICATION

According to the Office for National Statistics, in 2020, 8% of young people identified as 'lesbian, gay or bisexual' – ask about relationships openly, making no assumptions about the gender of any partners.

HINTS AND TIPS

Society's understanding of gender is evolving rapidly. You should respect the identity of a young transgender person, using the names and pronouns they are comfortable with.

Many people are coming out as nonbinary: any gender that is not exclusively 'man' or 'woman' – explore what this means to the young person in front of you and mirror the language they use.

NEONATAL HISTORY

When taking a neonatal history, more emphasis should be on the details of the birth. Many maternal conditions affect the newborn infant, and the details of delivery and resuscitation are essential.

Antenatal events

- Establish the results of antenatal ultrasound scans and invasive testing (amniocentesis or chorionic villus biopsy).
- Ask about antenatal blood tests for infection.
- Ask about any maternal illness during pregnancy, such as diabetes and hypertension.
- Ask about maternal smoking, alcohol and drug use during pregnancy.
- Ask about previous maternal pregnancies and outcomes.

Birth

Key facts about the birth:

- gestational age at delivery
- mode of delivery
- duration of rupture of membranes
- birthweight

RED FLAG

In a neonatal history, you should ask about and document any risk factors for sepsis in the newborn:

Red flag risk factor:

- Suspected or confirmed infection in another baby during multiple pregnancies.

Other risk factors:

- Invasive group B streptococcal infection in a previous baby or maternal group B streptococcal colonization, bacteriuria or infection in the current pregnancy.

- Preterm birth following spontaneous labour before 37 weeks gestation.
- Confirmed rupture of membranes for more than 18 hours before preterm birth.
- Confirmed prelabour rupture of membranes at term for more than 24 hours before the onset of labour.
- Intrapartum fever higher than 38°C if there is suspected or confirmed bacterial infection.
- Clinical diagnosis of chorioamnionitis.

Postnatal events

- Whether the baby needed any resuscitation.
- Any problems encountered after birth, for instance, admission to the neonatal unit, issues with feeding or jaundice.
- Whether the baby is breastfed or bottle-fed, establish how often they feed and what volume.
- Whether they passed meconium within 48 hours (if not, could be suggestive of Hirschsprung disease) and urine within 12 hours (if not, could suggest a genitourinary problem, e.g., posterior urethral valves in a baby boy).

HINTS AND TIPS

It is helpful to review the personal child health record (or 'Red Book') for all infants and young children concerning immunizations and growth development.

PAEDIATRIC EXAMINATION

The key to a successful paediatric examination is being flexible and opportunistic. If the child sits quietly on their parent's lap, that is an excellent time to auscultate their heart. If they are already crying or screaming, you might be able to examine their throat. Watching a child playing on the floor in front of you will give much information about their neurology. The parent/carer is often the best person to help you to examine their child.

COMMUNICATION

Play is an excellent way to help young children understand and overcome anxiety. Asking the child to help you examine their teddy bear first is one way of doing this.

General examination

1. Ideally, you would measure the weight and height and plot on a growth chart. While not feasible in objective structured clinical examinations (OSCEs), you should mention this.
2. Look at the observation chart and compare their values with the age-appropriate normal limits (Table 1.1).
3. Does the child look generally unwell to you? If the child happily plays, this tells you they are unlikely to be seriously ill. A child that does not interact or react much to you examining them is a worrying sign.
4. Look generally at the colour of the skin, any rashes or injuries, and at the face for any unusual (dysmorphic) features indicating an underlying condition.

Respiratory system

- Count the respiratory rate. Note the different normal values with age (Table 1.1). Measure oxygen saturations.

Inspection

- Are there any clues around the bedside (e.g., inhalers or sputum pots)?
- Note any cyanosis or finger clubbing (Table 1.2).
- Inspect the chest for any chest wall deformities (pectus excavatum, carinatum) or scars suggesting previous surgery.
- Look for signs of respiratory distress:
  - Nasal flaring.
  - Use of accessory muscles to breathe or head bobbing in an infant.
  - Intercostal, subcostal or sternal recession.
- During your initial inspection, listen for audible stridor (inspiratory), wheeze (expiratory) and any cough (a barking cough is suggestive of croup).

Table 1.1 Acute paediatric life support normal ranges for observations

Age (years)	Heart rate (beats/min)	Respiratory rate (breaths/min)	Systolic blood pressure (mmHg)
<1	110–160	30–40	70–90
1–2	100–150	25–35	80–95
2–5	95–140	25–30	80–100
5–12	80–120	20–25	90–110
>12	60–100	15–20	100–120

For heart rate, respiratory rate and systolic blood pressure (different health systems may use marginally different standardized values – which are used in Paediatric Early Warning Scores – to detect physiological deterioration)

Table 1.2 Causes of paediatric clubbing

Respiratory	Cardiovascular	Gastrointestinal
• Pulmonary abscess or empyema • Tuberculosis • Cystic fibrosis/other cause of bronchiectasis	• Cyanotic congenital heart disease • Infective endocarditis • Infected graft	• Inflammatory bowel disease (especially Crohn disease) • Coeliac disease • Chronic liver disease

Palpation

- Feel for chest expansion and whether it is symmetrical.
- Assess for a central trachea and the apex beat.

Percussion

- Percussion is more useful in children over 5 years and can give additional information to auscultation alone – are there any areas of dullness or hyperresonance?

Auscultation

- Auscultate the chest over the front and back for:
  - Understanding whether air entry is equal.
  - Ratio of inspiration to expiration.
  - Any additional sounds: bronchial breathing, wheeze or crepitations (in a coryzal child, you may hear transmitted upper airway noises).

Cardiovascular system

- Measure the heart rate and blood pressure and compare them with the normal values for age.

Inspection

- Are there any clues around the bedside (e.g., supplementary oxygen or medications)?
- Note any cyanosis, clubbing or peripheral signs of infective endocarditis (splinter haemorrhages, Osler nodes or Janeway lesions).
- Inspect the chest for scarring.

Palpation

- Feel whether the peripheries are warm and well-perfused.
- The brachial pulses are used rather than the radial pulses. Palpating the femoral pulses is essential as they can be absent in the coarctation of the aorta.
- Palpate the apex beat: in dextrocardia, it is on the right.
- Hepatomegaly is one of the signs of cardiac failure. In contrast to adults, children with cardiac failure usually do not show crepitations or sacral/peripheral oedema.

Auscultation

- Auscultate for heart sounds and added sounds and murmurs.
- See Chapter 3 for the murmurs heard in specific conditions.
- Innocent murmurs are common in children and should be distinguished from pathological murmurs (Box 1.1).

Gastrointestinal system

Inspection

- Are there any clues around the bedside (e.g., vomit bowls or nasogastric feeds)?
- Note any clubbing, nail changes (leukonychia [low albumin] or koilonychia [iron deficiency]) or jaundice.
- Inspect the abdomen for distension and scarring.

Palpation

- Watch the child's face for any sign of tenderness.
- Feel for masses and organomegaly: the liver is usually palpable until puberty. In a constipated child, you may feel hard stool.
- Peristalsis: this might represent obstruction or pyloric stenosis.
- Assess for hernias.

HINTS AND TIPS

While palpating the abdomen, ask the child questions to distract them. Genuine tenderness (e.g., from an inflamed appendix) will not be distractible.

Percussion

- Percuss for organomegaly or a distended bladder.

Auscultation

- Auscultate for bowel sounds. Absence suggests obstruction.

BOX 1.1 FEATURES OF INNOCENT HEART MURMURS; THE 7 S'S

- Soft
- Systolic
- Short
- Sounds (S1 and S2) normal
- Symptomless
- Special tests normal (X-ray, ECG)
- Standing/Sitting (vary with position)

Nervous system

Most children will give you much information in their play, and the examiner must observe how the child interacts with their surroundings.

Observe:

- the gait as the child walks in
- posture at rest
- level of alertness or conscious level

Assess tone, reflexes, power, coordination and sensation, cranial nerves and cerebellar function for an adult, adapting your examination to the child's age.

Assess primitive reflexes in infants less than one year of age. See Box 1.2.

> **HINTS AND TIPS**
>
> The plantar reflexes are predominantly extensor (down-going) in infants aged <6 months, and the transition to flexor might be asymmetrical.

BOX 1.2 PRIMITIVE REFLEXES

- Watching paediatricians assess these reflexes on infants on the ward may be helpful. These can form part of both neonatal and neurological examinations.
- Asymmetric tonic reflex: present from birth to 4–6 months. Abnormal if fixed in one position, to one side or if persists at 6 months of age.
- Grasp: present from birth to 4 months. As the reflex disappears, infants can grasp voluntarily.
- Moro: present from birth to 4 months. Abnormal if it persists beyond this.
- Stepping: present from birth to 6–8 weeks; reappears at 10–15 months when the child starts walking (voluntarily).
- Downward parachute: develops between 6 and 12 months of age and persists. Abnormal if not present by 12 months.

Ear, nose and throat

This is often done at the end because it causes the most distress to the child (Fig. 1.2). The examiner must be helped by a parent who can hold the child still. The neck should be palpated for lymphadenopathy, and the ears should be examined. The throat should be looked at the end because a wooden tongue depressor might be needed to visualize the throat.

Never examine the throat if upper airway obstruction is suspected (e.g., epiglottitis or severe croup).

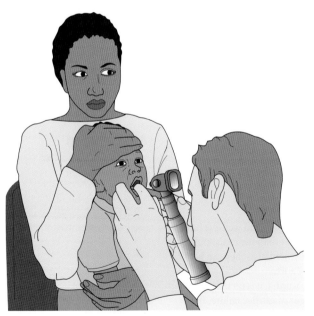

Holding a young child to examine the throat. The mother has one hand on the head and the other across the child's arms

Fig. 1.2 Throat examination. They are holding a young child to examine the throat. The parent has one hand on the head and the other across the child's arms. Remember to have a throat swab with you if pus or exudate is seen to avoid repeating the procedure.

THE NEONATAL EXAMINATION

All neonates should undergo a complete examination within 24 hours – a 'baby check' or newborn and infant physical exam (NIPE). This allows any abnormalities to be detected early and reassures parents of the numerous common normal variants found.

Begin by congratulating the new parents and asking whether there is any family history of congenital heart or hip problems. After a general inspection, a top-to-toe approach is usually helpful but if the baby is not crying, take the opportunity to auscultate the heart and lungs.

General inspection

- Assess the baby's colour, posture and activity. Look for any dysmorphic features.
- Measure the weight, length and head circumference.

Skin

- Many neonates show some jaundice. This becomes pathological if the level is above the treatment line or seen within 24 hours.
- Erythema toxicum is a benign condition affecting approximately 50% of all infants. It presents as macular lesions with a central yellow papule.
- Cyanosis can be challenging to detect and should be observed on the tongue and lips. Peripheral cyanosis without central cyanosis is not pathological (acrocyanosis).
- Pallor might represent anaemia or illness; plethora might be due to polycythaemia.
- Dermal melanocytosis (previously known as 'Mongolian Blue spots') must be documented because they appear identical to bruising. They are commoner in Afro-Caribbean babies and usually resolve by one year.
- Mottling is often seen in healthy infants (termed 'cutis marmorata') but must be distinguished from mottling in an unwell, septic infant.
- Vascular lesions such as infantile (strawberry) haemangiomas and port wine stains are relatively common. They are not concerning unless there are multiple, affecting function, ulcerated or they are on the face (Sturge Weber syndrome is discussed in Chapter 13).

HINTS AND TIPS

Note all grey naevi (=(Congenital) dermal melanocytosis – previously known as Mongolian blue spots or grey slate patches) for future reference, as they can be mistaken for bruises. These should also be documented in the child's health record (the red book).

Head and neck

Note the shape and size of the head and fontanelle. The sutures should be palpable, and head trauma from delivery may manifest as:

- Caput succedaneum: diffuse swelling that crosses the suture lines. It resolves in several days.
- Cephalohematoma: this never crosses the suture lines and is caused by subperiosteal haemorrhage; 5% are associated with fractures.
- Subgaleal haemorrhage: rare but potentially lethal neonatal condition where there is an accumulation of blood in the subaponeurotic space between the epicranial aponeurosis of the scalp and the periosteum. In term infants, this space can hold as much as 260 mL of blood, and a bleed can lead to severe hypovolemia.

Sternocleidomastoid tumours or thyroglossal cysts might be palpable as neck lumps in the midline. Palpable lymph nodes are found in 33% of all neonates.

Face

Observe for symmetry when the infant cries or yawns. Facial nerve palsy is common after forceps delivery and, in most cases, is self-limiting. This can suggest a rarer diagnosis such as CHARGE or Moebius syndrome, if persistent.

- Eyes: look for the red reflex (if absent, will need to exclude cataracts or neuroblastoma) and evidence of conjunctivitis. Occasionally the red reflex may be challenging to see, in which case it may be helpful to check the mother's red reflexes for comparison. Blue sclera is normal in babies aged <3 months.
- Ears: look at the position and for any skin tags.
- Mouth: loose natal teeth need removal. Palpate *and* look for cleft palate.

Chest

Commonly, periodic breathing can be seen, with pauses lasting less than 10 seconds. This is normal and more common in pre-term infants.

Auscultation for breath and heart sounds should be done when the infant is quiet.

- Breath sounds: listen for presence and symmetry.
- Heart sounds: listen for the quality and intensity of the heart sounds.
- Murmurs present after 24 hours of age should be re-assessed and an echocardiogram requested.

The femoral pulses should be palpated and, if weak or absent, might indicate coarctation of the aorta.

Abdomen

Many infants have a small degree of abdominal distension, a normal finding. Observe for:

- abdominal wall defects
- scaphoid abdomen suggesting diaphragmatic hernia

Examine for inflammation or discharge from the umbilicus. Separation should complete in 5 to 15 days.

Genitalia and anus

Girls: the clitoris and labia are usually enlarged, and vaginal bleeding might be observed. This is due to maternal oestrogen withdrawal and requires no treatment.

Boys: the testes should be palpable, and phimosis is normal. The foreskin should never be retracted. Check for hypospadias and good urinary stream in case of underlying renal pathology.

For the management of ambiguous genitalia, see Chapter 6.

Check for patency of the anus and that meconium is seen to be exiting from the anus to exclude any suspicion of a fistula; meconium should be passed in the first 24 to 48 hours. A delayed passage of meconium may indicate an underlying pathology (e.g., cystic fibrosis or Hirschsprung disease).

Limbs and spine

Examine all digits for palmar creases. Supernumerary digits (polydactyly) and abnormal fusion of the digits (syndactyly) are often familial.

The Barlow and Ortolani tests should be performed. In the Barlow test, backward pressure is applied to the head of each femur in turn; a subluxable hip is suspected based on palpable partial or complete displacement. The Ortolani test consists of forward pressure applied to each femoral head in turn in an attempt to move a posteriorly dislocated femoral head back into the acetabulum. Palpable movement suggests that the hip is dislocated or subluxed but reducible. Observe for leg length discrepancy and range of abduction; only gentle force is needed.

Palpate the vertebrae, looking for scoliosis. Any abnormal pigmentation, dimples or hairs over the lumbar region should raise suspicion of spina bifida. A sacral dimple is common and usually normal if the base is seen and <2.5 cm above the anus.

Neurology

The spontaneous movements of the infant (which should be equal in all limbs) should be observed, and then an examination of:

- tone: look for both hypotonia and hypertonia
- reflexes: both primitive and deep tendon reflexes

MEDICAL SAMPLE CLERKING

A sample medical clerking is shown in Fig. 1.3. It illustrates some of the points discussed earlier in this chapter.

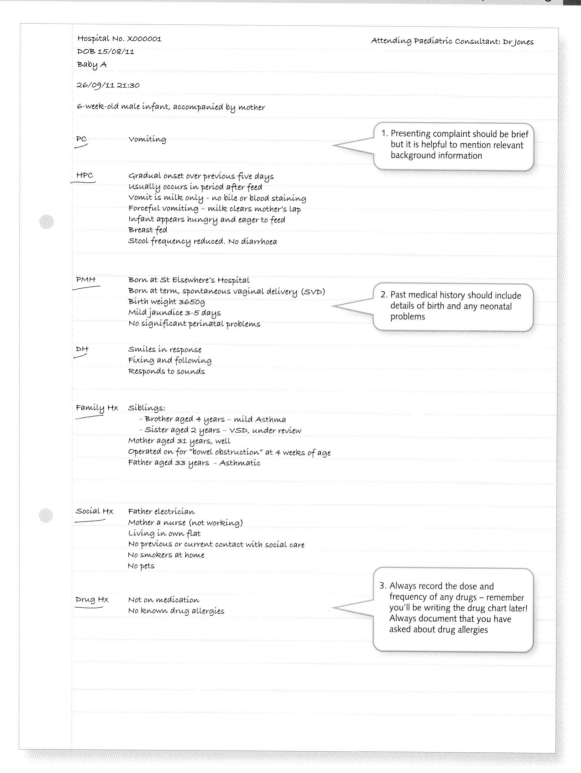

Hospital No. X000001   Attending Paediatric Consultant: Dr Jones
DOB 15/08/11
Baby A

26/09/11 21:30

6-week-old male infant, accompanied by mother

PC   Vomiting

> 1. Presenting complaint should be brief but it is helpful to mention relevant background information

HPC   Gradual onset over previous five days
            Usually occurs in period after feed
            Vomit is milk only - no bile or blood staining
            Forceful vomiting – milk clears mother's lap
            Infant appears hungry and eager to feed
            Breast fed
            Stool frequency reduced. No diarrhoea

PMH   Born at St Elsewhere's Hospital
            Born at term, spontaneous vaginal delivery (SVD)
            Birth weight 3650g
            Mild jaundice 3-5 days
            No significant perinatal problems

> 2. Past medical history should include details of birth and any neonatal problems

DH   Smiles in response
            Fixing and following
            Responds to sounds

Family Hx   Siblings:
               - Brother aged 4 years – mild Asthma
               - Sister aged 2 years – VSD, under review
            Mother aged 31 years, well
            Operated on for "bowel obstruction" at 4 weeks of age
            Father aged 33 years - Asthmatic

Social Hx   Father electrician
            Mother a nurse (not working)
            Living in own flat
            No previous or current contact with social care
            No smokers at home
            No pets

> 3. Always record the dose and frequency of any drugs – remember you'll be writing the drug chart later! Always document that you have asked about drug allergies

Drug Hx   Not on medication
            No known drug allergies

Fig. 1.3 Clerking.

Continued

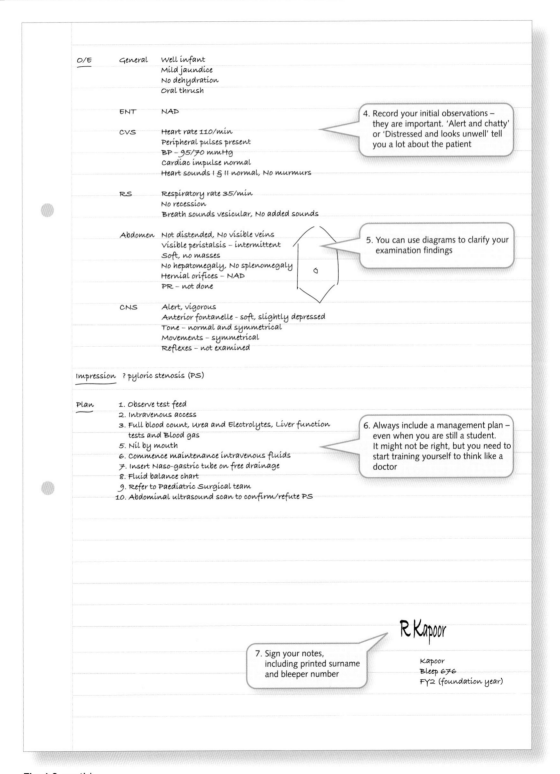

O/E   General   Well infant
                  Mild jaundice
                  No dehydration
                  Oral thrush

       ENT   NAD

       CVS   Heart rate 110/min
                  Peripheral pulses present
                  BP – 95/70 mmHg
                  Cardiac impulse normal
                  Heart sounds I & II normal, No murmurs

       RS   Respiratory rate 35/min
                  No recession
                  Breath sounds vesicular, No added sounds

       Abdomen   Not distended, No visible veins
                  Visible peristalsis – intermittent
                  Soft, no masses
                  No hepatomegaly, No splenomegaly
                  Hernial orifices – NAD
                  PR – not done

       CNS   Alert, vigorous
                  Anterior fontanelle - soft, slightly depressed
                  Tone – normal and symmetrical
                  Movements – symmetrical
                  Reflexes – not examined

Impression   ? pyloric stenosis (PS)

Plan   1. Observe test feed
         2. Intravenous access
         3. Full blood count, Urea and Electrolytes, Liver function
            tests and Blood gas
         5. Nil by mouth
         6. Commence maintenance intravenous fluids
         7. Insert Naso-gastric tube on free drainage
         8. Fluid balance chart
         9. Refer to Paediatric Surgical team
        10. Abdominal ultrasound scan to confirm/refute PS

R Kapoor

Kapoor
Bleep 676
FY2 (foundation year)

4. Record your initial observations – they are important. 'Alert and chatty' or 'Distressed and looks unwell' tell you a lot about the patient

5. You can use diagrams to clarify your examination findings

6. Always include a management plan – even when you are still a student. It might not be right, but you need to start training yourself to think like a doctor

7. Sign your notes, including printed surname and bleeper number

Fig. 1.3 cont'd

Chapter Summary

- You must be flexible and opportunistic with paediatric history taking and examination, adapting your approach to the child's age.
- Take a thorough social history, being aware of potential child protection issues.
- Always speak to adolescents on their own, as they may disclose things to you that they are not comfortable saying in front of their parents/carers.

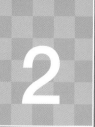
Investigations are often used to confirm, or refute, a clinical diagnosis or to monitor the progress of a disease or its treatment. In all cases, the clinician must consider the following:

- Will the results help inform or change patient management?
- Do the benefits outweigh the pain/discomfort to the child?

This chapter considers common and specialist investigations, focusing on the indications for doing them and how to interpret results.

URINE TESTS

A urine dipstick is a simple bedside test, which can look for protein, glucose, ketones, blood, pH, urobilinogen, leucocytes and nitrites. Results are obtained immediately and are not only useful in diagnosing urinary tract infections (UTIs; positive for leucocytes and nitrites) but also diabetes (glycosuria) and nephrotic syndrome (proteinuria). Methods of urine collection are discussed in Chapter 6.

BLOOD TESTS

Venous or capillary blood is usually satisfactory in children. Arterial blood sampling is only occasionally necessary for determination of oxygenation but pulse oximetry will often suffice. With experience, skill and local anaesthetic cream, blood can be obtained quickly and with minimal discomfort from most infants and children.

HINTS AND TIPS

Anaesthetic cream can be used in children over 1 month of age. It takes 30 to 40 minutes to take effect. Alternative analgesic options include ethyl chloride spray (cold spray) coupled with distraction techniques. Always take another person to help you take blood from a child.

Haematology

Full blood count

This provides information on:

- haemoglobin, Hb (g/L)
- total white cell count, white blood cell (WBC; $\times 10^9$/L)

- platelet count ($\times 10^9$/L)
- red cell indices: mean cell volume (fL), mean cell haemoglobin (pg), mean cell haemoglobin concentration (%)
- reticulocytes (%)
- differential white cell count: neutrophils, lymphocytes, eosinophils, monocytes (% or 10^9/L)

The examination of the film allows evaluation of:

- red cell morphology (Table 2.1)
- differential white cell count
- platelet numbers and morphology
- presence or absence of abnormal cells (e.g., blast cells)

See also Table 2.2, which shows important abnormalities that can be identified with full blood count (FBC).

HINTS AND TIPS

Haemoglobin concentration and white cell counts must be interpreted in relation to age:

- Hb concentration is high at birth (150–190 g/L) and falls to a nadir at 3 months (90–130 g/L).
- The total white blood cell is high at birth and rapidly falls to normal adult levels.

Haemoglobin electrophoresis

This detects variants in haemoglobin and is requested when a haemoglobinopathy is suspected. The pattern seen on haemoglobin electrophoresis varies at different ages (neonates vs. adults) and in different haemoglobinopathies (see Fig. 2.1).

Coagulation studies

This is requested to evaluate a bleeding disorder (Table 2.3), which is discussed in Chapter 8.

In addition to activated partial thromboplastin time (APTT) and prothrombin time (PT), fibrinogen is often measured. Low levels may indicate disseminated intravascular coagulopathy, severe malnutrition, end-stage liver disease or chronic hypofibrinogenaemia (rare). Fibrinogen is an acute-phase reactant, so it is raised in infection and inflammation.

Table 2.1 Red cell morphology

Appearance on blood film	Associated conditions
Normal red blood cell	Well child
Microcyte	Iron-deficiency anaemia
Macrocyte	Vitamin B12 and folate deficiency (megaloblastic anaemia)
Sickle cell	Sickle cell disease
Spherocyte	Hereditary spherocytosis
Target cell	Haemoglobinopathies Iron-deficiency anaemia Postsplenectomy
Schistocyte (fragments)	Disseminated intravascular coagulopathy Haemolytic uraemic syndrome

Table 2.2 Diagnostic indicators on full blood count

Abnormality	Differential diagnosis
Anaemia (Hb values age dependant)	Many causes (see Chapter 8), including: Iron deficiency (most common) Haemolysis Haemoglobinopathies Haemorrhage
Thrombocytopaenia (platelets <150 × 10^9/L)	Idiopathic thrombocytopaenic purpura (ITP) Malignancy (including Leukaemia) Disseminated intravascular coagulopathy (DIC) Hypersplenism
Neutropaenia (neutrophil values age dependent)	Immunodeficiency Infection (particularly in neonates)
Pancytopaenia	Malignancy (e.g., acute lymphoblastic leukaemia) Inherited causes of bone marrow failure (rare)
Neutrophilia (neutrophil values age dependent)	Bacterial infection
Lymphocytosis (lymphocyte values age dependent)	Viral infection (marked in *Bordetella pertussis*)

Biochemical analysis

Urea and electrolytes

Urea and electrolytes (U&Es) are the most commonly requested biochemical analysis and can be useful in a host of circumstances including:

- dehydration
- patients on intravenous fluids – monitoring electrolyte status
- diabetic ketoacidosis
- renal disease
- diuretic therapy

Sodium (Na$^+$)

Serum sodium levels reflect extracellular water shifts. It is important to avoid rapid changes in sodium concentration because cerebral oedema or myelinolysis might result.

- Hyponatraemia (either a result of excess water, i.e., overuse of hypotonic fluids, or sodium depletion, e.g., diuretic therapy).
- Hypernatraemia (either a result of water deficit/poor feeding in a neonate or sodium excess, e.g., salt poisoning).

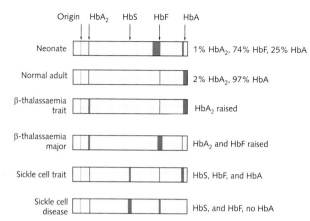

Fig. 2.1 Haemoglobin electrophoresis.

Neonate — 1% HbA$_2$, 74% HbF, 25% HbA
Normal adult — 2% HbA$_2$, 97% HbA
β-thalassaemia trait — HbA$_2$ raised
β-thalassaemia major — HbA$_2$ and HbF raised
Sickle cell trait — HbS, HbF, and HbA
Sickle cell disease — HbS, and HbF, no HbA

Origin HbA$_2$ HbS HbF HbA

Table 2.3 Interpretation of coagulation studies

Prothrombin time (PT)	Activated partial thromboplastin time (APTT)	Differential diagnosis
Prolonged	Normal	Liver disease Vitamin K deficiency Factor VII deficiency
Normal	Prolonged	Haemophilia A (factor VIII deficiency) Haemophilia B (factor IX deficiency) von Willebrand disease Factor XI/XII deficiency
Prolonged	Prolonged	Disseminated intravascular coagulopathy (DIC) Factor I, II, V or X deficiency Severe liver disease
Normal	Normal	Thrombocytopaenia Platelet dysfunction Minor factor deficiencies

---

> **HINTS AND TIPS**
>
> Concerning plasma sodium:
> - Artefactually low plasma Na$^+$ concentration can occur with hyperlipidaemia (e.g., in diabetic ketoacidosis, parenteral feeding).
> - A normal plasma Na$^+$ concentration might be found in salt depletion or overload if associated parallel changes in body water have occurred.
> - Rapid falls in plasma Na$^+$ can cause cerebral oedema.
> - In diabetic ketoacidosis, intracellular-extracellular fluid shifts can occur as hyperglycaemia is treated. This causes a rapidly rising serum sodium. Therefore, corrected sodium levels are often used.

See Chapter 21 for more details on causes and treatment.

> **RED FLAG**
>
> Electrocardiogram (ECG) changes and arrhythmias may occur with severe hyperkalaemia (Fig. 2.2). It is a potentially reversible cause of cardiac arrest.
>
> ECG changes in hyperkalaemia include:
> - Flattened P waves.
> - Broad QRS complexes.
> - Tented T waves.
> - Sine waves are a late sign.

Potassium (K$^+$)

Hypokalaemia is usually a result of potassium depletion (e.g., gastrointestinal loss) or inadequate intake (e.g., anorexia) or inadequate total parenteral nutrition constitution.

Hyperkalaemia is potentially dangerous, but children and neonates are less vulnerable to hyperkalaemia than adults. The most common cause is renal failure, which is an excretion problem, but it can also occur in severe acidosis, hypoaldosteronism and through prescribing errors.

See Chapter 21 for more details on causes and treatment.

Chloride (Cl$^-$)

Hypochloraemia is seen particularly in vomiting associated with pyloric stenosis and leads to a metabolic alkalosis.

Urea

Urea is a major metabolite of protein catabolism. It is synthesized in the liver and excreted by the kidneys. The plasma concentration is influenced by:

- state of hydration
- protein intake
- catabolism
- glomerular filtration rate (GFR)

The creatinine concentration is a more reliable indicator of renal function. The most commonly encountered cause of a raised plasma urea is dehydration.

Creatinine

Creatinine is a naturally occurring substance that is formed in muscles. The normal plasma concentration increases with age as muscle mass increases with growth. The plasma concentration of creatinine is a useful indirect measure of the GFR. In renal failure, the creatinine concentration increases steadily by more than 3 mmol/L per day.

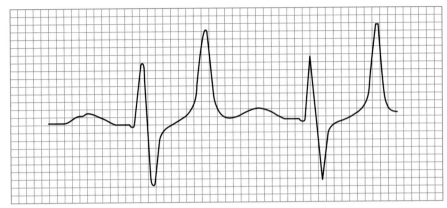

Fig. 2.2 This electrocardiogram demonstrates hyperkalaemic changes, with flat P waves, broad QRS complexes and tall, tented T waves.

Liver function tests

The basic biochemical tests of liver function include bilirubin, hepatic enzymes and albumin, and these are outlined in the following sections.

Bilirubin

Clinical evaluation of the severity of jaundice is unreliable, so it is important to measure plasma levels of bilirubin. If the unconjugated bilirubin is abnormally high, the conjugated fraction must also be measured. The normal proportion of conjugated bilirubin should not exceed 10% in infants. The causes of hyperbilirubinaemia are considered elsewhere (see Chapter 15).

Enzymes

- Transaminases (aminotransferases): Aspartate transaminase (AST) and Alanine transaminase (ALT).
- Alkaline phosphatase.
- γ-Glutamyltranspeptidase (GGT).

Transaminases (aminotransferases). These occur in many tissues including the liver, heart and skeletal muscle. Normal plasma levels reflect release of enzymes during cell turnover and their levels increase with tissue injury. Elevated aminotransferase activity is primarily seen in hepatocyte damage, for example, hepatitis (infection, drugs); however, it may also occur in other forms of hepatobiliary disease (e.g., biliary atresia, cholecystitis) and in nonhepatic conditions such as myocarditis and pancreatitis.

AST is the more sensitive indicator of liver injury, but ALT is more specific.

Alkaline phosphatase. Isoenzymes of alkaline phosphatase are widely distributed in many organs including the liver and bone. Normal activity levels change markedly throughout childhood, and reference ranges are both age and method dependent. Activity is increased in:

- Biliary obstruction: intrahepatic or extrahepatic.
- Hepatocellular damage.

- Increased osteoblastic activity (e.g., rickets, metabolic bone disease of prematurity and at times of normal growth spurts).

γ-Glutamyltranspeptidase (GGT). Serum activity is commonly raised in liver disease especially when there is cholestasis. It might also be raised in the absence of liver disease in patients taking certain drugs, for example, phenytoin, phenobarbital and rifampicin (as a result of enzyme induction).

Additional investigations, which are useful for evaluating hepatic function (and are therefore deranged in liver failure), include:

- Coagulation tests: PT, APTT.
- Ammonia.
- Glucose.

Albumin

Albumin is synthesized in the liver and is the main contributor to plasma oncotic pressure. It also has an important role as the protein to which many circulating substances are bound such as:

- bilirubin
- calcium
- drugs
- hormones

Albumin has a long half-life of about 20 days. Plasma albumin levels are a useful indicator of hepatic function. Low levels occur in several important clinical contexts (Table 2.4).

Prolonged hypoalbuminaemia (e.g., in nephrotic syndrome) is associated with oedema because fluid leaks into the extravascular space and hypovolaemia triggers renal salt and water retention.

Glucose

Blood glucose concentrations are normally maintained within fairly narrow limits, which are lower in the newborn. Blood glucose can be estimated very rapidly at the bedside using test sticks

Table 2.4 Causes of hypoalbuminaemia (albumin <30 g/L)

Mechanism	Cause
Decreased synthesis	Chronic liver failure
	Malnutrition
	Malabsorption
Increased losses	Nephrotic syndrome
	Burns
	Protein-losing enteropathy

BOX. 2.2 CAUSES OF HYPOCALCAEMIA AND HYPERCALCAEMIA

Hypocalcaemia	Hypercalcaemia
Rickets (low vitamin D and phosphate, high alkaline phosphatase)	Hyperparathyroidism
	William syndrome
Hypoparathyroidism (e.g., DiGeorge syndrome)	Iatrogenic (e.g., excess vitamin D or calcium supplementation)
Hypoalbuminaemia	

or by taking a blood gas, but values should be verified by laboratory investigation.

Common causes of hypoglycaemia and hyperglycaemia in children are listed in Box 2.1. Of note, diabetes mellitus type 2 is increasingly seen in children as obesity prevalence rises.

RED FLAG

Always measure the blood glucose urgently in a fitting or unconscious child as this is potentially reversible with a 10% dextrose bolus of 2 mL/kg.

Calcium and phosphate

Disorders of calcium and phosphate metabolism in childhood are uncommon and usually reflect abnormalities in the major controlling hormones, vitamin D and parathyroid hormone.

BOX 2.1 CAUSES OF HYPOGLYCAEMIA AND HYPERGLYCAEMIA

Hypoglycaemia	Hyperglycaemia
Endocrine: Hyperinsulinism (includes infant of diabetic mother), hypopituitarism, hypothyroidism, congenital adrenal hyperplasia	**Diabetes:** Type 1 diabetes mellitus (most common in children), Type 2 secondary causes (e.g., pancreatic insufficiency in cystic fibrosis, Cushing syndrome, obesity)
Metabolic: Medium chain acyl-CoA dehydrogenase deficiency (MCADD), organic acidaemia, ketotic hypoglycaemia, galactosaemia	**Post seizure**
	Sepsis
Toxic: Alcohol, insulin, oral hypoglycaemics, valproate	**Iatrogenic** (e.g., corticosteroids, sampling error, high glucose concentration in total parenteral nutrition)
Hepatic: Cirrhosis, hepatitis	
Systemic: Starvation, malnutrition, sepsis, malabsorption	

Laboratory estimations provide a measure of both total and ionized calcium. Changes in plasma albumin concentration affect total calcium levels independently of ionized calcium, leading to misinterpretation if serum albumin is outside the normal range. Therefore, the total calcium concentration needs to be corrected to give the expected value if albumin were in the normal range. Major causes of hypercalcaemia and hypocalcaemia are shown in Box 2.2.

RED FLAG

Calcium and magnesium levels should be measured in children with seizures (hypomagnesaemia can cause refractory hypocalcaemia until treated).

Blood gases and acid–base metabolism

Metabolism generates acid, which is eliminated via the lungs as carbon dioxide and via the kidneys as hydrogen ions. Acidosis, from whatever cause, is a much more common problem than alkalosis. Ideally, estimations of blood gas and acid–base status are made on an arterial sample, but in paediatrics capillary or venous blood is more commonly used as arterial sampling can be painful. Where the main concern is oxygenation, noninvasive pulse oximetry is a valuable alternative to arterial blood gas analysis.

The pattern of changes seen in different forms of acidosis and alkalosis is shown in Table 2.5. When compensation occurs, respiratory compensation will occur almost immediately whilst metabolic compensation is a slower process that indicates a more chronic cause.

The clinical contexts in which these disturbances occur are many; the common ones are:

- Respiratory acidosis: hypoventilation (e.g., respiratory distress syndrome or apnoea in preterm infants, life-threatening asthma, neuromuscular diseases).

Table 2.5 Acid–base disturbances

	pH	Partial pressure of carbon dioxide (PaCO$_2$)	HCO$_3^-$
Acidosis			
Respiratory	Low	High	Normal High (compensation)
Metabolic	Low	Normal Low (compensation)	Low
Alkalosis			
Respiratory	High	Low	Normal Low (compensation)
Metabolic	High	Normal High (compensation)	High

- Metabolic acidosis: diabetic ketoacidosis, diarrhoea, renal tubular acidosis, raised lactate (e.g., sepsis, hypoxic injury).
- Respiratory alkalosis: hyperventilation (e.g., hysteria in panic disorders or iatrogenic in ventilated patients).
- Metabolic alkalosis: pyloric stenosis, congenital chloridorrhoea, Bartter syndrome, Gitelman syndrome.

Immunology

Tests of the immune system carried out on the blood might be required in the following clinical contexts:

- infection: diagnostic serology, acute-phase reactants
- immunodeficiency
- autoimmune disease

Tests for immunodeficiency

Immunodeficiencies can be primary or secondary. The inherited primary deficiencies are rare; secondary causes are far more common.

Immunodeficiency should be suspected in the following clinical circumstances:

- family history of primary immunodeficiency
- recurrent severe infections
- infections with atypical organisms
- common infections with a severe or atypical clinical course
- failure to thrive

Basic screening tests of immune function should include:

- FBC including differential white cell count
- T lymphocyte subsets
- immunoglobulins (Igs)
- human immunodeficiency virus (HIV) test

CAUSES OF IMMUNODEFICIENCY

Primary

Combined (T-cell and antibody) deficiency disorders:

- Severe combined immunodeficiency (SCID)
- Wiskott-Aldrich syndrome
- Ataxia Telangiectasia

Major antibody deficiency:

- X-linked agammaglobulinaemia (XLA)
- Common variable immunodeficiency disorders (CVID)

Major neutrophil disorders:

- Severe congenital neutropaenia (SCN)
- Chronic granulomatous disease (CGD)
- Leucocyte adhesion deficiency (LAD)

Innate disorders:

- Familial haemophagocytic lymphohistiocytosis (HLH) syndromes
- Chediak-Higashi syndrome

Complement disorders:

- Classical pathway complement deficiencies
- Alternate pathway complement deficiencies
- Mannose-binding lectin (MBL) deficiency

Secondary

- Malnutrition
- Infections (e.g., human immunodeficiency virus, measles)
- Immunosuppressive therapy (e.g., steroids, cytotoxic drugs)
- Hyposplenism (e.g., sickle cell disease, splenectomy)

Immunoglobulins

Serum Ig levels vary with age. Maternally transferred IgG is present at high levels at birth but will mostly disappear by 6 months of age. This decline occurs before endogenous synthesis has fully developed, creating a physiological trough between 3 and 6 months of age. This is shown in Fig. 2.3.

IgG is the major Ig in normal human serum, accounting for about 70% of the total pool. There are four distinct subclasses (IgG-1 to IgG-4), which have different functions. Specific IgM changes are very useful in the diagnosis of viral infections (e.g., rubella).

HINTS AND TIPS

- Selective IgA deficiency is common (1:700 population) and might cause no symptoms.
- IgG2 is the most common subclass deficiency and might be associated with IgA deficiency. The total IgG level might be normal. It causes recurrent respiratory infections (e.g., sinusitis, pneumonia).

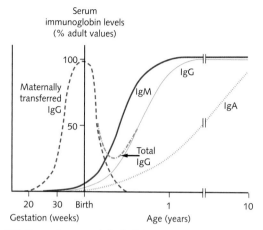

Fig. 2.3 Serum immunoglobulin (Ig) levels in fetus and infant.

Differential white cell count

Immunodeficiency caused by marrow-suppressive cytotoxic or immunosuppressive therapy is related to the absolute neutrophil count. Patients with absolute neutrophil counts below $1.0 \times 10^9/L$ are at increased risk of overwhelming bacterial infections and sepsis.

Lymphocyte subsets

Lymphocytes are further subdivided into T cells and B cells. T cells are categorized into:

- Cytotoxic T cells (TCs), which are mostly CD8+.
- Helper T cells (THs), which are mostly CD4+.

TCs recognize infected target cells and lyse them. THs secrete regulatory molecules (lymphokines) that affect other T cells and cells of various lineages.

Monitoring absolute numbers of CD4+ helper cells is useful in monitoring the progression of HIV-related diseases.

Autoantibodies

Autoimmune disease is uncommon in childhood but includes such entities as juvenile idiopathic arthritis (JIA), systemic lupus erythematosus (SLE) and Hashimoto thyroiditis. The following tests might be of value:

Antinuclear antibodies. Antinuclear antibodies are a broad group of antibodies present in 5% of normal children, but also induced by a wide spectrum of inflammatory conditions:

- SLE (raised in 95% cases)
- JIA (if raised is a risk factor for chronic anterior uveitis)

SLE is also associated with antibodies against specific nuclear antigens such as double-stranded DNA.

Rheumatoid factors. Rheumatoid factors are IgM autoantibodies against IgG. They should not be used to screen for JIA because they are neither sensitive nor specific. The majority of children with JIA are rheumatoid factor negative. Rheumatoid

factors can be useful as a prognostic indicator in polyarticular JIA (their persistent presence is a poor prognostic factor).

Thyroid antibodies. Antithyroid peroxidase (anti-TPO), TSH receptor (TRAbs) and thyroglobulin antibody titres should be measured in suspected autoimmune thyroid disease (e.g., Hashimoto thyroiditis and Grave disease).

Diagnostic serology

This is most widely used in the diagnosis of viral infections but is also of value in certain specific nonviral infections such as *Mycoplasma pneumoniae*, group A β-haemolytic streptococci and *Salmonella* spp.

Viral antibody tests

Serological diagnosis depends on the detection of virus antibody. Diagnosis of recent infection requires the demonstration of a rising titre of specific IgM between the acute phase and convalescence. Methods used include:

- immunofluorescence
- enzyme-linked immunosorbent assay
- radioimmune assay

Epstein–Barr virus. Specific Epstein–Barr virus serology is the most reliable diagnostic test. Antibodies to viral capsid antigen (VCA) are detected. IgG anti-VCA merely indicates a past infection. A positive IgM to VCA is diagnostic and is found early in the disease.

Tests for heterophile antibody, which agglutinates sheep red blood cells, are the basis of slide agglutination tests (monospot and Paul–Bunnell). However, this antibody does not appear until the second week or even later, and may not be produced at all in young children.

Mycoplasma pneumoniae. Diagnosis of infection with *M. pneumoniae* is most quickly established by acute and convalescent serology: a fourfold rise in complement-fixing antibodies is diagnostic.

Antistreptolysin O titre. Estimation of antibody to streptolysin O is a useful means of retrospectively diagnosing infection by group A β-haemolytic streptococci. The antistreptolysin O test is a valuable investigation in the evaluation of:

- suspected acute nephritis
- rheumatic fever
- scarlet fever

Acute-phase reactants

An inflammatory stimulus provokes the production of proteins in the liver known as the acute-phase reactants. This response is documented by the measurement of:

- C-reactive protein (CRP)
- erythrocyte sedimentation rate (ESR)

The response is nonspecific and does not help in identifying aetiology. However, if acute-phase reactants are elevated at the onset of disease, serial measurements are useful for monitoring progress.

The response times vary:

- CRP: elevated within 6 hours
- ESR: peaks at 3 to 4 days

Microbiology
Urine culture
Pus cells and bacteria are easily identified on microscopy; however, pyuria can occur with fever in the absence of UTI, and cell lysis might obscure pyuria if the sample is not examined immediately. The urine white cell count is not therefore a reliable feature in the diagnosis of UTI. Confident diagnosis of a UTI requires a bacterial culture of more than 10^5/mL colony-forming units of a single species in a properly collected specimen.

Microscopy can also be used to look for casts and red cells in suspected glomerular disease.

Blood culture
Blood is normally sterile. Transient asymptomatic bacteraemia can occur after dental treatment, or invasive procedures such as catheterization. However, bacteraemia leading to septicaemia and shock can accompany a number of important childhood diseases such as pneumonia and meningitis.

Blood culture should be taken under the following circumstances:

- pyrexia of unknown origin
- suspected sepsis
- fever in an immunodeficient child (e.g., sickle-cell disease, nephrotic syndrome, neutropenia) or in any patient with a central catheter

The most common pathogens affecting newborns are:

- group B streptococcus
- Staphylococcus aureus
- coagulase-negative staphylococci
- coliforms (e.g., enterococcus, Escherichia coli and Klebsiella)

These are primarily bacteria that are present in or around the birth canal. The organisms that typically affect older children include:

- Streptococcus pneumoniae
- Neisseria meningitidis
- S. aureus
- Salmonella spp
- Haemophilus influenzae type B

Most significant isolates will be obtained within 48 hours of inoculation.

Upper respiratory culture
- Nasopharyngeal aspirates are best for diagnosing viral respiratory tract infections. They are sent for immunofluorescence and results are usually back on the same day. Rapid antigen tests for COVID, influenza and respiratory syncytial virus are available and can offer a bedside diagnosis (point-of-care testing (POCT)).
- Throat swabs are useful to diagnose pharyngeal infections.
- A pernasal swab is used to diagnose pertussis infection.

CEREBROSPINAL FLUID

Cerebrospinal fluid (CSF) is obtained by performing a lumbar puncture (LP). This is the critical investigation for the diagnosis of meningitis (see Table 2.6). The CSF can be evaluated in several ways including:

- pressure (particularly in suspected case of idiopathic intracranial hypertension)
- appearance (clear or cloudy/turbid)
- microbiology: microscopy (white cell count, organisms – Gram stain or acid-fast), culture and sensitivity, polymerase chain reaction (PCR); typically N. meningitidis, S. pneumoniae, herpes simplex virus (HSV), varicella zoster virus (VZV), enterovirus and parechovirus biochemistry:

Table 2.6 Interpretation of cerebrospinal fluid (CSF) results in different types of meningitis

	Neutrophils (× 10^6/L)	Lymphocytes (× 10^6/L)	Protein (g/L)	Glucose (CSF:blood ratio)
Normal <1 month old	0	<22	<1.0	≥0.6 or CSF glucose ≥2.0 mmol/L
Normal >1 month old	0	≤5	<0.4	≥0.6 or CSF glucose ≥2.5 mmol/L
Bacterial meningitis	100–10,000 (but may be normal)	Usually <100	>1.0 (but may be normal)	<0.4 (but may be normal)
Viral meningitis	Usually <100	<10–1000	0.4–1.0 (but may be normal)	Usually Normal
Tuberculosis meningitis	Usually <100	50–1000 (but may be normal)	1.0–5.0 (but may be normal)	<0.3 (but may be normal)

protein glucose, lactate, glycine (raised in nonketotic hyperglycinaemia), oligoclonal bands (immunoelectrophoresis), neurotransmitters

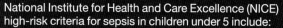
Appearance

Normal CSF is clear. If the cell count increases to more than $500 \times 10^6/L$ it becomes turbid. Typically, this occurs in bacterial meningitis. If the needle hits a blood vessel, the fluid may also be blood-stained.

Microbiology

Microscopy

Normally, a few ($<5 \times 10^6/L$) white cells can be found in CSF. In the early stages of meningitis, white cells might not be detectable but classically very high counts are found.

Spun CSF is routinely Gram stained:

- Gram-negative cocci: *N. meningitidis*
- Gram-positive cocci: *S. pneumoniae*
- Gram-negative coccobacilli: *H. influenzae*

Culture and sensitivity

This is always carried out even if the sample is clear and no white cells were detected on microscopy. Viral studies should be sent when encephalitis is suspected.

Biochemistry

Protein

Protein content of the CSF rises in bacterial meningitis. Note that in neonates the normal levels are high compared with older children and adults.

Glucose

Normal CSF glucose is approximately two-thirds of the blood glucose level. In bacterial meningitis, it drops to less than 40% of the blood glucose level. It is essential to take a capillary glucose sample at the time of the LP.

Polymerase chain reaction and DNA hybridization

New techniques that detect bacterial DNA and viral DNA or RNA are being used more frequently. They rely on the use of PCR techniques to amplify tiny amounts of DNA or RNA of pathogens. They can therefore detect pathogens without the need for culture and are reliable even after administration of antibiotics (e.g., 16S ribosomal DNA).

IMAGING

All the major imaging methods are used in paediatric practice:

- X-rays: plain or computed X-ray tomography and nuclear medicine
- ultrasound
- magnetic resonance imaging (MRI)

The main circumstances in which each of these tests can be used are described in the following sections.

X-rays

Most commonly requested are:

- chest X-ray (CXR)
- plain abdominal X-ray (AXR)
- skull X-ray
- computed tomography (CT)
- skeletal survey (for either safeguarding/child protection cases or genetic disorders)

Chest X-ray

When inspecting a CXR, adopt a systematic approach for viewing and presentation:

- check patient name, date, L/R orientation, posterior–anterior (PA) or anterior–posterior (AP)
- note any striking abnormalities
- heart and mediastinum
- lung fields and pulmonary vessels
- diaphragm and subdiaphragmatic areas
- bony thorax
- soft tissues

Indications for doing a CXR

Acute:

- complicated pneumonia
- severe bronchiolitis
- asthma: severe or first presentation
- cardiac failure
- foreign body inhalation

Nonurgent investigation of:

- cervical lymphadenopathy
- tuberculosis
- cystic fibrosis
- cardiac disease
- malignant disease

Abdominal X-ray

Supine AP is the standard plain film. There is wide variation in the normal appearance of these X-rays.

The checklist for an AXR includes:

- check patient name, date, erect or supine
- note striking abnormalities
- hollow organs: stomach, bowel and bladder
- solid organs: liver, spleen and kidneys
- diaphragm
- bones

Indications for doing an AXR

- suspected bowel obstruction
- suspected bowel perforation (request erect AP film to identify air under the diaphragm)
- refractory constipation or if there is diagnostic uncertainty

Skull X-ray

The most common indication for skull radiography used to be head injury, but CT scanning provides much more useful information. These days, its primary use is in the diagnosis of craniosynostosis, but CT is being used increasingly often.

Computed tomography

CT scanning uses multidirectional X-rays that, instead of falling onto film, are quantified by a detector and fed into a computer. Different readings are produced as the X-ray beam rotates around the body and the information is then presented as a two-dimensional image.

CT is a useful and widely available imaging modality for evaluating brain, chest and abdominal disorders. These include:

- Brain: intracranial haemorrhage (e.g., head injury), tumours, intracranial calcification (e.g., tuberous sclerosis).
- Chest: mediastinal masses (e.g., lymphoma), lungs (e.g., bronchiectasis).
- Abdomen: masses (e.g., neuroblastoma or Wilms), injury (e.g., splenic rupture).

CT accurately assesses the nature of a mass (e.g., fluid, fat, necrosis or calcification). Disadvantages include a lack of contrast between different organs. Intravenous contrast enhances the resolution between tissue planes. CT scans are a quick and readily available investigation, but less good for defining nonbony structures when compared with MRI scans.

Ultrasound

Ultrasound scanning (USS) uses ultra-high frequency sound waves to provide cross-sectional images of the body. In addition, Doppler ultrasound can be used for estimating the direction and velocity of blood flow.

The advantages of USS include:

- noninvasive – no ionizing radiation involved
- portable equipment

Body tissues reflect sound waves to different degrees and are therefore said to be of different echogenicity:

- hyperechoic tissues appear white (e.g., fat)
- hypoechoic tissues appear dark (e.g., fluid)

Ultrasound does not penetrate gas or bone and is therefore less useful for assessment of bony lesions. Intracranial contents are only accessible to ultrasound examination in young infants in whom the anterior fontanelle is still open.

The main applications include:

- antenatal ultrasound
- cranial ultrasound in the neonate
- abdominal and renal ultrasound
- hip ultrasound
- interventional radiology; vascular access line, biopsy

Antenatal ultrasound

Initial ultrasound screening is carried out at 12 weeks to confirm viability, followed by a more detailed scan at 18 to 20 weeks' gestation. Antenatal USS allows:

- estimation of gestational age (less than 20 weeks)
- identification of multiple pregnancies
- monitoring of fetal growth
- detection of structural malformations
- amniotic fluid volume estimation

Neonatal cranial ultrasound

This is useful for the detection and evaluation of intracranial pathology (Fig. 2.4), including:

- intracranial haemorrhage (e.g., intraventricular haemorrhage)

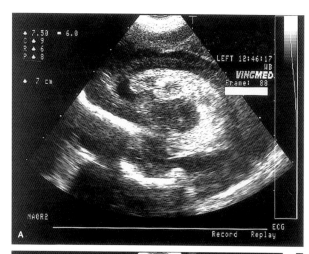

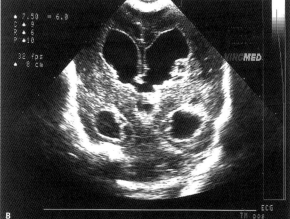

Fig. 2.4 (A) A parasagittal neonatal cranial ultrasound scan showing extensive intraventricular haemorrhage. (B) Coronal ultrasound scan of a neonatal brain with hydrocephalus.

- periventricular leucomalacia
- hydrocephalus
- cerebral malformations

> **HINTS AND TIPS**
>
> A cranial ultrasound is performed in all preterm babies under 32 weeks at birth and at serial intervals to look for haemorrhages and leucomalacia.

Abdominal and renal ultrasound

Abdominal ultrasound is useful in the evaluation of:

- acute abdominal pain: appendicitis, intussusception, pyelonephritis
- vomiting infant: pyloric stenosis
- liver disease: provides information on size and consistency of both the liver and spleen. The gall bladder and extrahepatic bile ducts can be visualized

Renal ultrasound is very useful in the investigation of disorders of the genitourinary tract (Fig. 2.5). It provides information on:

- kidney size
- structural abnormalities of the urinary tract (e.g., hydronephrosis, hydroureter or increased bladder size)
- gross renal scarring
- renal calculi
- tumours (e.g., Wilms)

See Chapter 6 for further guidance on how to investigate infants and children with confirmed UTIs.

Hip ultrasound

Ultrasound is a useful modality for the investigation of hip disease. It is the imaging method of choice for assessing neonatal

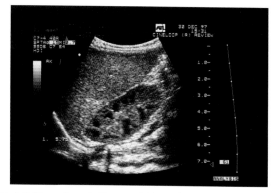

Fig. 2.5 Normal renal ultrasound. Normal prominent pyramids are demonstrated.

hip instability and is more reliable than plain radiography up to the age of 6 months. It allows evaluation of:

- acetabular morphology
- the degree to which the acetabulum covers the femoral head

Ultrasound is also useful in the investigation of suspected hip pathology in young children. Even small effusions can be detected, and needle aspiration can be carried out under ultrasound guidance.

Magnetic resonance imaging

MRI has several distinctive features that confer a number of useful advantages:

- no ionizing radiation
- images can be obtained in any plane
- excellent soft-tissue contrast

It is the imaging modality of choice for many disorders of the brain and spine (in which sagittal views are particularly useful). MRI is also helpful in the evaluation of musculoskeletal disorders. It has not replaced other approaches, such as CT or ultrasound, in the imaging of many thoracic and abdominal disorders. Its main disadvantage in children is the need for sedation or general anaesthesia to enable the child to remain still for a sufficient period.

Micturating cystourethrograms (MCUG)

This is sometimes indicated when there is a history of UTIs in children. It involves inserting a urinary catheter and filling the bladder with contrast medium. Serial fluoroscopic images are taken whilst voiding, which allows assessment of the renal tract anatomy, signs of vesicoureteric reflux and for posterior urethral valves.

Dimercaptosuccinic acid scans (DMSA)

This is a nuclear medicine scan, which is again indicated if there is a history of UTIs. It can provide information on structure, function and the presence of any renal scarring. It involves injecting a radioisotope intravenously and taking serial images of the renal tract.

● Chapter Summary

- Many important problems are identifiable using just a full blood count including anaemia, infection and signs of bone marrow failure.
- Assessment of fluid status when interpreting urea and electrolytes is crucial, and diabetic ketoacidosis can make interpretation of sodium and potassium difficult.
- Cerebrospinal fluid studies are key to diagnosing meningitis and results can differentiate between bacterial, viral and tuberculosis meningitis.
- Magnetic resonance imaging is better than computed tomography (CT) at imaging the brain and the musculoskeletal system; however, CT is more readily available at smaller hospitals and is quick, so often sedation can be avoided.

In developed countries, congenital heart disease (CHD) accounts for the majority of cardiovascular problems in infants and children, with Kawasaki disease being the leading cause of acquired cardiovascular problems. With improved cardiac surgery, 80% to 85% of children with congenital cardiac disease survive into adulthood.

Rare causes of cardiovascular disease in children include rheumatic fever, viral myocarditis, pericarditis and arrhythmias. In contrast to its incidence in adults, ischaemic heart disease is rarely seen.

CONGENITAL HEART DISEASE

CHD is the commonest cause of structural congenital malformations, affecting 6 to 8 of 1000 liveborn infants. A number of important associations are recognized (Table 3.1) but, in the majority of cases, the cause is unknown.

History

Cardiac symptoms vary with age. Parents of young infants may describe the following:

Table 3.1 Important associations with congenital heart disease

Genetic disorders	
Down syndrome	Atrioventricular septal defect
Turner syndrome	Coarctation of the aorta Bicuspid aortic valve
DiGeorge syndrome	Tetralogy of Fallot Truncus arteriosus Interrupted aortic arch
Williams syndrome	Supravalvular aortic stenosis
Noonan syndrome	Pulmonary stenosis
Teratogens	
Alcohol	Atrial septal defect Ventricular septal defect
Lithium	Ebstein anomaly
Infections	
Congenital rubella	Patent ductus arteriosus Pulmonary stenosis
Maternal conditions	
Diabetes mellitus	Transposition of the great arteries Truncus arteriosus

- poor feeding
- cough
- difficulty breathing
- sweating
- faltering growth
- recurrent chest infections

Older children may present with:

- syncope
- palpitations
- chest pain (although this rarely signifies cardiac disease)
- shortness of breath
- exercise intolerance

CHD may also present in a number of other ways, including:

- antenatal diagnosis by ultrasound
- incidental finding of a heart murmur
- cyanosis
- shock: low cardiac output

Examination

The major physical signs are:

- cyanosis
- murmurs
- signs of cardiac failure
- signs of cardiogenic shock
- finger clubbing (rare)

Cyanosis

Several varieties of CHD might present with central cyanosis (a 'blue' baby). This can present at the time of or soon after birth and is visible if the concentration of deoxygenated haemoglobin in the blood exceeds 5 g/dL.

- Central cyanosis describes blue lips and tongue and is always pathological.
- Peripheral cyanosis describes blueness of the hands and feet due to sluggish peripheral circulation. This can be a normal finding in newborn babies (acrocyanosis) within the first 24 hours of birth. It can also occur in babies who are cold, crying or unwell from some noncardiac cause. Table 3.2 summarizes all causes of cyanosis, including those of a noncardiac aetiology.

Differential cyanosis (measured as oxygen saturations) in the limbs indicates the presence of right-to-left shunting across the ductus arteriosus.

Table 3.2 Noncardiac causes of cyanosis in children

Respiratory	Neurological	Haematological
Upper airway obstruction	Seizures	Methaemoglobinaemia
Bronchiolitis	Oversedation	
Pneumothorax	Hypoxic Ischaemic Encephalopathy	
Pneumonia		
Asthma		
Pleural effusions		
Meconium aspiration		
Respiratory distress syndrome (RDS)		
Congenital diaphragmatic hernia		
Persistent pulmonary hypertension of the newborn (PPHN)		

HINTS AND TIPS

In suspected congenital cardiac disease, measure the preductal oxygen saturations (using the right hand) and compare with the postductal oxygen saturations (using the left hand or either foot). This will detect if there is abnormal mixing of deoxygenated systemic blood via a right-to-left shunt with oxygenated blood (i.e., via a patent ductus arteriosus in a duct-dependent critical cardiac defect).

Table 3.3 Grading a murmur

Grade	Description
1	Soft, barely audible
2	Soft but easily audible
3	Moderate but no cardiac thrill
4	Loud murmur with palpable cardiac thrill
5	Very loud (stethoscope barely on chest) with palpable cardiac thrill
6	Loudest murmur, audible with stethoscope off the chest wall

Murmurs

Cardiac murmurs are common in children of all ages. The majority of these are not associated with pathology (innocent murmurs) and clinical examination will allow most to be distinguished from structural cardiac disease.

A murmur is merely one component of the information obtained by examination of the cardiovascular system (CVS) and cannot be interpreted in isolation. Important features of a murmur include:

- *Timing*: Is it systolic or diastolic? (Most murmurs in children are systolic; diastolic murmurs are rare and always pathological).
- *Character*: Is it pansystolic or ejection systolic?
- *Loudness*: This is graded 1–6 (Table 3.3).
- *Radiation*: A murmur that radiates from its site of maximal loudness is more likely to be significant.

Innocent murmurs

The hallmarks of an innocent murmur are:

- an asymptomatic child
- a normal cardiovascular examination including normal heart sounds
- systolic or continuous

- no radiation
- variation with posture

Innocent murmurs are generated by turbulent flow in a structurally normal CVS. There are two main varieties of innocent murmurs: the ejection murmurs and the venous hums.

The ejection murmurs are:

- generated in the outflow tract of either side of the heart
- soft, blowing, systolic
- heard in the second or fourth left intercostal space

The venous hums:

- are generated in the head and neck veins
- are continuous low-pitched rumble
- are heard beneath the clavicle
- disappear on lying flat

RED FLAG

A diastolic murmur is always pathological and requires further investigation.

An innocent murmur is more likely to be noted during tachycardia (e.g., with fever, anaemia or exercise), and it is, therefore, important to reassess for the persistence of the murmur at a later stage following recovery of an acute illness.

Significant murmurs

A murmur with any of the following features is significant:

- symptoms: syncope, episodic cyanosis
- CVS signs: abnormal pulses, heart sounds, blood pressure or cardiac impulse
- murmur: diastolic, pansystolic, radiating to the back or associated with a thrill

Significant murmurs, which can be difficult to distinguish from an innocent murmur, include those caused by pulmonary stenosis (PS) and patent ductus arteriosus (PDA). Refer for echocardiography if in doubt.

Cardiac failure

Cardiac failure is less commonly seen in paediatric practice and is usually encountered during infancy.

COMMON PITFALLS

The clinical features of heart failure are different from those in adults. Feeding is the only exertion that infants undertake, hence they develop respiratory distress and become exhausted during feeds. Oedema is a rare finding and infants do not get ankle swelling as they are nonambulant. When assessing an infant with 'bronchiolitis' consciously consider whether the presentation might be of cardiac failure.

Clinical features

- Symptoms: poor feeding and breathlessness, faltering growth, excessive sweating and recurrent chest infections.
- Signs: tachycardia, cool periphery, tachypnoea and hepatomegaly. CVS signs can include a third heart sound, murmur and abnormal pulses.

Causes

This may be due to pressure overload (obstructive lesions) or volume overload (left-to-right shunts):

- Obstructive lesions typically present in neonates (e.g., severe coarctation of the aorta or hypoplastic left heart syndrome).
- Volume overload presents later in infancy. The left-to-right shunt increases (e.g., ventricular septal defects (VSDs), PDA) as the pulmonary vascular resistance falls.

Cardiac failure can be confused with the more common respiratory causes of tachypnoea, for example, bronchiolitis or wheezing associated with a viral infection. Less common causes

Table 3.4 Investigations in congenital heart disease

Investigation	Demonstrates
Chest X-ray	Cardiac shadow may be enlarged or abnormal in shape: • 'Boot shape' – tetralogy of Fallot • 'Egg on side' – transposition of great arteries
	Lung fields – pulmonary vascular markings may be: • Increased (plethoric): signifies left to right shunt, for example, ventricular septal defect • Decreased (oligaemic): signifies reduced pulmonary blood flow, for example, pulmonary stenosis
Electrocardiogram	Rate and rhythm of heart Mean QRS axis Hypertrophy of either ventricle
Echocardiogram	Precise anatomical abnormality
Cardiac catheter	Physiological/haemodynamic status rather than anatomy

of cardiac failure include supraventricular tachycardia and viral myocarditis.

Investigation

Initial evaluation should include a chest X-ray (CXR) and electrocardiogram (ECG), although these investigations do not usually provide a lesion diagnosis. Definitive diagnosis is usually achieved by echocardiography. Common investigations are shown in Table 3.4.

Classification

Although there are over 100 different cardiac malformations, a small number account for the majority of cases (Table 3.5). These are conveniently classified into:

- acyanotic forms
- cyanotic forms

Table 3.6 classifies congenital cardiac disease by acyanotic and cyanotic forms.

Acyanotic congenital heart disease

These conditions are caused by lesions that allow blood to shunt from the left to the right side of the circulation, or which obstruct the flow of systemic blood by narrowing a valve or vessel.

Left-to-right shunts (L to R)

Ventricular septal defect. Most are single, although multiple defects do occur and other heart defects coexist in about

Table 3.5 Common forms of congenital heart disease

Type	Name	Abbreviation	% of congenital heart disease
Acyanotic	Ventricular septal defect	VSD	32
	Patent ductus arteriosus	PDA	12
	Pulmonary stenosis	PS	8
	Atrial septal defect	ASD	6
	Coarctation of the aorta	COA	6
	Aortic stenosis	AS	5
Cyanotic	Tetralogy of Fallot	ToF	6
	Transposition of the great arteries	TGA	5

Table 3.6 Causes of cyanotic and acyanotic congenital heart disease (CHD)

Acyanotic	
Increased pulmonary blood flow	**Obstruction to ventricular blood flow**
ASD	CoA
VSD	Aortic stenosis
PDA	Pulmonary stenosis
AVSD	
Cyanotic	
Reduced pulmonary blood flow	**Mixed blood flow**
Tetralogy of Fallot	Transposition of the great arteries
Tricuspid atresia	Truncus arteriosus
	Total anomalous pulmonary venous connection
	Hypoplastic Left heart

one-third of affected children. The natural history and prognosis depend on the:

- size and position of the defect
- development of changes due to blood shunting from left to right through the defect. This includes narrowing of the right ventricular outflow tract and progressive, irreversible pulmonary hypertension

The clinical features, treatment and outcome are best considered separately for the different sizes of defect.

HINTS AND TIPS

A ventricular septal defect is the most common variety of congenital heart disease. It accounts for one-third of all cases.

Small VSD. The child is asymptomatic and the murmur is often first noted on routine examination. The only abnormality is a pansystolic murmur (sometimes with a palpable thrill) at the lower left sternal border.

Spontaneous closure might occur but if the murmur persists at 12 months, then an echocardiogram is warranted to look for any associated complications.

Medium VSD. These usually present with symptoms during infancy including slow weight gain, difficulty with feeding and recurrent chest infections. In time, symptoms might disappear due to the relative or complete closure of the defect.

On examination, there may be:

- an increased cardiac impulse
- palpable thrill
- harsh pansystolic murmur, loudest at the lower left sternal border

If the pulmonary blood flow is high, a mid-diastolic murmur occurs due to increased blood flow across the normal mitral valve.

A CXR will show moderate cardiac enlargement, a prominent pulmonary artery and increased vascularity of the lungs (pulmonary plethora). Echocardiography will show the position of the defect. The shunt is measured by Doppler studies.

Heart failure, if present, should be treated with diuretics and angiotensin-converting enzyme (ACE) inhibitors. Spontaneous improvement occurs in many childhood cases and surgical correction can be avoided. The decision to operate should be made on a case-by-case basis taking into account several factors (e.g., severity of cardiac failure and likely progression of cardiovascular disease).

Large VSD. Heart failure develops early on, especially if a chest infection occurs. The cardiac signs are similar to those of a medium VSD but it is worth noting that the systolic murmur might be soft in a very large defect. The defect tends to be larger than the cross-sectional area of the aortic valve.

Initial medical treatment of heart failure is required and surgical closure under cardiopulmonary bypass is usually necessary. In young infants with multiple defects, banding of the pulmonary artery allows a temporary respite until the child is big enough for definitive correction. An example of a VSD is shown in Fig. 3.1.

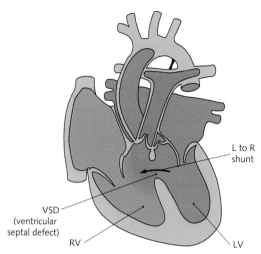

Fig. 3.1 Ventricular septal defect. *L to R shunt,* Left-to-right shunt; *LV,* left ventricle; *RV,* right ventricle.

Atrial septal defect. There are two types of atrial septal defect (ASD):

- Ostium secundum defect: The most common ASD (6 in 10,000 live births), is high in the atrial septum. It is more common in girls (female:male = 2:1) and accounts for 6% of all cases of CHD.
- Ostium primum defect: Much less common, occurring lower in the atrial septum (often associated with mitral regurgitation), and is a common defect in Down syndrome.

Secundum defects are usually asymptomatic in childhood. The left-to-right shunt develops very slowly, and pulmonary hypertension is extremely uncommon. It is important to distinguish ASDs from patent foramen ovale, which is present in one-quarter of all children. The patent foramen opens only in conditions of raised atrial pressure or volumes, whereas ASDs are large and always open.

Clinical features. The clinical features include:

- abnormal right ventricular impulse
- widely split and fixed second sound (S2)
- pulmonary flow murmur: soft, ejection systolic murmur in the pulmonary area
- tricuspid flow murmur: rumbling mid-diastolic murmur at the left sternal edge

No murmur is generated by low-velocity flow across an ASD. A significant left-to-right shunt generates flow murmurs at the tricuspid and pulmonary valves.

Diagnosis. The CXR shows pulmonary plethora and cardiomegaly, and the ECG shows right ventricular hypertrophy with incomplete right bundle branch block. Echocardiography is diagnostic without cardiac catheterization.

Management. Many small defects will close spontaneously in infancy and some moderate defects close spontaneously before school age. Treatment aims to prevent cardiac failure and arrhythmias in later life. Transcatheter closure of ASDs is now an established practice at most cardiac centres with successful implantation rates of more than 96% and this is best done at 3 to 5 years of age. Some larger defects may require surgical correction.

Atrioventricular septal defect. Atrioventricular septal defects (AVSDs) may be mild, moderate or severe and represent 4% of congenital cardiac defects. They are most commonly associated with Down syndrome; 40% of children will have CHD, of which 40% will have an AVSD (see Chapter 16 for more information on Down syndrome).

Left to right shunting results in atrial dilatation, ventricular loading and pulmonary hypertension. Clinical signs may include a loud pansystolic murmur at the LLSE and also a mitral regurgitation murmur at the apex. There may be signs of cardiac failure.

Treatment similarly aims to prevent heart failure and promote growth until complete surgical repair can be undertaken. Due to the risk of pulmonary hypertension, surgical correction occurs at a younger age than those with ASDs or VSDs.

HINTS AND TIPS

Faltering growth is often a feature in congenital heart disease, particularly in infants presenting with cardiac failure. Supporting growth and nutrition is vital, especially if an operation is planned. High-calorie milk or nasogastric tube feeds may be suggested by a dietician and is integral to their management.

Patent ductus arteriosus. The ductus arteriosus connects the aorta to the left pulmonary artery and this is a normal feature of foetal circulation (see Chapter 15). It usually closes within hours of delivery. A PDA is diagnosed if the duct does not close after 1 month of life. Risk factors include preterm infants, Down syndrome and high altitudes. PDA seen in preterm infants is a distinct clinical entity from congenital PDA in term infants.

HINTS AND TIPS

The risk of developing pulmonary vascular disease or infective endocarditis is higher in patent ductus arteriosus (PDA) than ventricular septal defect and surgical closure is recommended for all PDAs. This can be achieved by division, ligation or transvenous umbrella occlusion.

Clinical features. A PDA will result in a shunt between the aorta and pulmonary artery. The clinical features include:

- 'bounding' pulses
- wide pulse pressure
- continuous 'machinery hum' murmur: as pulmonary vascular resistance falls, a continuous run-off from the aorta to the pulmonary artery occurs

PDAs are commonly asymptomatic. If the duct is large and not corrected, features of cardiac failure will develop.

Diagnosis. CXR and ECG changes with a large symptomatic PDA are similar to those seen in a patient with a large VSD. The CXR is usually normal, but in large PDAs increased pulmonary markings and cardiomegaly are seen.

A PDA can be directly visualized by two-dimensional echocardiography and the ductal shunt can be confirmed and measured by Doppler ultrasound.

Management. Medical management is often attempted in preterm infants using a prostaglandin synthesis inhibitor (e.g., ibuprofen) or paracetamol. The duct can also be closed percutaneously via cardiac catheterization (within the first few months of life) or it can be ligated during open surgery (within the first year of life).

Obstructive lesions

Coarctation of the aorta. This accounts for about 10% of CHDs and has a male preponderance (male:female = 2:1). There is a narrowing of the aorta, which can be preductal or postductal. The site and severity of the coarctation determine the clinical features, which range from a severely ill newborn to an asymptomatic child, or adult, with hypertension.

HINTS AND TIPS

Every newborn baby should have their femoral pulses checked as part of their newborn check to rule out coarctation of the aorta. An urgent ECHO is warranted if they are weak or absent.

Preductal coarctation. This is often diagnosed antenatally but after birth, it presents as a sick neonate with absent femoral pulses. This is a 'duct-dependent' lesion as whilst the ductus arteriosus is open, the right ventricle can maintain adequate cardiac output to the systemic circulation. Once the duct closes, cardiogenic shock and cardiac failure are inevitable.

If critical coarctation is confirmed or even suspected, a prostaglandin infusion should be commenced to maintain ductal patency and the infant should be transferred to a cardiac centre for surgery.

Postductal coarctation. Although usually asymptomatic, there might be leg pains or headache. On examination, there is hypertension in the upper limbs compared with the lower limbs (if the coarctation is distal to the left subclavian artery) and weak or absent femoral pulses. There might be an ejection click (due to an associated bicuspid aortic valve) and a systolic ejection murmur audible in the left interscapular area.

In an older child, a CXR may demonstrate rib notching, which represents collateral blood vessel formation.
Surgical correction is required. Options include:

- balloon dilatation and stenting
- resection of the coarcted segment with end-to-end anastomosis

Aortic stenosis. This accounts for 5% of all CHDs and has a male preponderance (male:female = 4:1). Symptoms and signs depend on the severity of the stenosis:

- Mild or moderate stenosis presents a child with an asymptomatic murmur and a thrill often conducted to the aortic area and the suprasternal notch. There may also be an ejection systolic click.
- Severe stenosis can present with heart failure in the infant (a duct-dependent lesion) or with chest pain on exertion and syncope in older children.

Sustained, strenuous exercise should be avoided in children with untreated moderate to severe aortic stenosis. Surgical treatment depends on the severity and site of the stenosis. Balloon valvotomy is often attempted in critical stenosis; however, this results in aortic regurgitation and may require aortic valve replacement.

Pulmonary stenosis. This accounts for about 8% of CHD and might be valvular (90%), subvalvular (infundibular) or supravalvular. Infundibular PS occurs in association with a large VSD as part of the tetralogy of Fallot.

Most cases are mild and asymptomatic. The clinical features include:

- widely split S2, with soft pulmonary component (P2)
- systolic ejection click (valvular PS)
- a systolic ejection murmur maximal at the upper left sternal border, radiating to the back

Treatment options include transvenous balloon dilatation or pulmonary valvotomy.

Cyanotic congenital heart disease

There are two principal pathophysiological mechanisms for cyanosis in CHD:

- Decreased pulmonary blood flow with shunting of deoxygenated blood from the right side of the circulation to the left (systemic circulation). For example, tetralogy of Fallot.
- Abnormal mixing of systemic and pulmonary venous return, usually associated with an increased pulmonary blood flow. For example, transposition of great arteries.

HINTS AND TIPS

The 5 T's of cyanotic congenital heart disease:
- Transposition of the great arteries (TGA)
- Tetralogy of Fallot (TOF)
- Truncus arteriosus
- Tricuspid atresia
- Total anomalous pulmonary venous connection (TAPVC)

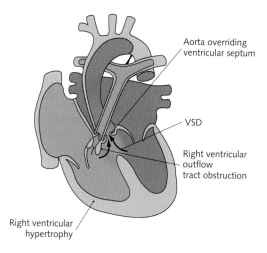

Fig. 3.2 Tetralogy of Fallot. *VSD,* Ventricular septal defect.

Tetralogy of Fallot
This represents 6% to 10% of all CHDs and is the most common cause of cyanotic CHDs presenting beyond infancy. The four cardinal anatomical features are shown in Fig. 3.2.

Clinical features. Most patients present with cyanosis in the first year of life, or sooner if the PS is severe. They may present with:

- cyanosis
- loud, single S2
- loud ejection systolic murmur maximal at the third left intercostal space
- clubbing (in older children, if uncorrected)

If uncorrected, children can experience hypercyanotic (or 'tet') spells, which are characteristic. These occur when systemic vascular resistance falls, for example, during crying or exertion, or can be triggered by emotion, hypothermia, dehydration or illness. During hypercyanotic spells, there is increased right-to-left shunting and poor oxygenation. Clinical signs may include:

- worsening and profound cyanosis or pallor
- distress/agitation
- hypotonia in infants
- children assuming a squatting position

Diagnosis. The ECG shows right-axis deviation and right ventricular hypertrophy but may be normal at birth. The CXR shows a characteristic 'boot-shaped' heart caused by right ventricular hypertrophy and a concavity on the left heart border where the main pulmonary artery and right ventricle outflow tract normally create a convexity. Pulmonary vascular markings are diminished. Congestive cardiac failure does not occur in tetralogy of Fallot.

Management. Most hypercyanotic spells are self-limiting and can be managed by soothing the child and increasing systemic vascular resistance by either bringing the infant's knees to their chest or getting a child to squat. Prolonged spells may require treatment. Approaches include:

- high-flow oxygen
- morphine – relieves pain
- intravenous fluids – increase systemic vascular resistance and ensure hydration
- sodium bicarbonate – corrects acidosis
- β-blockers – reduce tachycardia and relieve infundibular spasm
- intubation and ventilation, in severe cases

Definitive treatment of tetralogy of Fallot is surgical. Palliative procedures might be required in infants with severe cyanosis or uncontrollable hypercyanotic spells. Pulmonary blood flow is increased by creating a shunt between the subclavian and the pulmonary arteries (a modified Blalock–Taussig shunt). This would be followed by corrective total repair from 4 to 6 months of age. This involves patch closure of the VSD and widening of the right ventricular outflow tract.

Transposition of the great arteries
This accounts for about 5% of CHDs and is more common in males (M:F = 3:1). The condition involves:

- the aorta arising anteriorly from the right ventricle
- the pulmonary artery arising posteriorly from the left ventricle (Fig. 3.3)

Clearly, if completely separate, two such parallel circulations would be incompatible with life, but defects allowing mixing of the two circulations coexist. These include ASD, VSD or PDA.

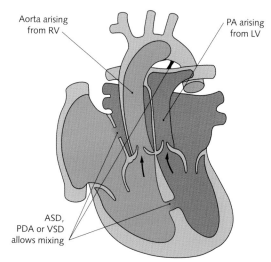

Fig. 3.3 Transposition of the great arteries. *ASD,* Atrial septal defect; *LV,* left ventricle; *PA,* pulmonary artery; *PDA,* patent ductus arteriosus; *RV,* right ventricle; *VSD,* ventricular septal defect.

Clinical features. Most cases present with severe cyanosis, often within the first day or two of life, particularly on closure of the ductus arteriosus resulting in reduced mixing of the systemic and pulmonary circulations. Hypoxia is unresponsive to oxygenation.

The second heart sound is single and loud. If the ventricular septum is intact, no heart murmur is audible. The systolic murmur of a VSD or PDA might be present.

Management. The immediate aim is to improve mixing of saturated and unsaturated blood. In the sick, cyanosed newborn, an infusion of prostaglandin E1 is started to reopen the ductus arteriosus. Emergency therapeutic balloon atrial septostomy is a lifesaving procedure. Definitive repair is usually achieved with an arterial switch procedure, which can be performed at a few weeks of age. The pulmonary artery and aorta are transected and switched over.

RHEUMATIC FEVER

Acute rheumatic fever is a sequela of group A β-haemolytic streptococcal infection, usually secondary to tonsillitis or pharyngitis. It is caused by an abnormal immune response that occurs in less than 1% of patients with streptococcal infection. Although the disease has largely been eradicated in developed countries with improved sanitation and the use of antibiotics for tonsillitis, it remains the most common cause of cardiac valvular disease worldwide. It mainly affects children aged between 5 and 15 years.

Clinical features

Most patients will have had a sore throat and coryzal illness in the preceding weeks. They may then go on to develop symptoms of rheumatic fever 2 to 6 weeks after the pharyngeal infection. Box 3.1 details the symptoms of rheumatic fever as determined by the Jones criteria. To fulfil the diagnosis the patient must meet the required criteria and either two major or one major and two minor criteria.

Erythema marginatum is an uncommon painless, early manifestation. It is a pink, macular rash seen on the trunk and limbs. Hard subcutaneous nodules occur on the extensor surfaces in a minority of cases.

Sydenham chorea is a late manifestation occurring 2 to 6 months after streptococcal infection in 10% of patients. There is emotional lability followed by involuntary, random, jerky movements lasting 2 to 3 months. Recovery is usually complete.

There is a pancarditis in 50% of patients:

- Pericarditis, which can cause a friction rub and pericardial effusion.
- Myocarditis, which can cause heart failure.
- Endocarditis, which commonly affects the left-sided valves leading to murmurs, for example, of mitral incompetence.

BOX 3.1 JONES CRITERIA FOR DIAGNOSING RHEUMATIC FEVER

Required criteria	Major criteria	Minor criteria
Evidence of streptococcal infection (e.g., positive bacterial throat swab or raised antistreptolysin O titre)	Polyarthritis (fleeting, mainly large joints)	Fever
	Erythema marginatum	Arthralgia
	Subcutaneous nodules	Raised erythrocyte sedimentation rate erythrocyte sedimentation rate/ C-reactive protein/ white cell count
	Carditis	Previous rheumatic fever
	Chorea	Prolonged PR interval

Diagnosis

The diagnosis is clinical and is based on the Jones criteria (see Box 3.1).

Laboratory investigations in a suspected case include:

- Erythrocyte sedimentation rate, C-reactive protein: elevated.
- Antistreptolysin O titre: might be elevated.
- Throat swab: usually negative at the time of presentation.
- ECG: prolonged PR interval.
- Echocardiography: might show evidence of carditis.

Management

The acute episode is treated by:

- Bed rest (depending on the severity of disease and joint involvement).
- High-dose aspirin to suppress fever and arthritis.
- Steroids for severe carditis.
- Diuretics and ACE inhibitors for heart failure.
- Antibiotics (both for acute illness and as prophylaxis, usually for 5 to 10 years, although lifelong prophylaxis has been advocated).

Complications

Rheumatic valvular disease is the most common form of long-term damage, with its severity increasing with the number of acute episodes. There is scarring and fibrosis of valve tissue, most commonly affecting the mitral valve. The commonest associated murmurs are mitral regurgitation and mitral stenosis.

CARDIAC INFECTIONS

These are uncommon and include:

- infective endocarditis
- myocarditis

Infective endocarditis

This may be defined as infection of the endocardium or endothelium of the great vessels.

Clinical features

Endocarditis should be suspected in any child with fever and a significant cardiac murmur. Clinical features include:

- Bacteraemia: fever, malaise and persistently positive blood cultures.
- Valvulitis: cardiac failure and murmurs due to the direct effect of pathogens circulating in the blood or damaging cardiac structures.
- Vascular or immunological phenomena causing embolic events. These include Roth spots, splinter haemorrhages, Janeway lesions, Osler's nodes, glomerulonephritis or a new stroke. Ischaemic emboli reflect vegetations (or part thereof) breaking into the systemic circulation; immune-mediated effects reflect a constant intravascular response to pathogens.

Noncardiac manifestations are less common in children than in adults. In a previously well child, this is a very rare diagnosis.

Diagnosis

It is important to stress that endocarditis is a clinical and laboratory diagnosis.

- Blood cultures: at least three should be obtained in the first 24 hours of hospitalization. The causative organism – most commonly *Streptococcus viridans* (α-haemolytic streptococcus) – is identified in 90% of cases.
- Transthoracic echocardiography; although this might confirm the diagnosis by the identification of vegetations, it cannot exclude it. Vegetations might persist after successful antibiotic treatment has been completed.
- Acute-phase reactants: elevated.

Management

Treatment comprises 4 to 6 weeks of intravenous antibiotics. Surgical removal of infected prosthetic material might be required.

Myocarditis

This uncommon disease primarily affects infants and neonates. Coxsackie and echoviruses, as well as varicella and influenza, have been associated with myocarditis. It can present acutely with cardiovascular collapse or slowly with a gradual onset of congestive cardiac failure.

Treatment involves supportive measures and managing heart failure. Most children recover but some develop a chronic dilated cardiomyopathy.

Kawasaki disease

Kawasaki disease is the most common cause of acquired cardiac disease in children. The underlying aetiological agent is at present unknown but it can result in coronary artery aneurysms. It is covered in detail in Chapter 10.

CARDIAC ARRHYTHMIAS

Sinus arrhythmia is more pronounced in children and shows as an increase in heart rate during inspiration and slowing during expiration. Normal sinus rhythm can be up to 210 beats/min and premature atrial and ventricular contractions are common and benign.

Supraventricular tachycardia

The child has a heart rate >220 beats/min and often is asymptomatic, although infants can develop cardiac failure. An accessory connection, for example, as seen in Wolff–Parkinson–White syndrome, can be present in up to 95% of all young children and infants.

Clinical features

Infants might present with signs of cardiac failure, such as poor feeding, sweating and irritability. Older children often feel unwell, describe palpitations, and may complain of chest pain, difficulty breathing and dizziness.

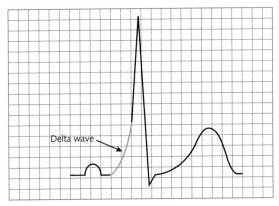

Delta wave

Fig. 3.4 Delta wave on electrocardiogram.

Diagnosis

The ECG usually shows a narrow complex tachycardia with P waves discernible after the QRS complex. In sinus rhythm, Wolff–Parkinson–White syndrome might be evident if there is an accessory bundle allowing premature activation of the ventricles. The PR interval is short and there is a wide QRS with a slurred upstroke (delta wave; see Fig. 3.4).

Management

An acute episode can be terminated and sinus rhythm restored by:

- Vagal stimulation: applying an ice-cold compress (or a bowl of ice cream!) to the face or carotid sinus massage.
- Intravenous adenosine: safe and effective.
- Synchronized direct current cardioversion: if the aforementioned options fail or if the child is haemodynamically unstable or shocked.

The prognosis is good in the majority of cases. About 90% of children will have no further episodes after infancy (>1 year old). Radiofrequency ablation of the bypass tract has been used for those with persistent, frequently recurring paroxysms. Some require antiarrhythmic medications.

RED FLAG

Syncope can be a manifestation of arrhythmia or cardiomyopathy. If syncope occurs whilst lying/sitting down, during exercise, with a family history of sudden death or prolonged QTc, suspect serious pathology and refer to a paediatric cardiologist.

Chapter Summary

- Congenital heart defects are the commonest type of structural congenital anomalies.
- Innocent murmurs tend to be soft, and systolic, vary with posture and do not radiate. Diastolic murmurs are always pathological.
- The commonest type of acyanotic heart disease is ventricular septal defects, which can be managed conservatively or surgically, depending on their size. Infants with a VSD may be asymptomatic with an audible murmur or present in cardiac failure depending on the size of the lesion.
- The commonest form of cyanotic heart disease is tetralogy of Fallot, which may present as cyanosis in the newborn period or later with hypercyanotic spells. A TOF comprises of right ventricular hypertrophy (RVH), ventricular septal defect (VSD), right ventricular outflow obstruction (RVOO) and an overriding aorta.
- Rheumatic fever is caused by group A β-haemolytic streptococcal infection and is diagnosed using the Jones criteria. The mitral valve is most commonly affected.
- The presence of fever and a murmur should prompt investigations for infective endocarditis. The likely causative agent is *Streptococcus viridians* which will require treatment with intravenous antibiotics.
- Wolff–Parkinson–White syndrome is a common underlying cause of supraventricular tachycardia in children and is characterized by a delta wave on an electrocardiogram.
- Acute episodes of supraventricular tachycardia (SVT) are treated with vagal stimulation in the first instance, escalating to intravenous adenosine or DC cardioversion if unsuccessful.

UKMLA Conditions
Down's syndrome

UKMLA Presentations
Congenital abnormalities
Cyanosis
Decreased/loss of consciousness

Infections of the upper and lower respiratory tract are extremely common in infants and children, and in winter, these conditions account for a high proportion of paediatric hospital admissions. Children are more susceptible to the effects of respiratory tract infections than adults for many reasons:

- their chest wall is more compliant than that of an adult
- fatiguability of the respiratory muscles
- increased mucous gland concentration
- poor collateral ventilation
- low chest wall elastic recoil
- narrower airways

While the majority of these infections will be viral and self-resolving, it is important to be aware of signs that indicate a bacterial infection. The other important diseases of this system include asthma and cystic fibrosis (CF).

PRESENTATION OF PAEDIATRIC RESPIRATORY DISEASE

The most common respiratory presentations are cough, stridor, wheeze and increased work of breathing.

Cough

In most instances, cough is due to an acute upper respiratory tract infection (URTI), but there are important causes of chronic cough (Box 4.1).

BOX 4.1 CAUSES OF COUGH

Acute cough	Chronic cough
Viral respiratory tract infection	Asthma
Croup	*Tuberculosis* (TB)
Bronchiolitis	*Pertussis* (whooping cough)
Pneumonia	Suppurative lung disease, e.g., cystic fibrosis, persistent bacterial bronchitis, bronchiectasis
Foreign body inhalation	

History

Key things to ask about:

- Duration of the cough: this is usually brief (e.g., <1 week). A chronic cough is defined as >3 weeks.
- Onset: abrupt onset of symptoms, sometimes with a history of choking, suggests an inhaled foreign body.
- Timing: a nocturnal cough can occur in asthma.
- Type of cough:
  - Whether dry or 'wet' (productive): a 'wet' cough raises the possibility of a lower respiratory tract infection (LRTI).
  - A 'barking' cough (think sea lion) is characteristic of croup.
  - A 'whooping' cough occurs in pertussis infection: there are paroxysmal prolonged bouts of coughing, sometimes ending in a sharp intake of breath (the 'whoop').
- Association with wheeze: occurs with bronchiolitis, viral-induced wheeze and asthma.
- Trigger factors: unwell contacts, cigarette smoke, contact with animals.
- Past medical history: including previous presentations of these symptoms, prematurity and other diagnoses.

HINTS AND TIPS

A productive cough is rare in children as sputum produced is swallowed.

HINTS AND TIPS

Note that children with neurological conditions (e.g., cerebral palsy) may have reduced ability to cough contributing to increased susceptibility to respiratory infections.

Stridor

Stridor is a harsh, inspiratory noise (can be biphasic) caused by upper airway obstruction, which can be life-threatening. The causes of stridor can be divided into acute and chronic (Fig. 4.1).

Wheeze

Wheeze is a high-pitched, whistling sound caused by collapse of the intrathoracic airways during expiration. In children aged <1 year, the tiny airways are easily narrowed by oedema and

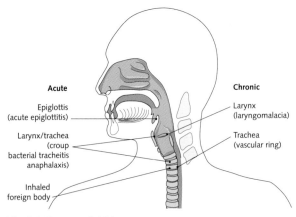

Fig. 4.1 Causes of stridor.

secretions, making wheeze a common feature of infections that involve the bronchi and bronchioles. In children aged >5 years, asthma is the most common cause of wheeze. In children younger than this, it can be difficult to distinguish asthma from the episodic wheezing induced by viral infections (viral-induced wheeze) and so a diagnosis should not be made hastily. Table 4.1 lists the differences between stridor and wheeze.

CAUSES OF WHEEZE	
Common	**Less common**
Bronchiolitis (<1 year)	Cystic fibrosis associated with failure to thrive and frequent chest infections.
Viral-induced wheeze	Laryngeal pathology: abnormal voice or cry.
Asthma	Gastro-oesophageal reflux: excessive vomiting.
	Inhaled foreign body: sudden onset, may be associated with choking.

Table 4.1 Differences between stridor and wheeze

Stridor	Wheeze
Extrathoracic airway (upper airway) narrowing	Intrathoracic airway narrowing
Usually worse on inspiration (extrathoracic airways naturally collapse)	Usually worse on expiration (intrathoracic airways naturally collapse)

> **COMMUNICATION**
>
> A parent will often find it difficult to distinguish between the sounds of stridor and wheeze. Do not be embarrassed to ask them to try and impersonate what their infant or child sounded like or to attempt to replicate the sounds yourself.

Respiratory distress and breathlessness

Respiratory distress or increased work of breathing presents differently in an infant compared with that in an older child. Signs specific to infancy are head bobbing and grunting.

- Head bobbing occurs due to contraction of the accessory muscles of breathing; weakness of the neck extensor muscles causes the head to bob up and down (Fig. 4.2).
- Grunting is caused by expiration against a partially closed glottis, which increases the peak end-expiratory pressure – older children may do this by breathing through pursed lips.
- Other signs of distress include subcostal and intercostal recessions, tracheal tug, tachypnoea and nasal flaring.

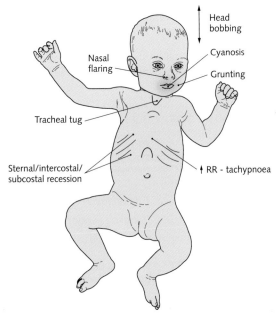

Fig. 4.2 Signs of respiratory distress in an infant. *RR,* Respiratory rate.

Tachypnoea (fast breathing) corresponds to a rate (in breaths/min) of:

- >60 in neonates
- >50 in infants
- >40 in children 1 to 5 years old
- >30 in older children
- >20 in older teenagers

The history is important in identifying whether the breathlessness has been a chronic ongoing problem or acute and will point you towards the correct underlying cause.

The most common cause of breathlessness in children is acute respiratory infections (viral or bacterial URTIs or LRTIs). Other respiratory causes include asthma, CF, bronchiectasis, foreign body inhalation, tonsillar hypertrophy and tracheomalacia. Nonrespiratory causes include anaemia and metabolic acidosis with compensatory hyperventilation (e.g., DKA). Cardiac failure can present with dyspnoea and can be secondary to a congenital cardiac lesion or acquired cardiomyopathy. Thorough examination with potential chest X-ray and blood gas if indicated will usually help delineate the cause.

HINTS AND TIPS

Respiratory distress may be due to a cardiac cause. History of an underlying heart problem, failure to thrive, presence of murmurs, abnormal position of the cardiac apex, hepatomegaly and cyanosis not improving despite 100% oxygen should alert to the possibility of a heart defect.

Apnoea

Apnoea is the cessation of breathing for at least 10 seconds or associated with a fall in heart rate. Its presence can signify significant respiratory disease, neurological disease or a Brief Resolved Unexplained Event (BRUE – replaced the previous term of acute life-threatening event – ALTE), especially in infants. It is common in preterm infants due to immaturity of the respiratory centres.

COMMUNICATION

Any respiratory admission can be seen as a potential 'teachable moment'. You should always ask about and address parental smoking. Remind parents that even if they smoke outside of the house, smoke will remain on their clothes and on their breath, which is harmful to their child as well as their own health.

UPPER RESPIRATORY TRACT INFECTIONS

Sore throat: pharyngitis and tonsillitis

These are commonly viral, especially in children under 3 years, but might also be caused by group A β-haemolytic streptococci (*Streptococcus pyogenes*). Epstein–Barr virus (infectious mononucleosis) is an important cause of exudative tonsillitis.

Clinical features

Children present with a sore throat, fever, lethargy and constitutional upset. It can be difficult to distinguish between a viral and bacterial infection clinically. Complications of bacterial URTI include:

- Retropharyngeal abscess.
- Peritonsillar abscess (quinsy) – may require incision and drainage.
- Scarlet fever.
- Poststreptococcal glomerulonephritis or rheumatic fever.

Management

Analgesia is the mainstay of treatment to enable drinking. Clinical prediction scores can be used to determine the likelihood of streptococcal infection.

HINTS AND TIPS

You can use either of the below scores to help determine the likelihood of streptococcal infection and, therefore, the need to prescribe antibiotics.

- The **FeverPAIN** criteria are:
  - **Fever** over 38°C.
  - **P**urulence (pharyngeal/tonsillar exudate).
  - **A**ttend rapidly (3 days or less).
  - Severely **I**nflamed tonsils.
  - **N**o cough or coryza.
  - Each of the criteria score 1 point. A score of 0 or 1 is associated with a 13% to 18% likelihood of isolating streptococcus. A score of 2 or 3 is associated with a 34% to 40% likelihood of isolating streptococcus. A score of 4 or 5 is associated with a 62% to 65% likelihood of isolating streptococcus.
- The Centor criteria:
  - Tonsillar exudate.
  - Tender anterior cervical lymphadenopathy or lymphadenitis.

- History of fever (over 38°C).
- Absence of cough.
- Each of the Centor criteria score 1 point. A score of 0, 1 or 2 is thought to be associated with a 3% to 17% likelihood of isolating streptococcus. A score of 3 or 4 is thought to be associated with a 32% to 56% likelihood of isolating streptococcus.

If streptococcal infection is suspected, a 5- to 10-day course of penicillin V can be given to prevent complications. Tonsillectomy is not performed as often as it used to be. It is reserved for children with severe recurrent tonsillitis; a frequency of more than seven episodes per year for 1 year, three per year for 2 years, or three per year for 3 years, and for whom there is no other explanation for the recurrent symptoms. Other indications may include recurrent quinsy or obstructive sleep apnoea (OSA).

HINTS AND TIPS

If amoxicillin is prescribed to children with EBV tonsillitis, a florid maculopapular rash may be seen.

Croup

Croup (acute laryngotracheobronchitis) is most commonly caused by the parainfluenza virus. Other causes include respiratory syncytial virus (RSV) and bacterial infection. It is most common in the second year of life and there is increased incidence during the winter months.

Clinical features

Symptoms of URTI (coryza, fever) are usually present for a day or two before the onset of a characteristic barking (sea lion) cough, hoarse voice and stridor (which is caused by subglottic inflammation and oedema). Symptoms typically start and are worse at night. Croup can be categorized into mild, moderate and severe disease based on the Westley scoring system.

Management

Most children are mildly affected and improve spontaneously within 24 hours, with symptoms lasting up to 3 days. The majority can be managed at home. About one in ten children require hospitalization because of:

- More severe illness.
- Young age (<12 months).
- Signs of fatigue or respiratory failure.

Glucocorticoids (steroids) reduce symptoms within 2 hours; dexamethasone tends to be used in preference to nebulized budesonide.

Nebulized adrenaline (epinephrine) can be used in more severe cases and provides transient improvement by constricting local blood vessels and reducing swelling and oedema. It should be given only under close supervision in hospital where it can provide rapid, if transient, relief of airway obstruction, allowing time for transfer to a high dependency or intensive care setting where intubation may be required if there is severe airway obstruction. Humidifiers and steam therapy are ineffective and the latter should also be avoided due to the risk of accidental burns.

RED FLAG

Impending upper airway obstruction can occur with conditions that cause acute stridor, e.g., croup, epiglottitis, bacterial tracheitis and foreign body inhalation.

Signs of impending airway obstruction include:

- Upright posture with neck hyperextension
- Drooling/inability to swallow saliva
- Moderate-severe respiratory distress
- Stridor at rest or continuously

It is important that these children do not become upset as this can precipitate obstruction. Avoid examining the child if it will cause distress and summon ENT and anaesthetic help early.

Acute epiglottitis

Acute bacterial epiglottitis is an uncommon, life-threatening emergency caused by infection with *Haemophilus influenzae* type B. It has become rare since the introduction of Hib immunization. It is most common in children aged 1 to 6 years.

Clinical features

The onset is rapid over a few hours with the development of an intensely painful throat. The characteristic picture is of an ill, toxic, febrile child who is unable to speak or swallow, with a muffled voice and soft inspiratory stridor. The child tends to sit upright with an open mouth and might drool saliva.

Management

It is vital to distinguish this illness from viral croup because the management is different:

- The child should be managed in the resuscitation room.
- No attempt should be made to lie the child down, to examine the throat or to do anything to upset the child such as taking blood, as these can precipitate total airway obstruction.

- Senior paediatric, ENT and anaesthetist help should be called.
- Examination under anaesthetic should be arranged without delay to allow confirmation of the diagnosis (cherry-red, swollen epiglottis on laryngoscopy) followed by intubation.
- Once the airway is secured, blood should be taken for culture and intravenous (IV) antibiotics started using a third-generation cephalosporin (e.g., ceftriaxone, cefotaxime). Intubation is not usually required for longer than 48 hours.

Bacterial tracheitis

This is an uncommon infectious disease in children but is more prevalent than acute epiglottitis. The usual pathogens are *Staphylococcus aureus, H. influenzae, Streptococcus* spp. and *Neisseria* spp. It often presents as an acute deterioration after a viral illness (e.g., croup). Children are often systemically unwell with high fever and respiratory distress. Stridor and hoarse voice are the predominant features but in contrast to acute epiglottis, there is no drooling. The management is very similar to that of acute epiglottitis (i.e., securing the airway followed by blood cultures and broad-spectrum IV antibiotics). See Table 4.2 for the differences between croup, epiglottitis and tracheitis.

> **COMMUNICATION**
>
> In a child with stridor, reduce distress by letting them sit in a position they are comfortable in, encouraging the parent/carer to soothe them and giving them a familiar toy. If oxygen masks cause more distress, oxygen can be wafted near to their face.

Diphtheria

This potentially fatal and highly infectious disease is caused by a toxin produced by *Corynebacterium diphtheriae* that usually affects the mucous membranes of the nose and throat. Diphtheria typically causes a sore throat, fever, lymphadenopathy (bull neck)

and respiratory distress (stridor). The hallmark sign is a thick, grey exudate covering the back of the throat. Its incidence has been greatly reduced by immunization but remains prevalent in unvaccinated and immigrant communities. Treatment is with diphtheria antitoxin; antibiotics (macrolides – clarithromycin or penicillin) should also be prescribed to reduce carriage and toxin production. Contacts are treated with erythromycin.

Whooping cough

Whooping cough is caused by the highly contagious Gram-negative bacterium *Bordetella pertussis*. It spreads by droplet infection and has an incubation period of 7 to 10 days. A case is infectious from 7 days after exposure to 3 weeks after the onset of the paroxysmal cough. Incidence has been greatly reduced by vaccination (including a single dose of acellular pertussis-containing vaccine during pregnancy).

Clinical features

The clinical course can be divided into catarrhal, paroxysmal and convalescent stages. It is characterized by paroxysms of coughing during expiration, followed by a sharp intake of breath (inspiratory 'whoop'); however, this can be absent in infants. Coughing (which is often worse at night) can cause vomiting, apnoea and cyanosis. Vigorous coughing can lead to nosebleeds and subconjunctival haemorrhage. Symptoms can persist for up to 3 months (the '100-day' cough).

Investigations

Although it is largely a clinical diagnosis, a marked lymphocytosis (>15–20 × 10^9/L) is characteristic. Specimens to corroborate the diagnosis (nasopharyngeal aspirate – NPA, pernasal swab) can be sent for culture or polymerase chain reaction (PCR) assay.

Management

Erythromycin given early in the disease eradicates the organism and reduces infectivity but does not shorten the duration of the disease. Management is largely supportive but 1% will need admission.

Complications

Complications, which include apnoea, seizures, pneumonia and bronchiectasis, are more common in infants under 6 months of age.

> **RED FLAG**
>
> Whooping cough is very dangerous to young infants (which is why maternal vaccination is offered during pregnancy). They should be admitted due to the risk of apnoea.

Table 4.2 Differences between croup, epiglottitis and tracheitis

Croup	Bacterial tracheitis	Epiglottitis
Systemically well	Toxic	Toxic
Barking cough	Barking cough	Mild/absent cough
Hoarse voice	Very hoarse voice	Muffled voice
Can swallow	Can swallow	Intensely sore throat – cannot swallow – drooling and cannot drink

LOWER RESPIRATORY TRACT INFECTIONS

LRTIs are much less common than URTIs, but they are more likely to be serious. Causative agents include viruses and bacteria. They vary with the child's age and the site of infection. Infection can occur by direct spread from airway epithelium or via the bloodstream. A number of well-defined clinical syndromes (determined by the predominant anatomical site of inflammation) are recognized (e.g., bronchiolitis and pneumonia) and often provide a clue to the likely pathogen. The term 'chest infection' should be avoided.

Bronchiolitis

Bronchiolitis is a common condition characterized by inflammation of the bronchioles, in response to a viral infection, most commonly RSV. Less common causes include adenovirus, influenza, parainfluenza and *Mycoplasma pneumoniae*. It is the major cause of lower respiratory tract infection in infants with increased risk if there is premature, congenital cardiac or respiratory disease, Down syndrome and exposure to cigarette smoke. Breastfeeding is protective. There are annual epidemics every winter.

Clinical features

A 1–3-day coryzal prodrome is followed by a cough with associated difficulty in breathing, which can lead to poor feeding and dehydration. Very young infants might develop apnoeic episodes. Examination may show:

- signs of respiratory distress (see Fig. 4.2)
- chest hyperinflation
- widespread wheeze and fine crackles
- clinical dehydration

Investigations

Bronchiolitis is a clinical diagnosis but if a chest X-ray is performed, it usually shows hyperinflation with patchy consolidation bilaterally and occasional collapse. RSV can be detected by immunofluorescence on an NPA, or with point-of-care PCR-based testing – performed to cohort inpatients together.

Management

Indications for admission include:

- Respiratory rate >70 breaths/min
- Oxygen saturations persistently <90%–92% in air
- Persistent severe respiratory distress
- Apnoeic episodes
- Reduced feeding <50%–75% of normal volume or clinical dehydration

A lower admissions threshold may be used for infants with congenital heart disease, ex-preterms, <3 months of age, neuromuscular disorders and immunodeficiency.

Management is supportive – oxygen is the mainstay of treatment and is given via nasal cannula or face mask. Some infants might be well enough to continue oral feeds, but many require fluids to be given either by nasogastric tube or intravenously. A minority of hospitalized infants require assisted ventilation (only 1%–2%). Secondary bacterial infection might occur, in which case antibiotic therapy is appropriate. For high-risk infants, a monoclonal antibody (palivizumab) can be given in the winter months to prevent RSV infection, and trials are ongoing considering possible routine monoclonal antibody vaccination to all infants (nirsevimab). However, neither offer protection against the many other viruses that can cause bronchiolitis.

Complications

Although most infants make a full recovery within 2 weeks, some have recurrent episodes of cough and wheeze over the subsequent few years. It is known that a subset of these infants will develop asthma.

Pneumonia

Pneumonia describes inflammation of the lung parenchyma with consolidation within the alveoli. It can be caused by viruses (more common in those under 2 years of age) and bacteria. Viruses:

    RSV
    Influenza
    Parainfluenza
    Adenovirus

Bacteria:

    Streptococcus pneumoniae (most commonly)
    S. aureus (typically post influenza and in children with CF)
    H. influenzae type B (in the unvaccinated)
    'Atypicals': *Mycoplasma*, *Chlamydia*
    Group B *streptococcus* (neonates)
    Pseudomonas (in children with CF)

Clinical features

There is a short history, often following a URTI, of fever, cough and breathlessness, often with reduced feeding. On examination, the patient will often be tachypnoeic and may show signs of respiratory distress. The classic signs of consolidation (decreased breath sounds, dullness to percussion, crackles and bronchial breathing) might be present, but they are difficult to detect in infants and young children. In bacterial pneumonia, pleural inflammation causing chest (or abdominal) pain and an effusion commonly develops.

Investigations

Diagnosis is largely clinical, and a chest X-ray is only indicated when there is a failure to respond to treatment or if complications are suspected. Blood tests looking for raised inflammatory markers, a blood culture, sputum culture and an NPA for viral isolation and PCR assay should be carried out in hospitalized children. Blood cultures are positive in just 10% of cases; using both NPA for culture and PCR testing increases identification of causative organisms to 30%.

It is often difficult to distinguish between viral and bacterial infections clinically. Young children and babies are not good providers of sputum and a definitive diagnosis of bacterial infection remains difficult. The following all suggest bacterial pneumonia:

- polymorphonuclear leucocytosis
- lobar consolidation
- pleural effusion

Mycoplasma infection can be diagnosed reliably by acute and convalescent serology or by demonstration of cold agglutinins.

Management

Where bacterial pneumonia is suspected, antibiotics will be given. The choice and route are dictated by the child's age, the severity of illness and local sensitivities. Oral amoxicillin is first line in most children; a macrolide is an alternative for penicillin-allergic children. In addition, if an atypical infection (*Mycoplasma, Chlamydia*) is suspected, a macrolide antibiotic should be given. Severely unwell children will need admission, supplementary oxygen and broad-spectrum IV antibiotics.

Complications

Rarely, pneumonia can be complicated by empyema; this should be evaluated by ultrasound and will need drainage via a chest drain. Other complications include septicaemia and metastatic spread, which can cause infective endocarditis, brain abscesses, osteomyelitis or septic arthritis. Recurrent or persistent pneumonia should raise the possibility of an inhaled foreign object or congenital abnormality of the lung, CF or tuberculosis.

ASTHMA

Asthma is a chronic inflammatory disorder of the airways characterized by episodic airway obstruction causing wheeze, cough, breathlessness and chest tightness. A key point is that symptoms are reversible with treatment, or in mild episodes, spontaneously.

Epidemiology

Asthma is the most common chronic respiratory disorder of childhood with a prevalence of 10% to 15% in the UK. It has increased in prevalence in the last decade. In early childhood, asthma is more common in boys than in girls, but by adulthood, the sex ratio is reversed.

Aetiology

Asthma is associated with a number of risk factors:

- personal or family history of atopy (asthma, eczema, hay fever, allergies)
- male sex
- exposure to cigarette smoke

Pathophysiology

The pathophysiology of airway narrowing in asthma includes chronic inflammation of the bronchial mucosa associated with mucosal oedema, secretions and the constriction of airway smooth muscle (Fig. 4.3).

Clinical presentation

The history should focus on:

- The pattern of symptoms (episodic or persistent, diurnal variation, symptoms on exercise).
- Triggers (viral URTI, cold weather, exercise, exposure to smoke/animal fur/pollen/dust).

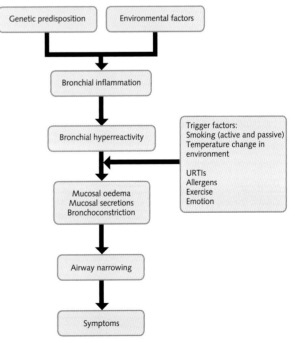

Fig. 4.3 Factors in the pathogenesis of asthma. *URTI,* Upper respiratory tract infection.

- Severity (exercise tolerance, night-time disturbance, school absence).
- Personal and family history of atopy.

On examination, there may be signs of chronic, severe asthma:

- hyper expansion
- pigeon chest (pectus carinatum)
- Harrison's sulcus

Auscultation of the chest is usually normal between attacks. For signs and management of acute asthma, see Chapter 20.

Investigations

Asthma can be diagnosed based on the history if symptoms are typical, in a child in whom asthma is likely (e.g., atopy, family history of asthma) and in whom other rarer causes (e.g., suppurative lung disease) have been excluded (Table 4.3) In children aged over 5 years, objective lung function tests should be attempted and the peak expiratory flow rate test can aid diagnosis if the child can carry this out reliably. Significant diurnal variability or decrease after exercise suggests bronchial hyper-reactivity. Spirometry in older children might demonstrate reversible airway obstruction. However, in the majority of children a diagnosis is made without lung function testing because this is too difficult to measure in young children; instead, an assessment of the child's response to a treatment is performed.

Management

The aim of asthma treatment is to have:

- no daytime symptoms or waking at night due to asthma
- no exacerbations
- no need for reliever therapy
- no limitations on activity
- normal lung function
- minimal side effects of therapy

Table 4.3 Differential diagnosis of asthma

Diagnosis	Clues
Cystic fibrosis	Growth faltering, productive cough and finger clubbing
Gastro-oesophageal reflux	Excessive vomiting
'Malacic' airways (tracheomalacia, laryngomalacia, bronchomalacia)	Inspiratory stridor with wheeze
Laryngeal problems	Abnormal voice
Inhaled foreign body	Sudden onset
Postviral wheeze	Recent respiratory infection in children under 2 years of age

Nonpharmacological management

Patient and parent/carer education and the provision of an individualized, written management plan are vital. There are also important lifestyle changes including smoking cessation advice, reduction of exposure to triggers and weight loss if obese.

Medication

The drugs used in the management of asthma in children can be classified into 'preventers' and 'relievers'.

> **HINTS AND TIPS**
>
> There is a colour code for asthma drug-inhaler devices:
> - 'Preventers' are mostly brown (e.g., inhaled corticosteroids). Other colours are purple, red, green and orange.
> - 'Relievers' are blue (e.g., inhaled salbutamol).

A stepwise approach to treatment has been devised (British Guideline on the management for asthma) and is summarized in Fig. 4.4. Patients should start treatment at the step most appropriate to the initial severity. Once control is achieved, treatment can be stepped down. A rescue course of oral prednisolone might be needed at any step. In children with marked seasonal variation in asthma severity, the treatment should be varied according to the season. Inhalation therapy is central to most asthma treatment. The basic systems available are considered in Table 4.4 and Fig. 4.5. The mode of action, indications for use and side effects of the most commonly used bronchodilator drugs are outlined in Table 4.5.

Steroid therapy in asthma

Glucocorticoids are key drugs in the management of asthma, both in prophylaxis and in the treatment of acute attacks. They can be given:

- by inhalation
- orally
- intravenously: in acute severe asthma

Inhaled corticosteroids are now the 'preventers' of choice in the management of childhood asthma. The lowest dose that achieves control should be used.

Inhaled corticosteroids (ICS):

- inhibit synthesis of inflammatory mediators (cytokines, leukotrienes and prostaglandins)
- reduce airway hyperresponsiveness
- reduce both the symptoms and frequency of attacks
- prevent irreversible airway narrowing

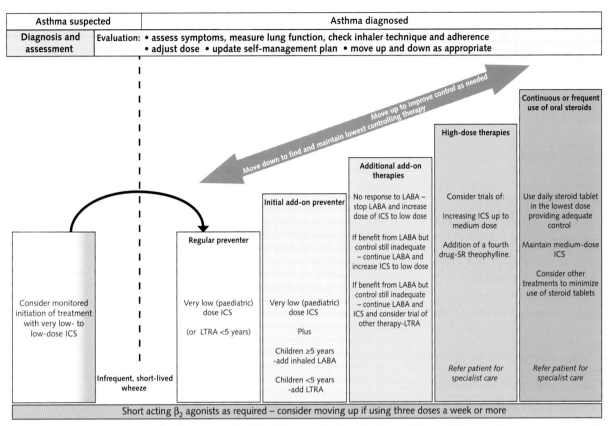

Fig. 4.4 Stepwise management of asthma as per the British Thoracic Society. Treat over 12-year-olds according to management of asthma in adulthood. *ICS,* Inhaled corticosteroid; *LABA,* long-acting β agonists; *LTRA,* leukotriene receptor antagonist.

Table 4.4 Administration of medication by inhalation

	Advantages	Disadvantages
Metered dose inhaler with spacer	Coordination not required Usable at all ages Effective for acute asthma unless needing oxygen	Bulky
Dry powder inhaler	Coordination unimportant Small and portable Easy to operate	Requires rapid inspiration Unsuitable for children <5 years of age
Nebulizer	Coordination unimportant Usable at all ages Can be driven by oxygen (useful for severe exacerbations, requiring oxygen therapy)	Expensive, noisy, cumbersome Treatment takes a long time, >5 minutes May not prompt and hence, delay hospital attention Frightens some infants

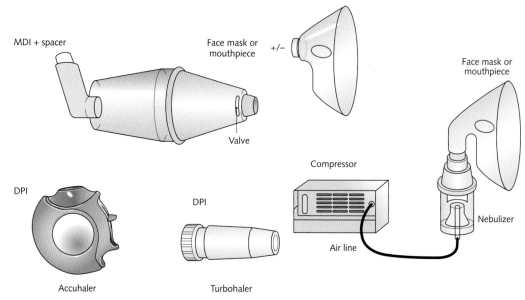

Fig. 4.5 Inhaler devices. *DPI,* Dry powder inhaler; *MDI,* metered dose inhaler.

Table 4.5 Asthma drug therapy: mode of action, indications and side effects of bronchodilators

Relievers (bronchodilators)	Mode of action	Use	Side effects
Short-acting β_2 agonists (e.g., salbutamol, terbutaline)	Smooth muscle relaxation	Relief of bronchospasm	Tachycardia Hypokalaemia Restlessness
Long-acting β_2 agonists (e.g., salmeterol)	Smooth muscle relaxation	Nocturnal asthma, exercise-induced asthma Trial alternative to high-dose inhaled steroids	
Theophylline	Phosphodiesterase inhibition	Oral theophylline for nocturnal asthma Intravenous aminophylline in acute severe asthma	Restlessness Diuresis Cardiac arrhythmias
Anticholinergics (e.g., ipratropium bromide)	Inhibit cholinergic bronchoconstriction; add-on to β_2 agonists in acute attack	In combination with short-acting β_2 agonists in severe asthma	Dry mouth Urinary retention
Magnesium sulphate	Smooth muscle relaxation, reduces inflammatory mediators, stimulates nitric oxide and prostacyclin synthesis	Severe asthma; either nebulized or IV (first-line IV treatment)	

Local side effects, such as oral thrush or dysphonia, are common- about 90% of the dose is deposited in the mouth and pharynx- but these side effects can be reduced by the use of a spacer (with metered dose inhalers) and mouth washing (with dry powder inhalers). High-dose treatments are used under specialist supervision; they can be associated with decreased growth and adrenal suppression. Children needing this management must have their height monitored closely.

COMMUNICATION

Parents, and sometimes children, can be anxious about the adverse effects of long-term inhaled steroids. Because the dose is low and is targeted at the lungs, systemic absorption is less and therefore systemic adverse effects are rare. While transient growth failure can occur, there is good evidence that the final height is not affected. In addition, asthma itself can lead to growth failure, which is probably worse than that due to steroids. Steroids can cause adrenal failure, but this is again rare unless high doses are used.

Short courses of oral steroids (typically 3 days) are indicated in severe acute exacerbations of asthma: prednisolone as a single daily dose is the drug of choice. Regular oral steroids are indicated only for the most severe asthma that cannot be controlled with high-dose inhaled steroids and regular bronchodilators. Alternate-day treatment is preferred to reduce systemic side effects.

Long-acting β_2 agonists (LABA)

This class of inhaled drug can be used as an add-on therapy in children over 4 years if control is poor with low-dose inhaled steroids. New combination inhaled steroid and long-acting β_2 agonists (Maintenance And Reliever Therapy, MART) are available.

Leukotriene receptor antagonists (LRTA)

This class of oral drug (e.g., montelukast) acts by inhibiting leukotrienes, which are released from mast cells, eosinophils and basophils, leading to increased secretions, inflammation and airway narrowing. They can be used in children including those under 5 years who cannot take an inhaled steroid or in children where a steroid inhaler has not controlled symptoms.

Theophylline

This oral drug can be used in difficult-to-treat asthma but its use is limited by side effects.

Anti-immunoglobulin E monoclonal antibody

More recent treatments include anti-immunoglobulin E (anti-IgE) monoclonal antibodies (e.g., omalizumab), which bind to circulating IgE, markedly reducing levels of free serum IgE. In children over 6 years of age, it is licensed in the UK for patients on high-dose inhaled steroids and LABA who have impaired lung function, are symptomatic with frequent exacerbations and have allergy as an important cause of their asthma. These are only prescribed in specialist centres.

Acute severe asthma

For the acute management of asthma, see Chapter 20, Emergencies.

Prognosis of asthma

The majority of children with asthma improve as they get older. Prognosis is better with earlier age at diagnosis. Children with poor pulmonary function testing and more frequent acute exacerbations are more likely to have recurrent wheeze in adulthood.

CYSTIC FIBROSIS

Incidence and aetiology

CF is the most common life-threatening genetic disease in Caucasians. It has a carrier rate of 1:25 and incidence of 1:2500 live births. CF is an autosomal recessive disease arising from mutations in a gene on chromosome 7 that encodes an adenosine triphosphate-binding cassette (ABC) transporter, the cystic fibrosis transmembrane regulator (CFTR) protein. The most common mutation is a three-base-pair deletion that removes the phenylalanine at position 508 (ΔF508). This is found in 90% of disease chromosomes, but nearly 2000 mutations have been identified so far. The mutations in the CFTR result in defective chloride ion transport across epithelial cells and increased viscosity of secretions, especially in the respiratory tract and exocrine pancreas. This predisposes to recurrent chest infections and pancreatic insufficiency. In addition, abnormal transport in sweat gland epithelium results in high concentrations of sodium and chloride in sweat, which form the basis of the most useful diagnostic test, the sweat test.

Clinical features

CF should be considered in any child with recurrent chest infection and failure to thrive. Viscid mucus in the small airways predisposes to infection with *S. aureus, H. influenzae* and *Pseudomonas* species. Repeated infection leads to bronchial wall damage with bronchiectasis and abscess formation.

There is a cough productive of purulent sputum and on examination, there might be:

- hyperinflation
- crackles
- wheeze
- finger clubbing (other causes listed in Box 4.2)

An example of typical chest X-ray changes is shown in Fig. 4.6.

In most children, deficiency of pancreatic enzymes (protease, amylase and lipase) results in malabsorption, steatorrhoea and

BOX 4.2 CAUSES OF CLUBBING

Respiratory	Cystic fibrosis, bronchiectasis, primary ciliary dyskinesia, fibrosing alveolitis, chronic empyema
Cardiac	Cyanotic heart disease
Gastrointestinal	Inflammatory bowel disease, liver disease
Infective	*Tuberculosis* (TB)

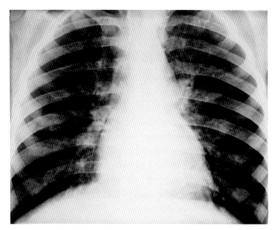

Fig. 4.6 Typical chest X-ray of a child with cystic fibrosis, showing bilateral severe lung pathology: hyperinflated lungs with bronchial wall thickening.

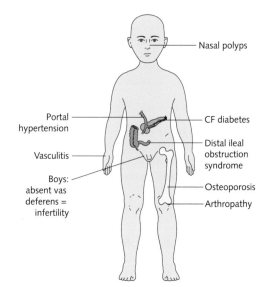

Fig. 4.7 Multisystem aspects of cystic fibrosis (CF).

failure to thrive. Stools are pale, greasy and offensive. About 10% of infants with CF present with 'meconium ileus' in the neonatal period, in which inspissated meconium causes internal obstruction. Another feature is delayed puberty and male infertility due to congenital absence of the vas deferens. Screening for CF-related diabetes is important.

HINTS AND TIPS

The CF PANCREAS mnemonic can be used to recall common clinical features associated with cystic fibrosis:

C – Chronic cough
F – Failure to thrive
P – Pancreatic insufficiency (exocrine)
A – Alkalosis and hypotonic dehydration
N – Nasal polyps, neonatal intestinal obstruction (meconium ileus)
C – Clubbing of fingers
R – Rectal prolapse
E – Electrolyte elevation (sweat)
A – Absence of vas deferens
S – Sputum with staph or pseudomonas

Investigations

Screening for CF is performed as part of the newborn blood spot test using immunoreactive trypsinogen with the aim of early diagnosis to preserve lung function. CF in this group (before symptoms manifest) is diagnosed by a positive newborn screening test, followed by both a sweat test & genetic studies. For those presenting with symptoms, diagnosis is either by genetic testing or the sweat test, using pilocarpine iontophoresis (rarely it is diagnosed by symptoms alone- if these two tests are negative). The sweat test demonstrates failure of the normal reabsorption of sodium and chloride by the sweat duct epithelium leading to abnormally salty sweat: chloride concentrations of 60 to 125 mmol/L are found (the normal value is <15 mmol/L). Two sweat tests showing a chloride of >60 mmol/L confirm CF.

Management

CF is a multisystem disease (Fig. 4.7) and management requires a multidisciplinary approach, which is delivered most effectively by a specialist centre. The main aims are to:

- prevent progression of lung disease
- promote adequate nutrition and growth

A team approach is required, involving paediatricians with an interest in CF, physiotherapists, dieticians, CF nurses, community nurses, psychologists, the primary care team and the child's parents or carers. Charities, like the Cystic Fibrosis Trust, play an extremely important role in supporting families.

CLINICAL NOTES

Cornerstones of cystic fibrosis treatment are:

- prevention of colonization and infection of the lungs
- effective mucociliary clearance
- nutritional support

Respiratory management

Physiotherapy (chest percussion with postural drainage, breathing exercises, positive expiratory pressure masks and flutter devices) is the mainstay of respiratory management. Many centres recommend continuous prophylactic antibiotics with oral flucloxacillin in the first 2 years of life, and if children are colonized with *Pseudomonas,* antipseudomonal nebulized antibiotics such as colomycin are used. Acute exacerbations require vigorous treatment, with IV antibiotics directed against the common bacterial pathogens (*H. influenzae, S. aureus* and *Pseudomonas aeruginosa*) and guided by recent sputum culture results if available. Use of indwelling vascular devices (e.g., Port-A-Cath) aids regular IV antibiotic courses. Mucolytics such as nebulized DNase or hypertonic saline to reduce sputum viscosity can help mucociliary clearance.

In the past few years, cystic fibrosis transmembrane conductance regulator (CFTR) modulator therapies have been used in specific patient subgroups and have shown very promising results. They are designed to correct the malfunctioning protein made by the CFTR gene. Lumacaftor–ivacaftor is used to treat children homozygous for the F508del mutation in the CFTR gene, the commonest mutation in the UK.

CF-associated severe lung disease may warrant referral to a lung transplantation centre and the child's local CF care team involved may discuss this option with the patient and family.

Nutritional management

The combined threats of malabsorption due to pancreatic insufficiency, poor appetite, increased metabolism due to chronic infection and increased respiratory work render nutritional management of vital importance in CF. The following supplements can be given:

- A high-calorie diet with vitamin supplements, especially fat-soluble vitamins A, D, E and K. Oral high-calorie diet alone may be inadequate in many children and enteral feeding via a gastrostomy is often needed in older patients.
- Pancreatic enzyme supplementation using enteric-coated microspheres in gelatin-coated capsules (e.g., Creon), which contain amylase, lipase and protease. This usually has a marked effect on steatorrhoea and allows 'catch-up' growth.

Prognosis

More than half of the present CF population are now expected to live beyond 40 years, and this will hopefully improve in the future. People with CF are at risk of a number of common complications; being underweight, upper airways complications (sinusitis and polyps), CF-related diabetes (uncommon in children under 10, but affect 50% of adults), liver disease (portal hypertension, biliary cirrhosis) and reduced bone mineral density.

Bronchiectasis

Bronchiectasis is at one end of a spectrum of disease characterized by bacterial airway infection causing a chronic cough and lung damage. At the other end of this continuum, protracted bacterial bronchitis is the commonest cause of chronic wet cough in children – but doesn't result in lung damage – evidenced radiologically (chest X-ray and/or CT chest).

Bronchiectasis in children is defined as the presence of abnormal bronchial dilatation on chest CT scan, in combination with a clinical syndrome of recurrent or persistent wet/productive cough, airway infection and/or inflammation. It is the end result of a variety of pathophysiologic processes that involve chronic or recurrent infection and airway obstruction and/or impaired mucociliary clearance. Early recognition in combination with aggressive treatment has led to better outcomes.

Aetiology

1. Postinfectious disease
   - Bacterial (*Pertussis*, TB, *Mycoplasma* and pneumonia-causing organisms)
   - Viral (measles, adenovirus, RSV)
2. Congenital
   - Cystic fibrosis
   - Structural airway and lung problems, e.g., congenital lobar emphysema
3. Immunodeficiencies
   - Acquired (HIV)
   - Congenital (hypogammaglobulinaemia and neutrophil function abnormalities)
4. Ciliary abnormalities
   - Kartagener syndrome and primary ciliary dyskinesia (PCD)
5. Mechanical
   - Foreign body
6. Aspiration (single episode or chronic)
7. Other
   - Inhalation of toxic gases
   - Idiopathic

Presentation

Symptoms include a chronic productive wet cough, haemoptysis, shortness of breath and failure to thrive. On examination, there may be coarse crepitations over the affected area, finger clubbing and chest deformity – hyperinflation, Harrison sulci and pectus carinatum.

Management

Initial imaging includes a chest X-ray and in severe cases, honeycombing may be seen. High-resolution CT scan is the gold standard investigation and may demonstrate the 'signet ring' sign.

Management is focused on treating the underlying causes and aggressively managing respiratory exacerbations with appropriate antibiotics (frequent sputum cultures are helpful). There is a role for chest physiotherapy, prophylactic/nebulized antibiotics and bronchodilators. These children require regular follow-up.

Pneumothorax

A pneumothorax is a collection of air in the pleural space (air leak) that results in a collapsed lung. This may occur due to positive pressure ventilation or trauma, but most are spontaneous and are primary in nature due to a ruptured subpleural bleb where there is no underlying lung disease. Less commonly, they may be secondary to respiratory causes such as CF, asthma, pneumonia and interstitial lung disease.

They are more common in adolescent males and thought to be due to the rapid growth of the thoracic cage leading to weakness in the pulmonary tissue at the peripheries.

Symptoms and signs include

Chest pain – sudden onset, pleuritic and stabbing
Tachycardia and tachypnoea
Unilateral hyperexpansion
Reduced or absent air entry on the affected side
Hyper-resonant percussion note on the affected side

Management

A chest X-ray is usually diagnostic though a small pneumothorax may be missed.

Treatment depends on important factors such as the degree and severity of symptoms, the size of the pneumothorax and whether it is a first pneumothorax, a recurrence or bilateral.

Options include:

- Observation and oxygen; many small pneumothoraces will heal without intervention.
- Needle thoracocentesis.
- Chest drain insertion.

HINTS AND TIPS

A tension pneumothorax occurs when there is continuous entry of air into the pleural space which cannot leave. This causes pressure on the heart, lungs, trachea and surrounding structures and will cause mediastinal shift. This is a medical emergency.

Clinical features include unilateral absent air entry/ hyper-resonant percussion note, acute shortness of breath, hypotension +/- shock, hypoxia and cyanosis, and tracheal deviation away from the affected side.

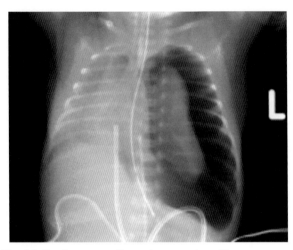

Fig. 4.8 Tension pneumothorax in a neonate on X-ray.

Urgent decompression with needle thoracocentesis is required (2nd intercostal space in the mid-clavicular line) and you should not wait to get a chest X-ray. If a chest X-ray is performed before needle decompression, Fig. 4.8 demonstrates the radiological signs.

EARS, NOSE AND THROAT (ENT)

There are key differences between the paediatric airway and the adult airway, meaning that airway obstruction is commoner in infants and young children (Fig. 4.9). Neonates are obligate nose

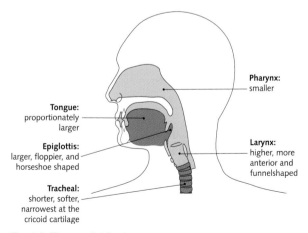

Pharynx: smaller

Tongue: proportionately larger

Epiglottis: larger, floppier, and horseshoe shaped

Larynx: higher, more anterior and funnelshaped

Tracheal: shorter, softer, narrowest at the cricoid cartilage

Fig. 4.9 The paediatric airway.

breathers until 5 months of age, although 40% of term babies will convert to oral breathing if nasal obstruction occurs.

Ears

Ear pain or discharge
Earache is usually caused by infection of the middle ear (otitis media). Less common causes include otitis externa, a foreign body or referred pain from the teeth. Ear discharge might be of wax or purulent material (from otitis externa, otitis media with perforation or a foreign body).

HINTS AND TIPS

Infants and small children are unable to localize pain to the ears or throat – ENT examination is important for all febrile children. Indications for ENT infection include toddlers pulling on their ears or refusing to feed.

Acute otitis media
Acute otitis media is an infection of the middle ear, which often occurs secondary to a viral URTI but can also be caused by a bacterial infection (e.g., *S. pneumoniae*, *Pneumococcus* spp., *H. influenzae*, *Moraxella catarrhalis*). It is very common in preschool children.

Clinical features
The presentation will often be nonspecific with fever, tachycardia, vomiting and distress, although older children may localize pain to the ear. On examination, otoscopy reveals a red, bulging eardrum with loss of the light reflex (Fig. 4.10). Perforation of the eardrum might occur, with a purulent discharge. Otitis media with effusion (OME) defines fluid in the middle ear, but

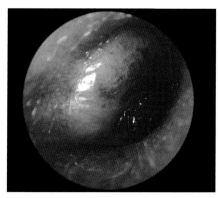

Fig. 4.10 Otoscopy: acute otitis media.

no signs of acute infection – often this follows acute otitis media. Mastoiditis and meningitis are now uncommon complications of acute otitis media.

Management
Symptomatic treatment is usually all that is needed. If bacterial infection is suspected, antibiotics can reduce the symptoms but not complications.

Hearing impairment
Hearing impairment is classified into two main types: conductive and sensorineural hearing loss. Conductive hearing loss is very common and is usually due to OME (also known as 'glue ear'). Sensorineural hearing loss is less common. Hearing impairment may present as speech delay or with behavioural problems.

CAUSES OF HEARING IMPAIRMENT	
Conductive	**Sensorineural**
Otitis media with effusion (glue ear)	Congenital • Hereditary causes (e.g., Alport syndrome) • Congenital infection (TORCH = toxoplasmosis, other infections, rubella, cytomegalovirus, herpes simplex) • Perinatal hypoxia • Neonatal jaundice (kernicterus)
Wax	Acquired • Meningitis • Ototoxic drugs (e.g., aminoglycoside antibiotics)
Foreign body	

Otitis media with effusion
OME or 'glue ear' is the commonest cause of conductive hearing loss in children. It occurs due to dysfunction of the eustachian tubes leading to persistent middle ear effusions. This can occur with recurrent URTIs but can also occur without a history of infections with increased incidence associated with Down syndrome, a cleft palate, enlarged adenoids, atopy and exposure to smoking. Over half of all preschool children have at least one episode of OME. A much smaller percentage will have persistent OME with hearing impairment.

Table 4.6 Tests of auditory function

Age	Test
Infant	Otoacoustic emission audiometry: Cochlear sounds are detected by a microphone in response to an auditory stimulus. Used for universal newborn hearing screening. Brainstem-evoked potential audiometry: Brainstem responses are detected by skin electrodes in response to an auditory stimulus.
Toddler	Conditioned response audiometry: Child trained to associate a visual reward or to perform a simple task when hearing a sound; sound volume/pitch varied to assess limits of hearing.
School-age children	Pure-tone audiometry: Child presses button in response to sound; sound volume/pitch varied to assess limits of hearing.
Any age	Impedance audiometry/tympanometry: measures eardrum compliance to detect middle ear effusions.

CLINICAL NOTES

Hearing thresholds (in decibels = dB):

- 70 dB = profound hearing loss.
- 20–70 dB = mild/severe hearing loss.
- <20 dB = normal hearing.

Speech uses frequencies of 400 to 4000 Hz.

HINTS AND TIPS

Parental suspicions about possible hearing loss should be taken seriously, with early referral for audiological testing. Other indications for referral are delayed speech development, behavioural problems or a history of repeated middle ear disease.

Assessment of hearing

Different age groups require different testing methods, summarized in Table 4.6. Universal newborn screening is now performed in the UK. Acquired hearing loss occurs after central nervous system infections (e.g., meningitis) and all affected children should have their hearing tested after the acute illness has resolved (Figs. 4.11 and 4.12).

Clinical features

Hearing loss can present as delayed speech, inattention and behavioural problems. Less common presentations include recurrent otalgia and loss of balance. Otoscopy is variable, the drum may be dull and may bulge or appear retracted (Fig. 4.13).

Management

The effusion and resulting hearing impairment is often transient but, if it is persistent, it can be an indication for surgical drainage of the middle ear with grommet insertion. A grommet is a

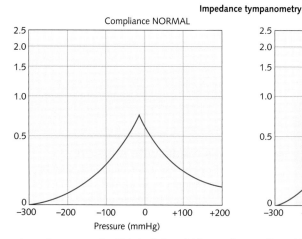
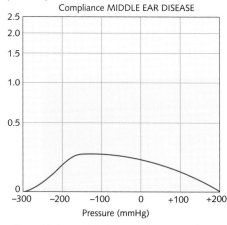

Fig. 4.11 Impedance tympanometry. This tests for middle ear disease. Sound is transmitted across the tympanic membrane if it is compliant (i.e., equal pressure on either side). The test measures reflected sound at different pressures. In serous otitis media, compliance is reduced at all pressures because of the fluid present, resulting in a flattened curve.

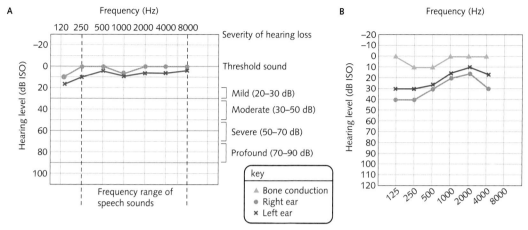

Fig. 4.12 Audiogram demonstrating: (A) normal hearing and (B) bilateral conductive hearing loss. In (B), there is a 20- to 40-dB hearing loss in both the right and left ears.

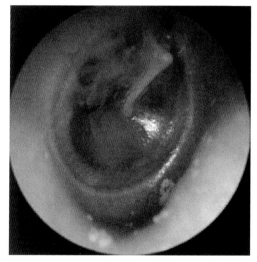

Fig. 4.13 Otoscopy: chronic otitis media (glue ear).

hollow plastic tube that ventilates the middle ear and remains effective only while patent. However, there is little evidence for the long-term benefits of grommets on hearing and speech development.

Nose

Nasal discharge and bleeding

The commonest cause of nasal discharge is a viral upper respiratory virus. A chronic discharge might be due to allergic rhinitis or a unilateral foreign body. Causes of epistaxis (nose bleeds) include:

- nose picking (most common)
- trauma
- bleeding disorders (especially thrombocytopenia)

Throat

Throat pathology may present with a sore throat, stridor or OSA.

Snoring and obstructive sleep apnoea

Snoring is a common symptom in children but in some is associated with significant OSA. History of apnoea with arousals during sleep and unusual sleep positions can indicate OSA. Daytime symptoms include chronic mouth breathing, behavioural problems and occasionally daytime headaches and sleepiness. Severe OSA can result in failure to thrive, right heart failure and corpulmonale. Children at high risk of OSA include those with craniofacial problems and Down's syndrome.

Chapter Summary

- Children are more susceptible to respiratory tract infections than adults, and therefore these are very common paediatric presentations.
- Remember that infections, including pneumonia/LRTI, are more commonly viral in children.
- Tonsillitis is commonly caused by a virus but prediction scores can help determine the likelihood of streptococcal infection and, therefore, the need to prescribe antibiotics.
- Epiglottitis is rare now due to immunization but remember not to examine and cause distress to a child if you suspect this diagnosis. Summon ENT and anaesthetic help early.
- Upper airway sounds are common in children, but stridor at rest (when undisturbed/not upset) can signify imminent airway obstruction and therefore should be acted upon urgently.
- Asthma is a very common childhood condition, more so in those with a personal or family history of atopy – treatment is stepwise, and you should follow the national BTS/SIGN guidelines.
- Cystic fibrosis is an autosomal recessive respiratory disease and has a carrier rate of 1:25. The gold standard diagnostic test is the sweat test. Newer CFTR modulator drugs are very promising and changing the way CF is managed.

UKMLA Conditions
Asthma
Bronchiectasis
Bronchiolitis
Croup
Cystic fibrosis
Epiglottitis
Lower respiratory tract infection
Obstructive sleep apnoea
Otitis media
Pneumothorax
Upper respiratory tract infection

UKMLA Presentations
Breathlessness
Cough
Stridor
Wheeze

Gastroenterology, hepatology and surgery 5

Both medical and surgical disorders of the gastrointestinal tract are common in paediatric practice. The range of pathological processes affecting the gastrointestinal tract is broad. It includes:

- congenital abnormalities
- infection
- immune-mediated allergy or inflammation

While jaundice in babies is very common (see Chapter 15, The newborn), liver disease in children is much less common but will be covered briefly at the end of this chapter.

PRESENTATION OF GASTROINTESTINAL DISEASE

Disorders of the gut present in a relatively limited number of ways which include abdominal pain, vomiting, diarrhoea, constipation and faltering growth.

Acute abdominal pain

There are many potential causes of acute abdominal pain. The key issue is to rapidly identify causes which require urgent surgical intervention Box 5.1.

BOX 5.1 CAUSES OF ACUTE ABDOMINAL PAIN

Surgical causes	Medical causes (abdominal)	Medical causes (systemic)
Acute appendicitis	Gastro-oesophageal reflux	Lower lobe pneumonia
Intestinal obstruction (e.g., Hirschsprung's, malrotation and volvulus)	Mesenteric adenitis	Diabetic ketoacidosis
	Gastroenteritis	Sickle cell disease
Meckel's diverticulum	Inflammatory bowel disease	Henoch–Schönlein purpura
Intussusception	Constipation	Addisonian crisis
Strangulated inguinal hernia	Urinary tract infection/pyelonephritis	Anaphylaxis
Volvulus	Renal colic	
	Pancreatitis (rare)	

BOX 5.1 CAUSES OF ACUTE ABDOMINAL PAIN (CONT.)

Surgical causes	Medical causes (abdominal)	Medical causes (systemic)
Boys: testicular torsion	Hepatitis/biliary colic (rare)	
Girls: Ovarian cyst pathology (e.g., rupture, torsion)		
Ectopic pregnancy		

History

In babies, abdominal pain is inferred from crying/screaming and drawing up of the legs. In older children, important features in the history are:

- Duration: pain lasting more than 4 hours is likely to be significant.
- Location: pain further away from the umbilicus is more likely to be significant (early appendicitis is an exception to this).
- Timing and character: constant aching or intermittent/colicky.
- Associated symptoms/signs:
  - vomiting (bilious suggests obstruction)
  - stools (bloody stools suggest intussusception in an infant, inflammatory bowel disease in older children)
  - anorexia (a normal appetite is reassuring)
  - dysuria [urinary tract infection (UTI)]
  - cough (pneumonia)

Examination

As well as examining the abdomen, a full systemic examination should be done.

- Fever: may be present in appendicitis, mesenteric adenitis, UTI and pneumonia.
- Jaundice: infectious hepatitis or biliary colic causes abdominal pain.
- Rash: the abdominal pain of Henoch–Schönlein Purpura might precede the characteristic purpuric rash.
- Respiratory examination for signs of pneumonia.
- Hernial orifices: is there a strangulated hernia?
- Genitalia: is there a torsion of the testis?

Investigations

- Urinalysis
  - Dipstick for nitrites/leucocytes (UTI) and glucose/ketones (diabetic ketoacidosis).
  - Send for microscopy and culture if indicated.
- Bloods: full blood count (FBC; looking for neutrophilia) and C-reactive protein (CRP) – raised inflammatory markers may be seen in acute appendicitis, pneumonia and a UTI. Liver function tests if jaundiced.
- Imaging
  - A plain abdominal film is rarely helpful unless obstruction/perforation is suspected.
  - Abdominal ultrasound is useful for some surgical causes of abdominal pain – it can diagnose intussusception and may show appendicitis (but cannot be used to rule it out).

Peritonitis

Peritonitis accounts for 1% to 3% of paediatric presentations with acute abdominal pain. It is reported to be more common in girls aged 4 to 9 years.

Peritonitis can be primary or secondary to inflammation of another intraabdominal organ (e.g., in appendicitis, colitis or a perforated organ/ulcer).

Primary peritonitis tends to occur as spontaneous bacterial peritonitis. Risk factors for this include presence of a VP shunt, peritoneal dialysis, chronic liver disease/ascites, nephrotic syndrome and immunodeficiency. Common organisms include *Streptococcus pneumoniae*, *Escherichia coli*, and *Klebsiella pneumoniae*.

Clinical features

Symptoms include abdominal pain, vomiting and fever which are common presenting features of many conditions. It is the examination that is specific for peritonitis: rigid abdomen, significant guarding, diffuse abdominal tenderness and rebound tenderness.

Investigations

Investigations may include a FBC, CRP and a blood culture, as well as abdominal imaging in secondary peritonitis such as an erect CXR if suspecting perforation of an abdominal organ or an USS if suspecting appendicitis or colitis.

Management

Treatment is directed at the underlying cause and administration of appropriate intravenous antibiotics. Laparoscopy and surgical treatment are common in secondary peritonitis.

Chronic and recurrent abdominal pain

The majority of cases of recurrent abdominal pain in children and adolescents do not have an organic cause and are functional in nature (Boxes 5.2 and 5.3). For this reason, the key is to take a detailed history exploring potential causes of underlying stress, as well as thoroughly examining the child to ensure there are no physical signs suggesting an underlying organic diagnosis.

Investigations

Investigations can be useful where possible organic causes are suspected. These may include:

- urine dipstick, microscopy and culture
- FBC, inflammatory markers, liver function tests
- *Helicobacter pylori* stool antigen

BOX 5.2 ORGANIC CAUSES OF RECURRENT ABDOMINAL PAIN

- Recurrent urinary tract infection.
- Urinary/renal calculi.
- *Helicobacter pylori* gastritis.
- Inflammatory bowel disease.
- Malrotation with intermittent volvulus.
- Gallstone disease.
- Recurrent pancreatitis.

BOX 5.3 FEATURES OF 'FUNCTIONAL' RECURRENT ABDOMINAL PAIN

- Pain usually periumbilical.
- No associated symptoms such as anorexia or change in bowel habits.
- On examination: thriving child with no physical signs.
- There may be a family history of recurrent abdominal pain, abdominal migraine, irritable bowel syndrome or migraines.
- Source of stress or anxiety identified on history taking.

- abdominal ultrasound
- other imaging such as magnetic resonance imaging or endoscopy (only after referral to a gastroenterologist if concerned there is an underlying organic pathology)

Normal investigations can be reassuring but it is important to avoid over investigating which can potentially contribute to child and parental anxiety.

Treatment

If a diagnosis of functional abdominal pain is made, it is important to emphasize that the pain is real and not 'faked', but does not have an identifiable physical cause. Management involves reassurance with an emphasis on continuing with activities. Psychological interventions like cognitive behavioural therapy or family therapy may be beneficial.

Vomiting

Vomiting can occur with a variety of serious conditions but can also be a normal finding in babies. It is important to differentiate normal milky possets from serious pathology. Vomiting may also indicate disease outside the gastrointestinal tract (Box 5.4). See also Chapter 15 for discussion on vomiting in the newborn.

History

Important points to establish include:

- Description of the vomit: volume, colour and whether it contains blood or bile. Biliary vomiting suggests intestinal obstruction until proven otherwise.
- Is it projectile? It is quite common for babies to posset and bring up small quantities of milk. Projectile vomiting, by

BOX 5.4 CAUSES OF VOMITING

Medical	Surgical

• Gastro-oesophageal reflux
 • Cow's milk protein allergy
 • Gastroenteritis
 • Systemic infections:
   - Urinary tract infection
   - Respiratory tract infection
   - Otitis media
   - Meningitis
 • Raised intracranial pressure
 • Inborn errors of metabolism
	• Pyloric stenosis
	 • Acute appendicitis
	 • Intussusception
	 • Intestinal obstruction

contrast, may indicate pyloric stenosis, particularly if the baby is hungry after vomiting.

- Duration: acute or persistent problem?
- Timing
  - Vomiting after feeds suggests overfeeding, gastro-oesophageal reflux or pyloric stenosis.
  - Early morning effortless vomiting suggests raised intracranial pressure.
- Associated symptoms: is vomiting accompanied by fever, headache, abdominal pain, constipation or diarrhoea?

Examination

Examine for the following:

- signs of dehydration (see Table 5.1)
- fever
- abdominal distension (visible peristalsis), tenderness or masses
- hernial orifices and genitalia

Table 5.1 Clinical features of dehydration and shock (adapted from NICE guidance).

Signs and symptoms	Not dehydrated	Dehydration	Shock
Sunken eyes or depressed fontanelle	Absent	Present (Red flag)	Present
Mucous membranes	Moist	Dry	Dry
Skin turgor	Normal	Reduced (Red flag)	Reduced
Alertness	Alert	Altered responsiveness (Red flag)	Lethargic
Heart rate and respiratory rate	Normal	Increased (Red flag)	Increased
Urine output	Normal	Reduced	Reduced
Skin colour	Unchanged	Unchanged	Pale or mottled
Extremities	Warm	Warm	Cool
Capillary refill time	Normal	Normal	Prolonged
Blood pressure	Normal	Normal	Hypotension is a preterminal sign which occurs in decompensated shock

'Red Flag' signs highlight those at increased risk of progression to shock.

Table 5.2 Causes of chronic diarrhoea

Cause	Examples
Infective causes	Giardiasis Amoebiasis
Food allergy or intolerance	Cow's milk protein allergy Lactose intolerance (primary or secondary to acute gastroenteritis)
Malabsorption	Coeliac disease Cystic fibrosis Pancreatic insufficiency
Inflammatory bowel disease	Crohn disease Ulcerative colitis

- Ask about recent travel considering infective causes.
- Any family history of inflammatory bowel disease?

Haematemesis

The differential diagnosis for vomiting blood varies with age. In the first few days of life it may be caused by swallowed maternal blood. Later on it can be due to oesophagitis and gastritis. Haematemesis can also occur due to a tear in the oesophageal mucosa as a result of forceful vomiting (Mallory-Weiss syndrome) or may be following a nosebleed due to swallowed blood.

Acute diarrhoea

Acute diarrhoea is most commonly caused by gastroenteritis (see later in this chapter). Bloody diarrhoea should raise suspicion of bacterial gastroenteritis and haemolytic-uraemic syndrome, as well as of noninfective conditions such as intussusception and inflammatory bowel disease.

Chronic diarrhoea

The most common cause of persistent loose stools in a well, thriving, preschool child is the so-called toddler diarrhoea. A maturational delay in intestinal motility causes intermittent explosive loose stools with undigested vegetables often present (peas and carrots). Chronic diarrhoea in a child who has faltering growth raises the possibility of several important diagnoses (Table 5.2).

History

- Define their usual bowel habit prior to this illness.
- A description of the stools might suggest steatorrhoea (pale, bulky and offensive), and the presence of blood or mucus suggests infective causes or inflammatory bowel disease.
- Any recent acute gastroenteritis? Watery diarrhoea with milk feeds suggests a transient secondary lactose intolerance which can last more than 2 weeks.

Examination

This includes assessment of dehydration (including weight) and then identifying the cause of diarrhoea. Look for any evidence of malabsorption – anaemia, poor weight gain, abdominal distension and buttock wasting. A thriving child with no associated symptomatology is unlikely to have significant disease.

HINTS AND TIPS

Faecal soiling due to constipation and overflow can be mistaken for diarrhoea.

Investigations

These are directed towards the suspected cause:

- stool microscopy and culture if bacterial cause suspected
- tests for reducing substances and faecal fats if considering malabsorption
- coeliac antibodies
- consider referral to a paediatric gastroenterologist if inflammatory bowel disease is suspected – they may do endoscopy and colonoscopy

Constipation

Constipation is a very common paediatric presentation – it refers to the delay or difficulty in passing stools for greater than 2 weeks. It might be accompanied by soiling caused by involuntary passage of faeces (overflow incontinence). The majority of cases are idiopathic (Box 5.5). Constipation might follow an acute febrile illness and can be prolonged if the hard stools cause a small, superficial anal tear. Fig. 5.1 shows the cycle of simple constipation.

BOX 5.5 ORGANIC CAUSES OF CONSTIPATION

- Coeliac disease.
- Food allergies (non-IgE mediated).
- Bowel obstruction.
- Hirschsprung disease.
- Cystic fibrosis.
- Neuromuscular disorders (e.g., cerebral palsy, spina bifida, spinal cord injury).
- Hypothyroidism.

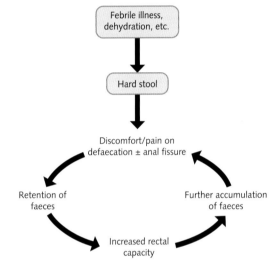

Fig. 5.1 The cycle of simple constipation.

RED FLAG

Constipation

- Starts in first few weeks of life.
- Meconium first passed at >24 hours of age.
- Abdominal distension or bilious vomiting (suggest bowel obstruction).
- Faltering growth.
- Delayed walking or lower limb neurology.
- Child protection concerns.

History and examination should be targeted at identifying any underlying organic causes. Always consider hypothyroidism and coeliac disease.

History

Enquire about:

- frequency and consistency of stools – hard, pellet-like stools are common

- presence of pain, needing to strain or blood on defaecation
- presence or absence of soiling
- any history of delay in passage of meconium

HINTS AND TIPS

Bowel habit varies enormously, and so a deviation from the norm is more of a concern than the actual frequency of defecation.

Examination

Check for the following:

- systemic signs of faltering growth
- abdominal distension, palpable descending colon
- presence of anal fissure

Digital rectal examination is not a routine part of the examination in idiopathic constipation and should only be performed if there is suspicion of an underlying disorder.

Management

Management involves a high fibre diet with adequate fluid intake. Prolonged treatment with laxatives may be needed – this may involve a disimpaction phase followed by a maintenance phase. Osmotic laxatives, commonly Macrogol (Movicol, Laxido), or lactulose tend to be used as a first line, using sufficient to produce a daily soft stool. Sometimes this may require a disempaction regime for severe cases. Treatment is often prolonged and in some cases requires psychological support.

HINTS AND TIPS

Laxatives work via different mechanisms and may be used in conjunction to help treat a child's constipation. There are:

- Bulk-forming laxatives – Fybogel (ispaghula husk)
- Osmotic laxatives – Macrogol, Movicol, lactulose
- Stool softeners – docusate, glycerol (suppositories) and arachis oil (enema)
- Stimulant laxatives – senna, bisacodyl, sodium picosulphate

In paediatrics, first line is an osmotic laxative and if this is unsuccessful, stimulants and/or stool softeners will be added.

Faltering growth

Faltering growth is used to describe a child who is not meeting their expected growth potential. It usually relates to weight gain but may also encompass linear growth. The rate of weight gain obtained by plotting serial weights on a centile chart over a period is more important, because a single observation is difficult to interpret. Remember that the birth weight is determined by the intrauterine environment, and the weight of a large infant may drop from its birth centile to a lower, genetically determined centile (catch down) in the first year.

The constitutionally small normal child should be recognized:

- small parents
- low birth weight for gestational age
- proportionally small: low centile for height, weight and head circumference
- normal height and weight velocities
- healthy child
- normal physical examination

COMMUNICATION

Poor weight gain is a common cause of parental anxiety. If the child's growth steadily follows the centile curve, it is likely to be normal. Reassure parents that normal small infants may have small appetites.

Globally, the most common cause of faltering growth is inadequate intake of food (i.e., starvation). In the UK, many cases have a nonorganic cause and are associated with psychosocial and environmental deprivation. Organic causes include inadequate food intake, defective absorption of food from the gastrointestinal tract (malabsorption) and increased energy expenditure (Table 5.3).

Following a thorough assessment, investigations should be targeted towards the most likely cause. A brief hospital admission to document weight gain on a measured dietary intake might be helpful (this is particularly important in cases of suspected neglect or factitious or induced illness).

IMPORTANT GASTROINTESTINAL CONDITIONS

Infantile colic

This is a common syndrome characterized by recurrent inconsolable crying often accompanied by drawing up of the legs. It usually occurs from around 2 weeks until about 4 months of age. It can occur several times a day, particularly in the evening. The differential diagnosis of inconsolable crying includes some important conditions that should be considered before a diagnosis of colic is made (Box 5.6). Infantile colic is benign and has a good prognosis, although it is a cause of great concern to parents and can be a risk factor for nonaccidental injury. A sympathetic explanation of the condition is helpful but there is no evidence for medication.

Gastro-oesophageal reflux

Gastro-oesophageal reflux is the involuntary passage of gastric contents into the oesophagus which occurs as a normal physiological finding in infancy. It is common in the first year of life due to transient lower oesophageal relaxation and a weak sphincter.

Table 5.3 Causes of faltering growth

Cause	Examples

Inadequate intake (must consider psychosocial deprivation, neglect and fabricated or induced illness within this category)	• Breastfeeding: insufficient milk supply or poor technique
	• Formula feeds: making feeds too dilute or not making up enough
	• Feeding problems
	  - Cleft palate
	  - Neurological (e.g., cerebral palsy)
	• Feeding aversion (e.g., secondary to severe gastro-oesophageal reflux)
	• Child with reduced appetite (e.g., underlying illness)

Malabsorption	• Coeliac disease • Cow's milk protein allergy • Short gut secondary to surgery • Cystic fibrosis (will also have increased requirements)

Increased requirements	• Any chronic disease
	  - Cystic fibrosis
	  - Congenital heart disease
	  - Chronic kidney disease

Infants at risk of severe gastro-oesophageal reflux include:

- preterm infants: especially those with chronic lung disease
- children with cerebral palsy
- infants with congenital oesophageal anomalies (e.g., after repair of a tracheo-oesophageal fistula)

Clinical features

The main symptom is posseting or vomiting. Some infants will be symptomatic with abdominal discomfort indicated by back arching and crying after feeds – this is usually worse when lying down; it may lead to feed aversion.

About 10% of infants with symptomatic reflux develop complications:

- bronchospasm and wheeze
- recurrent aspiration pneumonia
- oesophagitis (which may lead to haematemesis and anaemia)
- faltering growth

Investigations

Most reflux can be diagnosed clinically but several techniques are available for confirming the diagnosis and assessing the severity:

- twenty-four-hour oesophageal pH monitoring in older children or impedance studies in infants
- contrast (barium) studies: might be required to exclude underlying anatomical abnormalities
- endoscopy: indicated in patients with suspected oesophagitis

Management

In the majority of mildly affected infants, reassurance is all that is required and 95% will resolve by the age of 18 months. More troublesome reflux might respond to thickening the feeds.

The following drugs can be used in more severe reflux:

- drugs to reduce gastric acid secretion (H2 antagonists or proton pump inhibitors): especially if there is evidence of oesophagitis

- prokinetic drugs such as erythromycin and domperidone: these speed gastric emptying and increase lower oesophageal sphincter pressure; domperidone is less commonly used due to concerns of cardiac dysrhythmia

Surgery is required for very severe cases with complications. The most commonly used procedure is Nissen fundoplication in which the fundus of the stomach is wrapped around the lower oesophagus.

Gastritis and peptic ulcer disease

Gastritis is common in children, however, unlike in adults, it rarely leads to peptic ulcer disease.

H. pylori infection is the most common cause of gastritis in children which is also responsible for the majority of duodenal ulcers.

Other causes include:

- High-dose steroids and NSAIDs.
- Stress-related gastric injury due to trauma, burns, sepsis, intracranial disease, major surgery, or serious medical illness.
- Zollinger-Ellison syndrome (gastrin-secreting tumour).

Clinical features

The main presentation of children with gastritis is recurrent epigastric pain, dyspepsia (early satiety, bloating, belching, nausea) and/or vomiting.

These symptoms also occur in peptic ulcer disease. It is extremely difficult to differentiate between gastric and duodenal ulcers based on history alone. Classically, gastric ulcers present with epigastric pain shortly after meals and duodenal ulcers present with pain 2 to 3 hours afterwards. In practice, it is not this clear cut in paediatrics. Peptic ulcers can bleed so be aware of haematemesis, melena and symptoms of anaemia as presenting complaints.

Investigations

History, examination and investigations should be directed at establishing the underlying cause. In simple gastritis, no further investigations may be needed. If *H. pylori* is suspected, testing is often helpful to confirm this. Upper gastrointestinal endoscopy is the investigation of choice for children with suspected peptic ulcer disease.

Management

Treatment of simple gastritis may be with lifestyle interventions such as restricting irritants, such as spicy, fried or acidic foods and caffeinated drinks and can be managed with proton pump inhibitors.

In cases of *H. pylori* and peptic ulcer disease, triple therapy with a proton-pump inhibitor plus two antibiotics (amoxicillin and either clarithromycin or metronidazole) for two weeks will eradicate *H. pylori* and heal ulcers in the majority of cases.

Pyloric stenosis

Pyloric stenosis is due to hypertrophy of the smooth muscle of the pylorus and is an important cause of vomiting in babies. The incidence of pyloric stenosis is 1 to 5 per 1000 live births. It is five times more common in boys. It usually presents in the first 2 to 8 weeks of life.

Clinical features
It presents with persistent, projectile nonbilious vomiting after feeds. The infant remains hungry and eager to feed after vomiting. Weight loss, constipation, dehydration and mild jaundice develop after a few days.

Investigations
Diagnosis is clinical and is made by palpation of the hypertrophied pylorus during a test feed. Peristaltic waves might be visible. Ultrasound of the abdomen can confirm diagnosis, demonstrating the hypertrophied pylorus. In addition, a characteristic electrolyte disturbance develops with a hypochloraemic hypokalaemic metabolic alkalosis due to the loss of acidic gastric contents and the kidneys retaining hydrogen ions at the expense of potassium.

Management
Correction of fluid and electrolyte abnormalities is vital prior to surgical correction. The definitive treatment is the Ramstedt pyloromyotomy, in which the hypertrophied pyloric musculature is divided.

Acute appendicitis

Acute appendicitis is inflammation of the appendix secondary to obstruction (usually by a faecolith) or lymphoid hyperplasia. It is the most common surgical emergency and can occur at any age, although it is rare in infancy when the lumen of the appendix is wider and well drained.

Clinical features
The classical presentation of appendicitis is abdominal pain which initially starts as poorly localized, periumbilical pain (inflammation of the visceral peritoneum only) that then becomes sharper and localized to the right iliac fossa over a period of hours (once the inflammation affects the parietal peritoneum). The pain is usually severe and worse on movement, therefore the child may lie still. Common associated symptoms

include anorexia, nausea, vomiting and diarrhoea or constipation. On examination, there may be:

- low-grade fever
- tachycardia
- signs of dehydration
- right iliac fossa tenderness or tenderness over McBurney point (one-third of the way from the right anterior superior iliac spine to the umbilicus). A positive Rovsing sign is when palpation of the left iliac fossa causes pain in the right iliac fossa
- signs of peritonism if the appendix has perforated

Atypical presentations with poorly localized pain are common in young children and if the appendix lies in retrocaecal or pelvic orientations(common anatomical variants).

RED FLAG

A perforated gangrenous appendix can cause peritonitis. Suspect this if there is a high fever (>40°C), profuse vomiting, severe abdominal tenderness/guarding or absent bowel sounds.

Investigations
The diagnosis is usually made clinically. If there is diagnostic uncertainty, useful investigations include:

- FBC and CRP: neutrophilia and raised CRP may be seen but these can be normal in early appendicitis so cannot be used to exclude it.
- Abdominal ultrasound may show an appendicitis or other abdominal pathology; however, it cannot be used to exclude an appendicitis.
- Investigations to consider other differentials (e.g., urine dipstick and pregnancy test, chest X-ray).

Management
Management is by appendicectomy which may be done laparoscopically or as an open procedure with intravenous (IV) antibiotic cover. Where there is diagnostic uncertainty, a period of observation may be indicated although progression to peritonitis can occur within a few hours in young children. Other complications include sepsis, appendiceal abscess and appendiceal mass. An abscess requires surgical drainage. Conservative management (with antibiotics)is given for an appendiceal mass with elective appendicectomy carried out 6 weeks later.

Mesenteric adenitis

Mesenteric adenitis describes inflammation of intra–antiabdominal lymph nodes following a viral infection, usually an upper respiratory tract infection or gastroenteritis. The acute pain can mimic appendicitis; however, there will not be peritonism or guarding on examination. There may be a history of recent infection or signs on examination (e.g., a red throat or cervical lymphadenopathy). Observation in hospital is often required due to the difficult diagnosis. The symptoms are self-limiting. Management is conservative with analgesia.

HINTS AND TIPS

Persistent right iliac fossa tenderness warrants surgical exploration to rule out appendicitis.

Intussusception

Intussusception is a condition in which one segment of the bowel telescopes into an adjacent distal part of the bowel. The peak age of occurrence is between 5 and 10 months. It most commonly begins just proximal to the ileocaecal valve (the ileum invaginates into the caecum–ileocolic). It usually occurs after a viral infection, with enlarged lymphatics (Peyer patches) forming the lead point of the intussusception. It can, rarely, occur due to a pathological lead point, such as a polyp, lymphoma or with a Meckel diverticulum. This is more likely to be present in an older child.

Clinical features
The classical presenting 'triad' is:

- Paroxysmal colicky abdominal pain – a typical history of episodic screaming, during which the infant draws up the legs and becomes pale.
- An abdominal mass – typically a 'sausage-shaped' mass in the right upper quadrant.
- 'Redcurrant jelly' stool – this is a late sign where compromise in the blood supply to the bowel results in blood and mucus mixed in with the stool.

    Other important signs are of vomiting which becomes bilious, and signs of intestinal obstruction and shock.

Investigations
Ultrasound is the imaging modality of choice: the typical finding is the 'doughnut' sign which shows bowel within the bowel.

Management
Intussusception is a life-threatening condition which can lead to perforation – it warrants immediate transfer to a paediatric surgical unit. Air or barium enemas are often sufficient to reduce the

intussusception but if this fails, laparoscopy or laparotomy will be needed.

Meckel's diverticulum

This remnant of the foetal vitello-intestinal duct occurs in 2% of the population. It is usually 2 inches (5 cm) long and found 2 feet (60 cm) proximal to the ileocaecal valve (the rule of twos). It contains ectopic gastric mucosa. The majority are asymptomatic but the most typical presentation is painless rectal bleeding due to peptic ulceration. Treatment is surgical.

Hirschsprung disease (congenital aganglionic megacolon)

This is a rare inherited disorder where there is an absence of ganglion cells in the myenteric and submucosal plexuses for a variable segment of bowel extending from the anus to the colon. The aganglionic segment is narrow and contracted. It ends proximally in a normally innervated and dilated colon. It is more common in males and in children with Down syndrome.

Clinical features
Infants with the disease usually present in the neonatal period with:

- delayed passage of meconium (>48 hours of life)
- subsequent intestinal obstruction with abdominal distension and bilious vomiting

Older children present with:

- chronic, severe constipation present from birth
- an absence of faeces in the narrow rectum
- abdominal distension

Investigations
A barium enema might demonstrate a transition zone where the bowel lumen changes in diameter. Confirmation of the diagnosis is made by demonstrating the absence of ganglion cells on a suction biopsy of the rectum.

Management
Surgical resection of the involved colon is required. An initial colostomy is usually followed by a definitive pull-through procedure to anastomose normally innervated bowel to the anus.

Bowel obstruction and Ileus

Bowel obstruction can occur anywhere along the length of the bowel. This is often associated with abdominal distension and no bowel motions, and may progress to bilious vomiting.

Causes of small bowel obstruction include:

- duodenal atresia (associated with Down syndrome)
- malrotation with volvulus
- strangulated inguinal hernia
- meconium ileus due to cystic fibrosis

Causes of large bowel obstruction include:

- Hirschsprung disease
- imperforate anus or rectal atresia

Abdominal X-ray will help differentiate between small and large bowel obstruction and may give a clue to the underlying cause. Treatment is directed at establishing and correcting the underlying cause; surgery may be required. Medical management includes 'drip and suck'; keeping nil by mouth, insertion of a wide-bore NG on free drainage and IV fluids.

Ileus is a temporary lack of the normal muscle contractions of the intestines causing gut stasis without mechanical obstruction. Causes include drugs (opiates and TCAs), postabdominal surgery, sepsis, inflammatory bowel disease, colitis and electrolyte disturbance. This usually resolves without intervention when the underlying cause is treated.

Gastroenteritis

Gastroenteritis is an infection of the gastrointestinal tract which presents with a combination of diarrhoea and vomiting. In developed countries it is usually mild and self-limiting (affecting 1 in 10 children under the age of 2 years) but in the developing world approximately 2 million children under 5 years of age die from gastroenteritis each year.

Causes

In about half of cases, no pathogen will be found even with full investigation. In the UK, the majority of cases are viral, with rotavirus being the most common causative virus. Other causes are bacterial and parasitic (Box 5.7).

Clinical features

- Viral infection can cause a prodromal illness followed by vomiting and diarrhoea. The vomiting might precede diarrhoea and is not usually stained with bile or blood.

- Abdominal pain and blood or mucus in the stool suggest an invasive bacterial pathogen.
- If the child appears toxic with high fever, a bacterial cause is more likely.

Examination is necessary to assess the presence or absence of dehydration and shock (Table 5.3).

Investigations

Most children will not require investigations. Plasma urea, electrolytes and glucose should be measured if IV therapy is used or hypernatraemic dehydration suspected. Stool culture is indicated if the stool is bloody or if the child is septic or immunocompromised.

> **RED FLAG**
>
> With bloody diarrhoea, you need to consider the differential of haemolytic-uraemic syndrome (see Chapter 6 for more details) – check renal function and blood pressure.

Management

The key to management is rehydration with correction of the fluid and electrolyte imbalance.

If the child shows no signs of dehydration, then encourage parents to continue with normal fluid intake with oral rehydration salts (ORSs) as supplemental fluid if the condition worsens.

If there is evidence of clinical dehydration, give 50 mL/kg ORS over 4 hours in addition to maintenance fluids as ORS. If there is evidence of shock (decreased conscious level, poor perfusion, hypotension), give a bolus of 10 mL/kg 0.9% sodium chloride intravenously rapidly and repeat if necessary; may warrant transfer to a high dependency area. Then continue IV rehydration including the deficit.

To calculate maintenance fluids:

- 100 mL/kg/24 h for 0–10 kg bodyweight
- 50 mL/kg/24 h for 10–20 kg bodyweight
- 20 mL/kg/24 h for >20 kg bodyweight

BOX 5.7 CAUSES OF GASTROENTERITIS		
Viral	**Bacterial**	**Parasites**
Rotavirus	*Campylobacter* spp.	*Giardia lamblia*
Astrovirus	*Escherichia coli*	*Entamoeba histolytica*
Adenovirus	*Salmonella* spp.	
Norovirus (Norwalk virus)	*Shigella* spp.	*Cryptosporidium parvum*
	Vibrio cholerae	

HINTS AND TIPS

It is important to emphasize <u>oral</u> rehydration. Unless the child has persistent vomiting, oral fluid is the best means of rehydration. Smaller, more frequent sips may be better tolerated and should be encouraged. Another method of enteral hydration is via a nasogastric tube, which is preferable to IV fluids if tolerated by the child and parents.

There is no role for antidiarrhoeal medication in gastroenteritis. Antibiotics are rarely indicated except for specific bacterial infections, such as invasive salmonellosis or severe *Campylobacter* infection, and amoebiasis or giardiasis.

Inflammatory bowel disease

Inflammatory bowel disease describes chronic, relapsing and remitting inflammation of the intestine, with a number of associated symptoms. Up to one-quarter of cases of inflammatory bowel disease have their onset during childhood or adolescence, with Crohn disease (CD) being twice as common as ulcerative colitis (UC) in the paediatric setting (Box 5.8).

Aetiology

The precise aetiology of these conditions is unknown but it is thought to involve a complex interaction of environmental triggers (possibly infection; smoking is a risk factor in CD but is protective in UC) in a genetically susceptible host (there is an increased risk with HLA-B27 and with a positive family history). The resulting immune dysregulation causes damage to the bowel.

Pathophysiology
Clinical features

Inflammatory bowel disease may present with:

- abdominal pain (typically 'cramping' in UC)
- bloody diarrhoea with mucus
- weight loss/faltering growth
- UC: more likely to be systemically unwell with malaise, fever and tachycardia
- CD: more likely to see aphthous ulceration and perianal disease (skin tags, fissures, abscesses and fistulae)
- extraintestinal features might be present – see Fig. 5.2

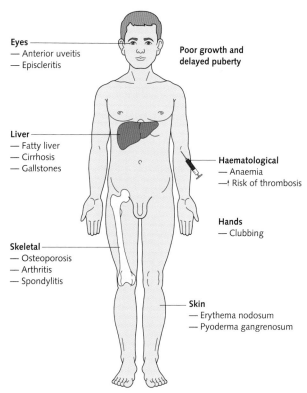

Fig. 5.2 Extraintestinal presentation of inflammatory bowel disease.

Complications of CD include intestinal strictures, abscesses and fistulae. Long term, they have a five to six times increased risk of developing colorectal cancer.

Complications of UC include toxic megacolon, risk of primary sclerosing cholangitis and cholangiocarcinoma and a 20 to 30 times increased risk of developing colorectal cancer over 30 years.

Investigations

Diagnosis is by colonoscopy with biopsy, looking for typically macroscopic and microscopic features. Crohn disease results in transmural inflammation (affects all layers of the bowel wall) whereas UC affects only the mucosa/lining. Other features of Crohn's include cobblestone mucosa (clustering of ulcers that resembles a cobblestone street), skip lesions (normal bowel between areas of disease), and 'Rose thorn ulcers' (deep, linear ulcers; strictures and fistulae).

In addition, blood tests should involve an FBC (looking for inflammation and anaemia), CRP/erythrocyte sedimentation rate (increase with disease activity), renal function and liver function. Stool samples should be sent for culture to

BOX 5.8 COMPARISON OF CROHN DISEASE WITH ULCERATIVE COLITIS

Crohn disease	Ulcerative colitis
Occurs anywhere from mouth to anus (skip lesions)	Continuous disease which always involves the rectum and can spread proximally
Full-thickness 'transmural' inflammation	Mucosa inflamed only
Granulomatous inflammation – "cobblestone mucosa"	Nongranulomatous inflammation

exclude a bacterial gastroenteritis which could present similarly and for faecal calprotectin which is a marker of inflammation in the gut.

Management

The focus of management is to induce and maintain remission and to support normal growth.

CD is managed initially with an elemental diet for 6 to 8 weeks; for severe or refractory disease, steroids will be needed to induce remission. For maintenance, immunosuppressive agents are needed, such as mesalazine and azathioprine, followed by antitumour necrosis factor antibodies such as infliximab. Surgery is an option for failure of medical treatment or for complications.

UC is treated initially with aminosalicylates or steroids, topical or systemic depending on the severity of disease. Maintenance agents will be needed. Surgery may be used when medical treatment has failed: a subtotal colectomy and ileostomy can be curative.

Coeliac disease

Coeliac disease is an autoimmune disease in which gluten (present in wheat, barley and rye) ingestion results in damage to the mucosa of the proximal small intestine with subsequent atrophy of the villi and loss of the absorptive surface. The incidence varies between 0.5% and 3% in children. There is a familial predisposition with approximately 10% of first-degree relatives affected. HLA-DQ2 is found in 95% of affected individuals. It is more common in Caucasian people. There is an association with other autoimmune disease (e.g., type 1 diabetes mellitus and autoimmune thyroid disease), Down syndrome and Turner syndrome.

Clinical features

The classic presentation is of faltering growth, steatorrhoea and abdominal distension; however, features may be more subtle. They include:

- abdominal pain
- diarrhoea
- constipation
- fatigue
- iron- or folate-deficiency anaemia
- aphthous ulcers
- short stature
- amenorrhoea

Investigations

The first-line test is for immunoglobulin A tissue transglutaminase (TGA-IgA) which should be done in conjunction with total IgA (in IgA deficiency, IgG antibodies can be used). If this result is more than 10 × the upper normal value, and endomyseal antibodies are present (EMA-IgA) a biopsy is not required to diagnose coeliac disease. Otherwise, a definitive diagnosis will be made by taking a duodenal or jejunal biopsy, which will show a flat mucosa that then improves after gluten withdrawal from the diet.

A diet free of gluten-containing products should be adhered to for life. Multidisciplinary care is required with support from a dietician. Complications include an increased risk of small bowel malignancy (especially lymphoma) and osteoporosis. Lifelong follow-up is required to monitor for these conditions. A strict gluten-free diet reduces the malignancy risk.

Food intolerance

Adverse reactions to specific foods or food ingredients are not uncommon and can be transitory or permanent. The majority are immune-mediated reactions, usually to proteins, and are properly referred to as food allergies. However, nonimmune-mediated intolerance also occurs (e.g., lactose intolerance due to intestinal disaccharidase deficiency).

Lactose intolerance

Lactose is the predominant disaccharide in milk and requires the intestinal brush-border enzyme lactase for its digestion. Lactase deficiency is most commonly encountered as a secondary and transient phenomenon after gastroenteritis but can occur as a congenital deficiency. Accumulation of intestinal sugar results in watery diarrhoea and bacterial production of organic acids, which lowers stool pH and causes excoriation of the perianal region. Lactose is a reducing sugar and may therefore be detected in the stool by the Clinitest method. Treatment is with a diet free of products containing lactose.

LIVER DISEASE

Liver disease is relatively uncommon in childhood. It usually manifests as jaundice or hepatomegaly, but, rarely, can cause acute liver failure or with chronic liver disease/cirrhosis, requiring liver transplant.

Jaundice

Jaundice is a yellow discolouration of the sclerae, skin and mucosae, caused by an increase in circulating bilirubin. The bilirubin can be unconjugated or conjugated, depending on the aetiology (Fig. 5.3). Jaundice is most commonly seen in the neonatal period (see Box 5.9 and Chapter 15) but can occur in older children too.

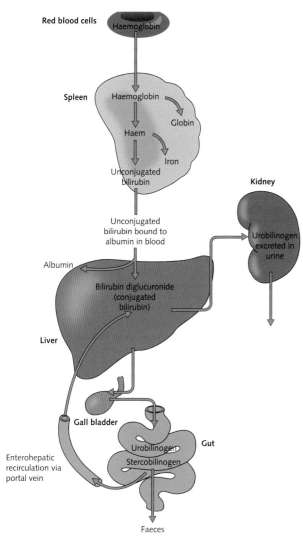

Fig. 5.3 Bilirubin metabolism.

Causes of jaundice after infancy

Jaundice in childhood usually has an infective cause. Infective hepatitis can be caused by:

- hepatitis viruses: hepatitis A is the most common cause of jaundice after the neonatal period
- Epstein-Barr virus
- malaria or bilharzia

Liver injury can be caused by a variety of drugs (e.g., sodium valproate, halothane) and, in overdose, paracetamol and iron are toxic to the liver. Jaundice with pallor suggests a haemolytic episode (e.g., glucose-6-phosphate dehydrogenase deficiency, sickle cell disease or haemolytic-uraemic syndrome).

Hepatomegaly

Isolated hepatomegaly is uncommon. In association with jaundice, the causes include biliary atresia and infective hepatitis. In young children, hepatomegaly is an important feature of cardiac failure. Hepatosplenomegaly can occur in malaria, in advanced liver disease and in a number of important haematological diseases (e.g., leukaemia, sickle cell disease and thalassaemia) and rare storage disorders (e.g., mucopolysaccharidosis).

Chapter Summary

- Although functional abdominal pain is the most common cause of abdominal pain in children, it is vital to rule out potentially life-threatening organic causes, such as appendicitis.
- The key to the management of paediatric vomiting and diarrhoea is the clinical assessment of dehydration and management by rehydration.
- In cases of bloody diarrhoea, consider the possibility of haemolytic-uraemic syndrome.
- Constipation is a common problem but if poorly managed can lead to pain, encopresis and poor school attendance. Start with an osmotic laxative and add in a stimulant or stool softener if required.
- Pyloric stenosis occurs in the first few weeks of life and presents with projectile vomiting and hypokalaemic hypochloraemic metabolic alkalosis.
- Failure to pass meconium in the first 48 hours of life is a red flag and warrants investigation for anorectal malformations, Hirschsprung disease and obstruction.
- 25% of cases of inflammatory bowel disease present in adolescence. Always consider this diagnosis in chronic abdominal pain and weight loss. A simple initial investigation may be faecal calprotectin but gold standard diagnosis is colonoscopy.
- Red flags requiring further investigation are weight loss, blood in the vomit or stool, jaundice or hepatomegaly.

UKMLA Conditions
Appendicitis
Biliary atresia
Coeliac disease
Constipation
Gastro-oesophageal reflux disease
Hernias
Inflammatory bowel disease
Intestinal obstruction and ileus
Intussusception
Peptic ulcer disease and gastritis
Peritonitis
Pyloric stenosis
Viral gastroenteritis
Volvulus

UKMLA Presentations
Acute abdominal pain
Chronic abdominal pain
Diarrhoea
Coeliac disease
Food intolerance
Infant feeding problems
Jaundice
Vomiting

Paediatric renal and genitourinary conditions can present in various ways, from antenatal diagnosis on ultrasound scan to late presentation in adulthood with chronic kidney disease (CKD). Some of the important symptoms and signs of disease within this system are as follows.

Important symptoms:

- Polyuria or increased urinary frequency: suggests urinary tract infection (UTI) or diabetes mellitus. Polyuria means increased urine output due to a diuresis (diabetes mellitus, diabetes insipidus) or due to increased water intake, whereas frequency does not necessarily mean an increased urine output.
- Dysuria: suggests UTI.
- Oliguria: suggests dehydration or acute kidney injury (AKI).
- Discoloured urine (Fig. 6.1).
- Fever with or without rigors: rule out UTI or pyelonephritis.

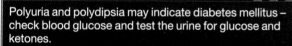

RED FLAG

Polyuria and polydipsia may indicate diabetes mellitus – check blood glucose and test the urine for glucose and ketones.

HINTS AND TIPS

Polyuria and frequency can present as secondary enuresis – organic causes of these should be considered as part of the assessment of enuresis.

Important signs are:

- Haematuria (see later).
- Proteinuria (see later).
- Hypertension (upper limit of normal varies with age and height): suggests renal disease, cardiovascular disease or endocrine diseases – always warrants further investigation.
- Oedema: suggests nephrotic syndrome.
- Palpable bladder or kidneys suggests anatomical abnormalities or malignancy.

HAEMATURIA

Haematuria can be divided into visible (frank) haematuria and nonvisible (microscopic) haematuria. Glomerular disease usually causes nonvisible haematuria with pathognomonic red

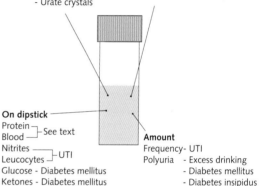

Fig. 6.1 Information available from urine. *UTI,* Urinary tract infection.

blood cell casts on urine microscopy. Haematuria detected on urine dipstick should be confirmed by urine microscopy.

Causes

- Intense exercise.
- Glomerulonephritis.
- UTIs (e.g., acute bacterial UTI, tuberculosis, schistosomiasis).
- Trauma (e.g., catheter associated).
- Renal calculi.
- Malignancy (e.g., Wilms' tumour).
- Congenital obstructive lesions.
- Heritable conditions (e.g., Alport syndrome [haematuria and deafness]).
- Bleeding disorders.
- Transient, benign haematuria can occur but is a diagnosis of exclusion.

History

Find out the following:

- duration
- associated dysuria and urinary frequency: suggest UTI

67

- associated loin pain: suggests pyelonephritis (if associated with fever) or renal calculi (especially if the pain is colicky)
- recent sore throat or skin infection: suggests post–streptococcal glomerulonephritis
- recent foreign travel: suggests schistosomiasis
- family history: suggests heritable conditions (e.g., Alport syndrome)

COMMUNICATION

Orange or red urate crystals in the nappy are a normal finding in the newborn – reassure parents who may be concerned that this is blood.

Examination

Examine for:

- fever: suggests UTI
- hypertension: suggests acute nephritis or CKD
- oedema: suggests nephrotic syndrome. In nephritis, oedema is usually mild if present
- typical rash and joint swelling: suggests Henoch-Schönlein purpura
- bruises and purpura: suggests idiopathic thrombocytopenic purpura
- abdominal mass: suggests Wilms' tumour

Investigations

The choice of investigations depends on the renal pathology suspected:

- urine dipstick
- midstream urine for microscopy, culture and sensitivity (MC&S)
- haematology: full blood count, coagulation screen and sickle cell screen
- biochemistry: urea and electrolytes (U&Es), Ca^{2+}, PO_4^{3-} and urate
- evidence of streptococcal infection: throat swab, antistreptolysin O titre (ASOT)
- complement: C3, C4
- hepatitis B antigen
- imaging: ultrasound scan (usually first line) and further imaging including nuclear medicine

A renal biopsy might be indicated in the following situations:

- persistent haematuria for >6 months
- unexplained abnormal renal function
- chronic glomerulonephritis

PROTEINURIA

Normal children produce <60 mg/m^2/24 hours of protein in the urine.

Definition of proteinuria

- Early morning urine protein:creatinine ratio >20 mg/mmol.
- Greater than 5 mg/kg in a 24-hour urine sample.

Causes

Transient, mild proteinuria frequently occurs in children with viral infections and is self-limiting. By contrast, nephrotic syndrome causes persistent, heavy proteinuria.

Causes of transient proteinuria:

- fever
- exercise
- orthostatic proteinuria – not seen first thing in the morning after lying flat all night

Causes of persistent proteinuria:

- nephrotic syndrome
- glomerulonephritis
- UTI

Examination

Physical examination should include evaluation for signs of renal disease (especially nephrotic syndrome). Signs to look for include:

- oedema: especially ankle, periorbital and scrotal
- ascites
- pleural effusions (unusual)
- blood pressure: low or high

Investigations

The investigations include:

- urine dipstick (Table 6.1)
- midstream urine for MC&S
- early morning protein: creatinine ratio
- U&Es

Table 6.1 Albustix values

Stix reading	Albumin concentration (g/L)
+	0.3
+ +	1.0
+ + +	3.0
+ + + +	>20

- complement: C3, C4
- plasma albumin and lipids
- evidence of streptococcal infection: throat swab, ASOT

Peripheral oedema and ankle swelling

Peripheral oedema has several multisystem causes but is considered here due to its strong association with nephrotic syndrome.

Causes include:

- Cardiac failure
- Nephrotic syndrome
- Hepatic failure
- Malnutrition in, e.g., kwashiorkor
- Protein-losing enteropathy
- Connective tissue disease
- Syndromic aetiology, e.g., Noonan and Turner syndrome
- Congenital lymphoedema (Milroy disease)
- Side effects of ACE inhibitor drugs

A full history and examination should be undertaken. The presence of GI symptoms may point towards an enteropathy. The presence of poor feeding, tachypnoea and a murmur may signify a cardiac cause.

Initial investigations include urine dipstick and MC+S, laboratory bloods including FBC, U+Es, LFTs and a CXR. An echo may help demonstrate an underlying cardiac cause.

Management

This should be directed at treating the underlying cause. Symptomatic relief can be obtained by bed rest and elevation of the legs, sodium restriction and use of diuretics.

URINARY TRACT ANOMALIES

Structural anomalies of the kidney and urinary tract are relatively common, occurring in about one in 400 foetuses. Many of these will be identified on antenatal ultrasound screening or they may present later in infancy or childhood, for example, with recurrent UTIs.

Congenital anomalies of the urinary tract include:

- renal anomalies
- obstructive lesions of the urinary tract
- vesicoureteric reflux (VUR)

Renal anomalies

Anomalies of the renal parenchyma include:

- Renal agenesis – if bilateral, this presents with Potter syndrome (oligohydramnios due to a lack of foetal urine leading to pulmonary hypoplasia and typical facies of beaked nose and low set ears) and death.

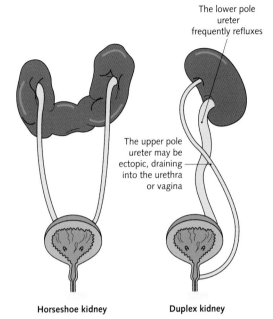

Fig. 6.2 Urinary tract anomalies.

- Abnormalities of ascent and rotation – result in ectopic kidneys.
- Duplex kidney (Fig. 6.2) – duplex systems are commonly associated with other abnormalities such as renal dysplasia and VUR. The upper pole ureter might be ectopic (draining into the urethra or vagina) and the lower pole ureter often refluxes.
- Horseshoe kidney (Fig. 6.2).
- Cystic disease of the kidney – caused by multiple conditions including autosomal recessive polycystic kidney disease (infantile form), autosomal dominant polycystic kidney disease (adult type) and tuberous sclerosis (see Chapter 16).
- Renal dysplasia.

HINTS AND TIPS

Pain arising from an ectopic kidney can be misleading due to its atypical site.

Obstructive lesions of the urinary tract

The site of obstruction may be at the pelviureteric junction, the vesicoureteric junction, the bladder or the urethra (Fig. 6.3). These can often be detected on antenatal ultrasound scans as they can cause hydronephrosis (abnormal dilatation of the renal pelvis ± renal calyces). If not detected before birth, the patient can present with:

- UTIs
- urinary calculi

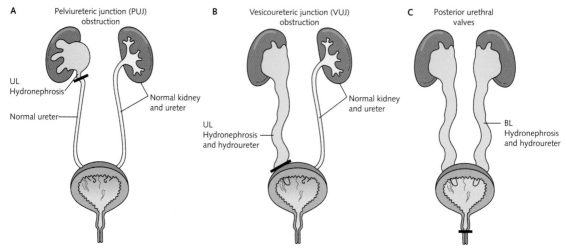

Fig. 6.3 Sites of urinary tract obstruction and dilatation. *BL*, bilateral; *UL*, unilateral.

- haematuria
- abdominal or loin pain
- a palpable bladder or kidney
- reduced renal function
- hypertension

Pelviureteric junction obstruction

Obstruction at the point where the renal pelvis joins the ureter is the commonest cause of antenatal hydronephrosis. It can be caused by a narrow lumen or external compression by a fibrous band or blood vessel, and varies from partial to almost complete obstruction (with gross hydronephrosis and minimal remaining renal tissue). Mild degrees of obstruction can resolve spontaneously but severe obstruction requires surgical treatment with conservation of renal tissue wherever possible.

Vesicoureteric junction obstruction

Obstruction at the point where the ureter joins the bladder can be due to stenosis, kinking or dilatation of the lower part of the ureter (ureterocoele). It can be unilateral or bilateral. There is a combination of hydroureter and hydronephrosis. As with pelviureteric obstruction, it may resolve spontaneously but severe cases require stenting and/or surgery.

Posterior urethral valves

Posterior urethral valves occur in male infants only and are abnormal folds of the urethral mucous membrane which block the urethra. They impede the flow of urine with backpressure on the bladder, ureters and kidneys leading to bladder hypertrophy and bilateral hydroureteronephrosis. In very severe cases, there can be Potter syndrome with oligohydramnios, renal failure and pulmonary hypoplasia. Less severe cases may present later with

poor urinary stream, UTIs and declining renal function. Posterior urethral valves are often diagnosed antenatally. Management involves initial catheter drainage followed by endoscopic valve ablation, as soon as the child is stable.

> **RED FLAG**
>
> Although antenatal hydronephrosis is common and usually resolves spontaneously after birth, if bilateral, it warrants urgent investigation due to the possibility of posterior urethral valves.

Vesicoureteric reflux

This is a condition in which there is retrograde flow of urine up the ureter during voiding, predisposing to ascending infection. This can lead to scarring (reflux nephropathy) and a gradual decline in renal function. It is a major cause of paediatric CKD. Primary VUR is caused by a developmental anomaly of the vesicoureteric junction. With normal development, the ureters enter the bladder at an angle, with a large section of the ureter within the muscular wall, which is compressed with bladder contraction. In primary VUR, the ureters enter perpendicularly, meaning that the segment of the ureter within the bladder wall is abnormally short and there is inadequate ureter closure during voiding. There is a spectrum of severity which is graded I–V (Fig. 6.4). VUR is often associated with other genitourinary anomalies and may be secondary to bladder pathology (e.g., a neuropathic bladder).

Clinical features

VUR is often asymptomatic. If not diagnosed antenatally, it may present with recurrent UTIs or pyelonephritis. If not

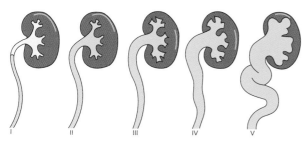

Fig. 6.4 Grades of vesicoureteric reflux.

treated early, progressive renal scarring can cause CKD and hypertension.

Investigation

VUR is diagnosed by a micturating cystourethrogram (MCUG) which allows visualization of the whole urethra.

Management

Mild VUR resolves spontaneously (10% each year) but prophylactic antibiotics (e.g., trimethoprim) may be given to prevent infection in more serious cases.

Surgery is indicated if there are recurrent UTIs or grade IV–V VUR.

> **HINTS AND TIPS**
>
> The siblings of children with vesicoureteric reflux should be investigated as there is a strong genetic component.

URINARY TRACT INFECTION

UTIs are common in childhood. About 3% to 5% of girls and 1% to 2% of boys will have a symptomatic UTI during childhood. Boys outnumber girls until 3 months of age, they occur equally in boys and girls from 3 to 12 months and girls outnumber boys from age 1 year upwards.

Causes

In children, most infections are caused by *Escherichia coli* originating from the bowel flora. Other pathogens include *Proteus* (especially in boys), *Klebsiella, Pseudomonas* and *Enterococcus* species. Risk factors for UTIs:

- poor hygiene
- urinary stasis secondary to habitual infrequent voiding and constipation
- VUR

- obstructive lesions of the urinary tract: congenital lesions and secondary to stones
- neuropathic bladder (e.g., spina bifida)

Clinical features

In infants and young children, presentation is often nonspecific with a fever, lethargy, vomiting or poor feeding. UTI should be considered in all children with an unexplained fever and it accounts for 4% to 5% of fever in infants. Jaundice might occur in those under 3 months of age. Preverbal children may show signs of abdominal or loin pain/tenderness. Those aged 5 years and over are more likely to present with classic symptoms/signs of dysuria, urinary frequency and enuresis. Offensive-smelling urine and haematuria can occur at any age.

Diagnosis

Obtaining an uncontaminated urine sample from infants and young children is not easy (Table 6.2). Urine dipstick positive for nitrites and leucocytes is sufficient to confirm a UTI in well children over 3 years old. Urine should be sent for MC&S:

- in all children under 3 years of age
- in systemically unwell children
- where there is a single positive result for nitrites or leucocytes
- recurrent UTI
- UTI unresponsive to treatment

Confirmation of diagnosis requires culture of a pure growth of a single pathogen of at least 10^5 colony-forming units/mL of urine.

> **HINTS AND TIPS**
>
> A urine sample should be cultured from:
>
> - An infant with a fever and no obvious clinical source.
> - Any child with recurrent or prolonged fever.
> - Any child with unexplained abdominal pain.
> - Any child with dysuria, frequency, enuresis or haematuria.

Table 6.2 Collecting a urine sample

Method	Indication
Clean catch	Method of choice for obtaining sample
Bag or pad sample	If clean catch not obtainable
Suprapubic aspirate (with ultrasound guidance)	If an urgent sample required and noninvasive technique not practical
Catheter	Only fresh samples valid for infection

Treatment of the acute infection

Prompt treatment with antibiotics is indicated to prevent serious illness and reduce the risk of renal scarring. A urine sample for MC&S should be taken before treatment but antibiotics should not be delayed in an unwell child. Treatment can be modified when culture results are available and stopped if negative. Asymptomatic bacteriuria is common in school-age girls and does not need treatment. Choice and length of treatment depends on the age of the child, whether signs or symptoms of an upper UTI (pyelonephritis) are present and will be according to local microbiology guidance.

- Children <3 months of age: a full septic screen is often needed and management is by broad-spectrum intravenous (IV) antibiotics.
- Children >3 months of age with uncomplicated, lower UTI: oral antibiotics for 3 days.
- Children >3 months of age with signs of pyelonephritis/ complicated UTI: IV antibiotics as needed for 2 to 4 days, oral antibiotics for 7 to 10 days.

Further investigation

Further investigation depends on:

- The age of the child.
- Whether episodes are recurrent (2 upper UTIs, 1 upper UTI + 1 lower UTI or >3 lower UTIs).
- Presence of any atypical features (non-*E. coli* UTI, failure to respond to treatment in 48 hours, sepsis, abnormal renal function).

Investigations aim to identify structural renal abnormalities (ultrasound scan), reflux (with MCUG) or renal scarring (with nuclear medicine radioisotope scan – first line is a static scan, dimercaptosuccinic acid (DMSA)).

The recommended imaging schedules (National Institute for Health and Care Excellence (NICE) guidelines 2022) are shown in Tables 6.3–6.5.

Simple advice should be given concerning measures, which can reduce recurrence risk such as:

- increasing fluid intake
- regular unhurried voiding

Table 6.3 Imaging schedule for infants younger than 6 months of age

Test	Responds well to treatment within 48 hours	Atypical urinary tract infection (UTI)	Recurrent UTI
Ultrasound during acute infection	No	Yes	Yes
Ultrasound within 6 weeks	Yes (if abnormal consider MCUG)	No	No
DMSA scan 4–6 months following acute infection	No	Yes	Yes
MCUG	No	Yes	Yes

Table 6.4 Imaging schedule for children aged 6 months to 3 years

Test	Responds well to treatment within 48 hours	Atypical urinary tract infection (UTI)	Recurrent UTI
Ultrasound during acute infection	No	Yes	No
Ultrasound within 6 weeks	No	No	Yes
DMSA scan 4–6 months following acute infection	No	Yes	Yes
MCUG	No	No	No

Table 6.5 Imaging schedule for children older than 3 years

Test	Responds well to treatment within 48 hours	Atypical urinary tract infection (UTI)	Recurrent UTI
Ultrasound during acute infection	No	Yes	No
Ultrasound within 6 weeks	No	No	Yes
DMSA 4–6 months following acute infection	No	No	Yes
MCUG	No	No	No

- good perineal hygiene
- avoiding constipation

ACUTE NEPHRITIS

Glomerulonephritis describes inflammation of the glomeruli and nephrons which can present clinically in a number of different ways, including acute nephritis (nephritic syndrome) and nephrotic syndrome. These syndromes describe the clinical presentation rather than the underlying pathology.

Acute nephritis is characterized by:

- haematuria
- reduced renal function
- hypertension
- there may also be proteinuria and oedema, but these are usually less prominent than in nephrotic syndrome (Table 6.6)

Causes

In children the majority of cases are due to a postinfectious glomerulonephritis and occur 10 to 14 days after a throat or skin infection with group A β-haemolytic streptococci. Less common causes include:

- Henoch–Schönlein purpura
- IgA nephropathy
- systemic lupus erythematosus
- mesangiocapillary glomerulonephritis
- haemolytic-uraemic syndrome

Table 6.6 Comparison of acute glomerulonephritis and nephrotic syndrome

Feature	Acute nephritis	Nephrotic syndrome
Aetiology	Most often poststreptococcal	Usually minimal change disease
Gross haematuria	Very common	Unusual
Hypertension	Common	Less common
Oedema	Less prominent	Prominent, generalized oedema
Urinalysis	Red cell casts, proteinuria +	Proteinuria +++
Serum C3 and C4	Usually decreased	Usually normal
Anti-DNase B/ antistreptolysin O titre (ASOT)	May be positive	Negative
Treatment	Supportive	Steroids

Clinical presentation

The presenting history will be of haematuria/discoloured urine (with postinfectious glomerulonephritis, urine will typically be described as 'cola' coloured). Physical examination may reveal hypertension and oedema. Other features may be present depending on the underlying cause.

Investigation

The urine should be dipped for blood and protein, microscopy performed to look for red cell casts and renal function assessed. Abdominal imaging may be required to exclude other causes of haematuria. Investigations to determine the underlying aetiology include throat swab, anti-DNase B, complement levels and renal biopsy if there is severe renal involvement.

Management

Management centres around:

- Careful control of fluid and electrolyte balance.
- Use of diuretics and antihypertensives as required.
- Treatment of underlying cause as appropriate.
- For postinfectious glomerulonephritis, oral penicillin can be given to reduce spread to others, but it does not alter the course of the nephritis. The prognosis of poststreptococcal nephritis is good and 95% make a full recovery. Rarely, a rapidly progressive glomerulonephritis with renal failure occurs, especially with nephritis from other causes.

NEPHROTIC SYNDROME

Nephrotic syndrome is characterized by the triad of proteinuria (see Table 6.1), hypoalbuminaemia and oedema. In addition, there is often hypertriglyceridaemia.

Causes

The majority of childhood nephrotic syndrome is minimal change disease which can be classified into steroid sensitive (90%) or steroid resistant (10%). Less common causes are focal segmental glomerulosclerosis and membranous glomerulonephritis.

Clinical features

The usual presenting feature is oedema, which manifests as facial puffiness (especially around the eyes), swelling of the feet and legs and, in severe cases, gross scrotal oedema, ascites and pleural effusions.

Several serious complications may occur including:

- Hypovolaemia (manifested by oliguria, peripheral vasoconstriction, a raised packed cell volume and hypotension).

- Thrombosis.
- Secondary infection, typically with *Streptococcus pneumoniae*.

Investigation

Diagnosis is confirmed by documentation of proteinuria and hypoalbuminaemia. Baseline investigations should be carried out including urine dipstick, urine protein-to-creatinine ratio, urine MC&S, U&Es, C3, C4, ASOT, anti-Dnase B and hepatitis serology.

The following features should prompt consideration of renal biopsy to identify rarer causes:

- age: <1 year or >12 years
- renal failure
- hypertension
- frank haematuria
- low C3
- failure to respond to steroid therapy

Management

If the clinical features are consistent with minimal change disease, treatment is begun with 4 weeks of high-dose oral steroids (60 mg/m^2) followed by a gradually reducing regimen. Steroid resistance is defined as no remission (i.e., continued proteinuria) after 4 weeks and is associated with CKD. Fluid balance must be closely monitored with daily weighing and salt restriction. Penicillin V prophylaxis is given in the acute phase to prevent secondary infection and pneumococcal vaccination is recommended. Relapses (2+ or greater proteinuria on dipstick for 3 or more days) occur in up to 70% of children; these are treated with steroids. With frequent relapses (two relapses in the first 6 months of diagnosis, or 4 relapses in any 12-month period), additional immunosuppressants such as levamisole, cyclophosphamide or ciclosporin may be needed.

HINTS AND TIPS

- The mnemonic HOP and HIT can be used to help remember the key features of nephrotic syndrome
- **H**ypoalbuminaemia
- **O**edema
- **P**roteinuria (heavy)
- **H**yperlipidaemia
- **I**nfection
- **T**hrombosis

ACUTE KIDNEY INJURY

AKI is a rapid reduction in renal function which occurs over hours to days, leading to a failure in maintenance of normal fluid, electrolyte and acid–base homeostasis. It is defined as a recent increase in creatinine greater than 1.5 times the previous result or upper limit of the normal. It is usually associated with a fall in urine output (<0.5 mL/kg/hour for 8 hours). AKI is less common in paediatric patients but as with adults, causes can be divided into prerenal, renal and postrenal. AKIs can be graded Stage 1 to 3 depending on the degree of increase in serum creatinine from baseline.

Aetiology

As mentioned above, AKI causes can be divided into the following categories:

Prerenal

- Hypovolaemia secondary to sepsis, major burns, haemorrhage, dehydration
- Hepato-renal syndrome

Renal

- Glomerulonephritis
- HUS, HSP
- Interstitial nephritis
- Drugs
- Acute tubular necrosis (ATN)
- Tumour lysis syndrome

Post renal

- Posterior urethral valves
- Bilateral ureteric obstruction (trauma, calculi)
- Urethral obstruction (trauma, calculus)

Investigations

All patients with an AKI should have a urine dip and urinalysis for MC+S. Blood tests should include U&E, FBC, bone profile and blood gas. A renal ultrasound should be requested.

Management

It is important to treat underlying causes of renal impairment. For example, giving intravenous antibiotics if there is a prerenal AKI due to sepsis.

AKI management should include a strict fluid balance with urine output, daily weights and U+Es. Adequate fluid resuscitation and maintenance are key, as is ensuring nephrotoxic medications are withheld. Depending on the duration and severity of renal impairment, children with an AKI should be followed up in clinic.

Haemolytic-uraemic syndrome

This is the most common cause of AKI in a previously healthy child and is associated with diarrhoea from Shiga-toxin-producing *E. coli* O157:H7. This toxin results in red blood cell fragmentation (glomerular microangiopathic haemolytic anaemia) and thrombocytopenia. The kidney vasculature becomes thrombosed and infarcted. Management is supportive and 90% of children recover full renal function. Antibiotics are contraindicated as they induce expression and release of Shiga toxin.

CHRONIC KIDNEY DISEASE

CKD involves a progressive impairment of renal function and can be classified by the glomerular filtration rate.

Important paediatric causes of CKD:

- congenital dysplasia
- inherited renal disease (e.g., autosomal recessive polycystic kidney disease and Alport syndrome)
- reflux nephropathy
- chronic glomerulonephritis (e.g., IgA nephropathy)

Clinical presentation is relatively nonspecific but includes poor growth, fatigue, malaise, weakness, as well as signs of the complications of CKD. The complications include uraemia, hyperkalaemia, metabolic acidosis, hypertension, anaemia and renal osteodystrophy. Treatment is initially supportive with careful fluid and electrolyte management through a restricted diet and supplementation. Once the glomerular filtration rate (GFR) is less than $15 \text{ mL/min/1.73 m}^2$, renal replacement therapy is required, which involves dialysis or renal transplantation.

URINARY INCONTINENCE

Enuresis

Enuresis is the involuntary discharge of urine at an age after continence has been reached by most children. Urinary continence is achieved by most girls by age 5 years and boys by age 6 years. Children with primary enuresis have never been continent for a period of at least 3 months.

Secondary enuresis is incontinence after a prolonged period of bladder control. About 85% of children are only incontinent at night (nocturnal enuresis).

Organic causes are uncommon but include:

- UTI
- polyuria due to diabetes mellitus or CKD
- neuropathic bladder
- faecal retention causing bladder neck dysfunction

History

The history should establish the frequency (50% or more wet nights over 2 weeks is severe) and time of night that wetting occurs. The presence of any daytime urgency or wetting should be established as this suggests an underlying cause. A family history might be present and an assessment should be made of any emotional stresses either at school or at home.

Examination

Physical examination must include:

- A review of growth and measurement of blood pressure to identify unrecognized renal failure.
- Careful abdominal palpation to exclude an enlarged bladder.
- Inspection of the genitalia.
- The spine and overlying skin should be inspected for any deformity, hairy patch or sinus and the neurology of the lower limbs examined thoroughly.

Investigations

Investigation is usually not indicated but may include urinalysis if features of diabetes or UTI are present.

Management

A supportive and nonpunitive attitude is key. Reassuring the child that it is a common problem and not shameful can help. A description of how the bladder works can also be useful. Simple measures such as cutting down fluid intake and caffeine in the evening and ensuring the bladder is completely emptied prior to bed help. Parents often employ techniques such as 'lifting' to reduce wet beds. This involves taking the child to the toilet while still asleep halfway through the night. This should be discouraged as the child will learn that voiding while in a drowsy state is normal and may perpetuate the problem.

First-line treatments involve star charts focusing on helpful behaviours like going to the toilet before bed rather than rewarding dry nights. A bell and pad alarm can be tried which wakes the child at the onset of wetting if over 5 years of age. The child should be encouraged to go to the toilet to complete voiding. Gradually the child learns to wake before voiding starts. Desmopressin can also be trialled which increases the levels of antidiuretic hormone and therefore reduces the volume of urine produced. These are particularly useful if the child wants to sleepover at a friend's house or go on a school trip.

GENITAL CONDITIONS

Inguinoscrotal swellings

Undescended testis

The testes develop intraabdominally and migrate through the inguinal canal to the scrotum in the third trimester. The testes are therefore usually in the scrotum in term neonates, but are frequently undescended in preterm infants. Undescended testes are the most common congenital genitourinary anomaly. Undescended testes may be along the normal pathway or, in <1% of cases, ectopic and found elsewhere within the abdomen or pelvis.

Examination

The testes should be examined during the Newborn & Infant Physical Examination (NIPE) within 72 hours of birth and at 6 to 8 weeks. Referral to a surgeon should be made if an ectopic testis is found or if either testis is impalpable at the 6- to 8-week check.

Investigation

Bilaterally undescended testes in the newborn always warrant investigation to rule out congenital adrenal hyperplasia (see Chapter 24). Further investigations may include:

- ultrasound ± MRI
- laparoscopy
- endocrine and genetic investigations

Management

Undescended testes carry an increased risk of malignancy, sub-fertility and torsion. Treatment is by orchidopexy if the testes have not descended by 6 months. Orchidectomy is indicated for a unilateral intraabdominal testis that is not amenable to orchidopexy.

Inguinal hernias and hydroceles

The testis descends into the scrotum, taking with it a connecting fold of peritoneum (the processus vaginalis), which normally becomes obliterated at or around birth. Failure of the processus vaginalis to close results in a hydrocele or an inguinal hernia (Fig. 6.5).

Hydroceles

If there is a patent processus vaginalis, a hydrocele may form; this is a fluid-filled swelling which is painless and transilluminates. On examination, it is possible to get above the swelling, which cannot be reduced. Spontaneous resolution by the age of 12 months is common and treatment during the first 2 years is not required unless the hydrocele is extremely large. If they are still present at 2 years of age or recurrently enlarge and become tense then they may be considered for repair via ligation of the processus vaginalis

Inguinal hernias

Inguinal hernias are more common in boys, premature babies and infants with a positive family history. A minority are bilateral. Parents may notice an intermittent swelling in the

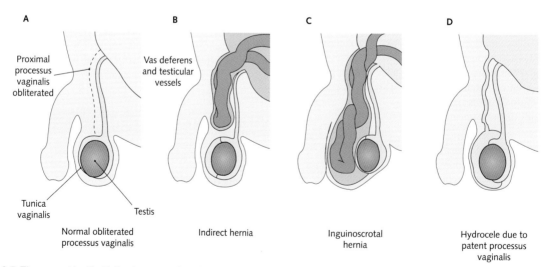

Fig. 6.5 The normal testis. Following normal testicular descent, the processus vaginalis, an evagination of the parietal peritoneum between the internal inguinal ring and testis, disappears leaving only the tunica vaginalis around the testis. Persistence of the processus vaginalis results in an inguinal hernia (B, C) or a hydrocele (D).

groin or scrotum. The main concern is the risk of incarceration and strangulation, which is higher in young infants (up to 30% in ex-premature infants). On examination, there will be a palpable groin mass which is not possible to get above but should be reducible. A prompt outpatient referral to paediatric surgeons should be made and these should be repaired surgically.

Varicocele

A varicocele is an abnormal dilatation of the pampiniform plexus of veins. This is classically described as feeling like a 'bag of worms'. It is more common in adolescent boys and on the left side as the testicular vein drains into the left renal vein. It is important to exclude other causes of obstruction at this level (e.g., renal tumour, renal vein thrombosis). They may be managed conservatively if not causing problems. Indications for repair include persistent symptoms of pain, heaviness or testicular atrophy.

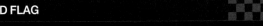

RED FLAG

Danger signs requiring urgent surgical referral are:
- An irreducible hernia.
- Hardness.
- Tenderness.
- Vomiting.

These signs indicate possible incarceration and strangulation. Urgent reduction of the hernia is required.

HINTS AND TIPS

- Testicular cancer is very rare in children but can present as a firm, painless testicular mass. In all cases, an ultrasound scan should be requested to confirm the diagnosis.

The acute scrotum

Acute pain and swelling of the scrotum is an emergency because of the possibility of testicular torsion. The three major causes of acute scrotal pain are testicular torsion, epididymo-orchitis, and torsion of the testicular appendage. Table 6.7 delineates the key differentiating features of the three conditions.

Other differentials include:

- Referred pain from a strangulated or incarcerated inguinal hernia
- Varicocele
- Trauma

In the history, it is important to elicit the onset and duration of symptoms, the location of pain, the presence of urinary symptoms and fever. A past history of urinary tract abnormalities and recurrent UTIs may point to a diagnosis of epididymo-orchitis. In some adolescents, it may be appropriate to take a sexual history.

Testicular torsion

Torsion occurs where there is inadequate fixation to the tunica vaginalis allowing the testis to rotate and occlude its vascular supply resulting in ischaemia. It can occur at any age but is most common in the neonatal period and at puberty. It typically presents with sudden onset severe unilateral pain, often associated with nausea or vomiting. An ultrasound with Doppler studies can assist in diagnosis but surgical exploration must not be delayed, as the testis might become nonviable; this is a surgical emergency. The defect is commonly bilateral, so the contralateral testis should also be fixed at surgery.

Epididymo-orchitis

Epididymo-orchitis is inflammation of the epididymis and testes, usually caused by infection secondary to UTIs or sexually transmitted infections (STIs), although in many cases it is not clear. In the infant, anatomical urinary tract abnormalities need to be excluded with ultrasound. The onset of symptoms is subacute and the scrotum tends to be swollen, hot and red. A history of urinary symptoms, urethritis and penile discharge should be sought to clarify the underlying cause. Treatment is always with antibiotics; the choice depends on whether there is suspicion of an STI.

HINTS AND TIPS

Don't forget that mumps orchitis is a cause of scrotal swelling and pain. It tends to occur 7 to 10 days after infection.

Torsion of the testicular appendage (hydatid of Morgagni)

The testicular appendage is a small embryological remnant at the upper pole of the testis. Torsion can occur spontaneously and results in pain secondary to ischaemia of the cyst. A torted testicular appendage (cyst of Morgagni) most commonly occurs in prepubertal boys. Clinical features are shown in Table 6.7. Many of these patients may undergo surgical exploration as testicular torsion may not be confidently excluded on examination alone. If there is confidence in the diagnosis, some children may be managed with analgesia alone.

Table 6.7 Comparison of clinical features of the common causes of acute scrotal pain

Clinical Feature	Testicular torsion	Epididymo-orchitis	Torsion of testicular appendage
Age	Neonate or adolescent	Adolescent	Prepubertal (typically age 9–11)
Symptom onset	Acute	Subacute	Subacute
Site of tenderness	Not localized	Diffuse/epididymis	Upper pole
Cremasteric reflex	Absent	Present	Present
Other features	Possible high riding testis	Scrotum may be warm, red and swollen. Fever	'Blue dot' sign positive

Penile conditions

Hypospadias

A spectrum of congenital abnormalities of the position of the urethral meatus occurs, ranging from mild displacement to a urethral opening within the scrotum or perineum. The foreskin is incompletely closed giving a dorsal hooded appearance. Severe forms are associated with chordee (ventral curvature of the penis), and may lead to problems with continence and fertility. Management depends on severity; urological assessment is required.

HINTS AND TIPS

Infants with hypospadias must not be circumcised as the foreskin may be needed for surgical correction.

Phimosis and paraphimosis

The foreskin is nonretractile in young children up to 6 years of age and forcible attempts to retract the foreskin should not be made. Ballooning of the prepuce during urination is not uncommon and this usually resolves as the prepuce becomes more retractile. Phimosis refers to adhesion of the foreskin to the glans penis. Mild degrees can be managed with periodic, gentle retraction. Paraphimosis is irreducible retraction of the foreskin beyond the glans. It leads to venous congestion and permanent damage if not reduced.

Circumcision

Medical indications for circumcision include recurrent balanitis (infection of the glans) and balanitis xerotica obliterans (lichen sclerosis), which causes a thickened, scarred, white prepuce that is fixed to the glans. Most circumcisions are performed for religious or cultural reasons.

Complications of circumcision can include:

- haemorrhage
- infection
- damage to the glans

Ambiguous genitalia

Approximately 1 in 2000 babies will be born with ambiguous genitalia. The most common underlying cause is congenital adrenal hyperplasia (see Chapter 7) with virilization of an infant with an XX genotype. Examine the child and measure the blood pressure (may be raised in congenital adrenal hyperplasia). Important investigations include measurement of electrolytes, endocrine investigations, chromosomal analysis and ultrasound imaging of the abdomen and pelvis. Best practice management is to reassure and support families so that any decision about genital surgery can be delayed until the child is old enough to decide for themselves (see Ethics).

ETHICS

Until recently, babies with ambiguous genitalia underwent surgery they could not consent to, which attempted to 'normalize' their genitalia. Complications included lifelong sexual dysfunction, incontinence and pain.

COMMUNICATION

Many families of children with ambiguous genitalia have reported that the way in which they are told about this is vital. It is important to provide appropriate support and reassurance, opportunities to ask questions and to explain any investigations being done. Remember that families are often under pressure to tell relatives and friends the sex of the baby and to choose a name.

Chapter Summary

- In any febrile child, consider a urine dipstick – it is an easy-to-use and cheap bedside test.
- Although urinary tract infections are a common childhood presentation, further investigations may be required to look for an underlying condition, depending on the age of the child and their clinical presentation – follow the National Institute for Health and Care Excellence (NICE) guidance.
- In the acute scrotum, obtaining an ultrasound should not delay surgical exploration.
- A firm, painful, irreducible hernia should be referred to the on-call paediatric surgeon for potential strangulation/incarceration.
- Nephrotoxins should be stopped in all children with an AKI and an underlying cause sought.

UKMLA Conditions
Acute kidney injury
Chronic kidney disease
Epididymitis and orchitis
Hernias
Testicular torsion
Urinary tract infection

UKMLA Presentations
Acute kidney injury
Haematuria
Peripheral oedema and ankle swelling
Scrotal/testicular pain and/or lump/swelling
Urinary incontinence
Urinary symptoms

Endocrinology and growth 7

The endocrine system involves a series of glands that secrete hormones (chemical messengers) which bring about effects in target organs through their interactions with receptors. Endocrine conditions can present in many different ways, from antenatal presentation to development of disease only at puberty or later in adulthood.

HYPOTHALAMUS AND THE PITUITARY GLAND

The pituitary gland is divided into the anterior and posterior lobes. These have different embryonic origins and separate hormonal functions, summarized in Fig. 7.1. The pituitary gland is under the control of the hypothalamus.

Anterior pituitary disorders

A deficiency of the anterior pituitary hormones is more common than an excess and it can be specific to individual hormones only or generalized (panhypopituitarism).

Hypopituitarism in children can be caused by:

- congenital defects (e.g., septo-optic dysplasia and agenesis of corpus callosum)
- tumours (e.g., craniopharyngioma)
- trauma/surgery and radiation
- idiopathic hormone abnormalities

Growth restriction is a common feature, together with thyroid, adrenal and gonadal dysfunction depending on the pattern of deficiency. These conditions are discussed in more detail in the following sections.

Posterior pituitary disorders

The posterior lobe (neurohypophysis) secretes antidiuretic hormone (ADH) and oxytocin. Key pathologies are those related to ADH release or response: diabetes insipidus and syndrome of inappropriate secretion of ADH (SIADH).

Diabetes insipidus

Diabetes insipidus is caused by either a decreased release of ADH (central diabetes insipidus) or a decreased response to ADH (nephrogenic diabetes insipidus – this is rare and in most cases hereditary). It might occur as an isolated idiopathic defect or in association with anterior pituitary deficiency (e.g., due to tumours, infections or trauma). It presents with polydipsia and polyuria (the passage of large volumes of dilute urine). Several conditions can mimic diabetes insipidus, including diabetes mellitus, psychogenic polydipsia, chronic kidney disease and hypercalcaemia. Diagnosis is by a water deprivation test, and central diabetes insipidus can be treated with a synthetic version of ADH, desmopressin (1-deamino-8-D-arginine vasopressin).

Syndrome of inappropriate secretion of ADH

SIADH involves the oversecretion/increased release of ADH resulting in a very small volume of concentrated urine being passed, leading to low plasma osmolarity. This is a common stress

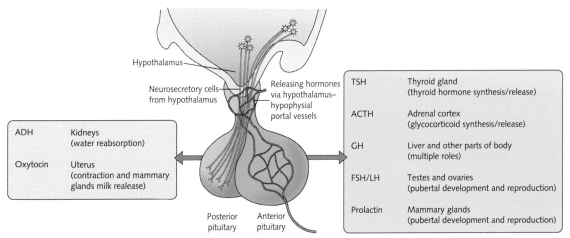

Fig. 7.1 The hypothalamic–pituitary axis. *ACTH,* Adrenocorticotrophic hormone; *ADH,* antidiuretic hormone; *FSH,* follicle-stimulating hormone; *GH,* growth hormone; *LH,* luteinizing hormone; *TSH,* thyroid-stimulating hormone.

response and might be caused by several underlying conditions including central nervous system disease (e.g., meningitis, brain tumours or head trauma) and lung disease (e.g., pneumonia, bronchiolitis). Symptoms occur due to effects of water intoxication: these include vomiting, behavioural changes and seizures.

Diagnosis consists of:

- low serum osmolality with hyponatraemia
- high urine sodium and osmolality
- normal or increased volume status
- normal renal, thyroid and adrenal function

Treatment involves targeting the underlying cause and fluid restriction, usually to 2/3 maintenance.

GROWTH

Four phases of growth are recognized:

1. Infantile phase (birth to 1 year): dependent on nutrition. Insulin and thyroxine also play key roles.
2. Childhood phase (1 year to 5 years): dependent on growth hormone and thyroxine.
3. Mid-childhood phase (5 years to puberty): increased levels of adrenal androgens influence growth. The growth rate in mid-childhood is 5 to 6 cm per year.
4. Pubertal phase: growth spurt caused by increased levels of sex steroids. This is the period of peak growth velocity. On average, children grow 30 cm during puberty.

Growth is assessed by measuring three specific parameters:

- height (or length in children <2 years)
- weight
- head circumference

There are centile charts showing the normal range of values for these measurements from before birth to adulthood. The 50th centile corresponds to the population median. In preterm infants the corrected age (chronological age minus number of weeks preterm) should be used until 2 years of age. An approach to the evaluation of 'short stature' is presented here. Problems with inadequate weight gain (faltering growth) and abnormal head growth (microcephaly and macrocephaly) are considered elsewhere.

Short stature

A pragmatic definition of short stature requiring further evaluation is:

- A height below the 0.4th centile for age.
- A predicted height less than the mid-parental target height.
- An abnormal growth velocity as indicated by the height changing by more than the width of one centile band over 1 to 2 years.

Causes

The causes of short stature are shown in Box 7.1.

The most common causes are familial short stature and constitutional delay of growth (±puberty).

History

This should elicit information about:

- birth weight, length and head circumference
- a timeline of how they have grown and whether there has been any pubertal development
- early childhood illness and systemic disorders

BOX 7.1 CAUSES OF SHORT STATURE

Familial short stature: the child's height centile is appropriate when the mid-parental height is calculated. There is no delay in bone age.

Constitutional delay of growth (± puberty): there may be a positive family history. There is a delay in bone age – the growth potential is reached later than peers.

Intrauterine growth restriction.

Endocrine disorder:

- growth hormone deficiency: can be primary or secondary to hypopituitarism (e.g., due to a tumour)
- hypothyroidism: delayed bone age
- Cushing syndrome

Genetic causes:

- Achondroplasia – mutation in the *GFGR3* gene resulting in disproportionately short stature as well as other skeletal abnormalities including macrocephaly and trident hand configuration (all fingers nearly equal in length).
- Mucopolysaccharidosis: short stature, coarse facial features and associated learning difficulty.
- Syndromes:
  - Turner syndrome: 45 × 0 karyotype, short stature, other features include shield-shaped chest and a webbed neck, may be associated endocrine disease and coarctation of the aorta.
  - Down syndrome.
  - Prader-Willi syndrome: short stature, hyperphagia and hypogonadism.
  - Russell-Silver syndrome: short stature which starts antenatally, associated with other skeletal abnormalities.

Malabsorption (e.g., cystic fibrosis or coeliac disease).

Any chronic disease (e.g., congenital heart disease, chronic kidney disease).

Psychosocial deprivation/neglect.

- parental height: the genetic height potential is estimated by calculating the target centile range from the mid-parental height
- family history: inherited skeletal dysplasias
- dietary and social history

A way of explaining a height centile to parents is to say, 'your son is on the 25th centile – this means that if there were 100 boys with the same birthday lined up, then 75 would be taller than him'.

Examination

Examine the following:

- height: measure accurately with a wall-mounted, calibrated stadiometer (under 2-year-olds should be measured supine). Calculate growth velocity in centimetre/year: requires a minimum of two measurements, 6 months apart
- weight
- head circumference
- stage of puberty
- dysmorphic features: might identify a syndrome
- visual fields and fundi: might indicate a pituitary tumour

Parents may be unable to remember exact birth weights and lengths – ask whether they have the red book available and look at the growth charts yourself.

To estimate the adult height potential:
1) Calculate the mid-parental height:
   - Boys: add 7 cm
   - Girls: subtract 7 cm
   - Father's height plus mother's height divided by 2
   - Then adjust for the sex of the child:
2) Identify the mid-parental centile (the centile nearest the mid-parental height):
   - Boys can deviate from this by 10 cm either way
   - Girls can deviate by 8.5 cm either way

Alternative: plot parental heights directly onto the 'mid-parental centile comparator' on the World Health Organization (WHO) growth chart.

An approach to the evaluation of short stature is shown in Fig. 7.2.

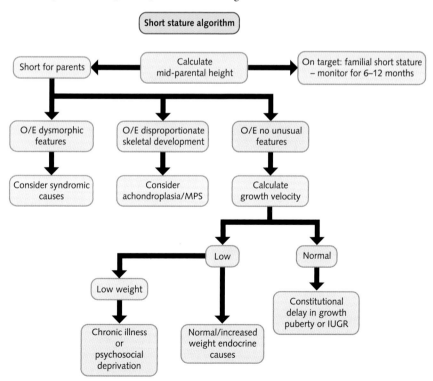

Fig. 7.2 Short stature algorithm. *IUGR,* Intrauterine growth restriction; *MPS,* mucopolysaccharidosis; *O/E,* on examination.

Management

Investigations that might be of value include the following:

- Bone age: estimated from X-rays of the left wrist (delayed skeletal maturity in constitutional growth delay and endocrine causes).
- Endocrine investigations: thyroid function tests (T_4, thyroid-stimulating hormone (TSH)) and growth hormone (secretion is pulsatile so a provocation test, e.g., insulin-induced hypoglycaemia or glucagon stimulation, is necessary to identify deficiency).
- Karyotype: chromosomal analysis to identify Turner syndrome (45X0) in girls with significant short stature.
- Skeletal survey: in disproportion (skeletal dysplasias).
- Magnetic resonance imaging (MRI) head for suspected craniopharyngioma/pituitary tumours.

Height should be monitored over 6 to 12 months in response to parental concern regardless of current centile. Treatment may involve growth hormone injections for deficiency – it can also be given in cases of intrauterine growth restriction if there is no catch-up growth by the age of 4 years. Short courses of androgens can be given to start puberty in constitutional delay.

RED FLAG

Do not assume short stature in girls is due to a constitutional delay – all girls whose height is lower than expected for their mid-parental height should be tested for Turner syndrome.

PUBERTY

Abnormalities of the hypothalamic–pituitary–gonadal axis can cause variations of sex differentiation and disorders of puberty.

Variations of sex differentiation

While we tend to think of sex as a binary (either male or female) determined by looking at a baby's genitals, the evidence shows that sex is determined by multiple biological factors including chromosomes, hormones, gonads and secondary sex characteristics, as

Table 7.1 Endocrine causes of variations in sex differentiation

Chromosomes and phenotype	Causes
46XY chromosomes, testes, with reduced virilization/masculinization	- Inborn errors of testosterone synthesis - 5α-reductase deficiency - Androgen-insensitivity syndrome
46XX chromosomes, ovaries, increased virilization/masculinization	- Congenital adrenal hyperplasia - Maternal androgen exposure - Ovarian or adrenal tumour

well as external genitalia. Variations of sex differentiation (intersex conditions) can occur due to a difference in any of these factors (Table 7.1). These conditions may represent completely healthy and functioning variants, which do not require any medical intervention. Some of these conditions will result in ambiguous genitalia (see Chapter 6 for more information).

Puberty

During puberty, secondary sex characteristics are acquired and reproductive capacity is attained. Puberty usually starts between 8 and 13 years in females, and between 9 and 14 years in males. Puberty can be divided into stages by the Tanner system (Fig. 7.3).

Precocious puberty

This refers to the development of secondary sexual characteristics before the age of 8 years in girls or 9 years in boys. There is an associated growth spurt. The causes of precocious puberty are shown in Table 7.2. In females, it is usually due to early onset of normal puberty (idiopathic central puberty). In boys, it is more likely to be pathological.

Investigations include hormone levels, karyotyping and imaging to look for a brain or peripheral tumour.

Treatment depends on the cause. Gonadotrophin-releasing hormone analogues can be used to prevent puberty from progressing – these only work for gonadotrophin-dependent causes.

Precocious puberty should be differentiated from:

- Premature thelarche: isolated breast development in a very young girl. A nonprogressive, benign condition.

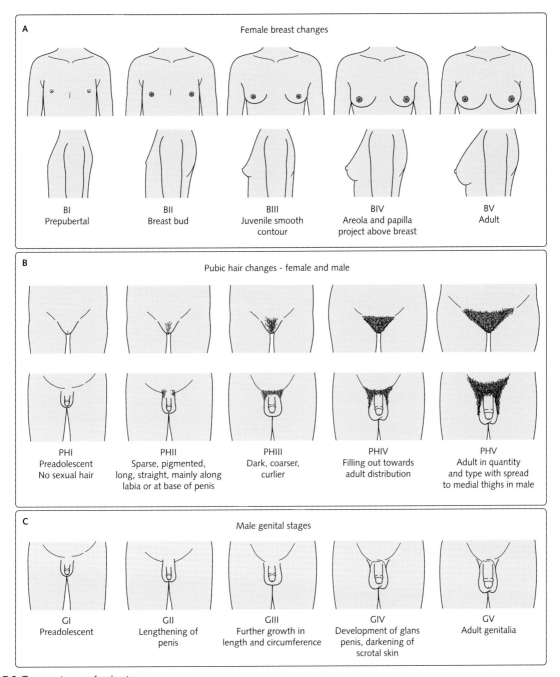

Fig. 7.3 Tanner stages of puberty.

- Premature adrenarche: isolated early appearance of pubic hair. A benign, self-limiting condition due to early maturation of adrenal androgen secretion, although an adrenal tumour might need to be excluded.

Delayed puberty

This can be defined as the absence of secondary sex characteristics at 13 years of age in girls or 14 years of age in boys. The problem is more common in boys and the majority of adolescents affected are normal. The causes are summarized in Table 7.3.

Table 7.2 Causes of precocious puberty

Type of precocious puberty	Causes
Gonadotrophin-dependent (central) precocious puberty. There is premature activation of the hypothalamic–pituitary–gonadal axis → consonant puberty (normal pattern of puberty but earlier).	• Idiopathic – common in girls • Central nervous system abnormalities: arachnoid cyst, hydrocephalus, brain tumour or secondary to surgery or irradiation
Gonadotrophin-independent precious puberty. There is disconsonant puberty (abnormal pattern).	• Congenital adrenal hyperplasia • Cushing syndrome • Sex steroid-secreting tumours, for example, of ovaries, liver or adrenals • McCune-Albright syndrome: autosomal dominant condition with skeletal abnormalities and multiple endocrinopathies including precocious puberty

Assessment should include pubertal staging and examination to exclude systemic disease. If indicated, helpful investigations are:

- Karyotype.
- Measurement of gonadotrophin levels, sex steroid levels and thyroid function.
- Ultrasound to identify gonads if variation of sex differentiation suspected.

Treatment is often not required for constitutional delay, but hormone therapy (e.g., oxandrolone or low-dose testosterone) can be used to accelerate growth and induce secondary sexual characteristics in boys. Oestrogen therapy can be used in girls but care must be taken to prevent premature closure of the epiphyses.

RED FLAG

Precocious puberty in girls is usually physiological. Precocious puberty in boys is nearly always pathological and requires investigation, in particular, to rule out a central nervous system tumour.

Conversely, delayed puberty in boys is usually physiological but delayed puberty in girls requires investigation to rule out Turner syndrome which may not present with the typical features.

ADRENAL DISORDERS

The adrenal glands are made up of the cortex and the medulla. The cortex is divided into three zones (the zona glomerulosa which produces mineralocorticoids, the zona fasciculata which produces glucocorticoids and the zona reticularis which produces sex steroids). Cortisol, the major glucocorticoid, is stimulated by pituitary adrenocorticotrophic hormone (ACTH) under a negative feedback loop. Aldosterone is the principal mineralocorticoid and is controlled by the renin-angiotensin system. The major sex steroids produced by the adrenal glands are androgens. Disorders of the adrenal cortex can result in deficiency or excess of adrenocortical hormones. The medulla produces catecholamines (adrenaline and noradrenaline). Disorders of the medulla (e.g., pheochromocytoma) are very rare.

Table 7.3 Causes of delayed puberty

Type of delayed puberty	Causes

Hypogonadotropic hypogonadism (central delayed puberty)	• Constitutional delay in puberty – common in boys
	• Hypothalamic/pituitary disorders (e.g., congenital panhypopituitarism), secondary to tumour (e.g., craniopharyngioma) or surgery
	• Syndromes:
	  – Kallmann syndrome: Gonadotrophin-releasing hormone deficiency, associated with anosmia
	  – Prader-Willi syndrome
	• Systemic disease/stress/starvation
	• Hypothyroidism

Hypergonadotropic hypogonadism (gonadal failure)	• Variations of sex differentiation
	• Syndromes:
	  – Turner syndrome (45X0) – associated with rudimentary 'streak' ovaries
	  – Klinefelter syndrome (47XXY) – delayed puberty, long arm span and psychiatric associations
	• Testicular/ovarian damage:
	  – trauma or surgery
	  – postchemotherapy/irradiation
	  – testicular torsion or following orchitis in boys

Table 7.4 Causes of Cushing syndrome	
Type of Cushing syndrome	**Causes**
Endogenous	Primary (adrenocorticotrophic hormone (ACTH) independent): • adrenal tumour: usually adenoma • McCune-Albright syndrome Secondary (ACTH dependent): • ACTH-secreting pituitary adenoma (Cushing disease) Ectopic ACTH production
Exogenous/iatrogenic	Long-term steroid use

Table 7.5 Primary and secondary adrenocortical insufficiency	
Type of Addison	**Causes**
Primary – destruction of adrenal cortex (Addison disease)	• Autoimmune disease • Haemorrhage and infarction (Waterhouse-Friderichsen syndrome associated with meningococcal septicaemia) • Tuberculosis (common worldwide)
Secondary – decreased adrenocorticotrophic hormone (ACTH) production	Long-term steroid use leading to suppression of pituitary ACTH production

Cushing syndrome

Cushing syndrome is the clinical state produced by glucocorticoid excess, which can be due to either endogenous overproduction of cortisol or exogenous treatment with pharmacological doses of corticosteroids. The causes are listed in Table 7.4.

HINTS AND TIPS

- Cushing syndrome and Cushing disease are often used interchangeably in error. Cushing syndrome is the clinical state produced by excess glucocorticoids. Cushing disease is the presence of an ACTH-secreting pituitary adenoma causing the clinical state of excess steroids.

Clinical presentation

The clinical features include:

- faltering growth
- truncal obesity, 'buffalo' hump, rounded 'moon' facies
- signs of virilization, striae and skin thinning
- hypertension
- hyperglycaemia
- mood and behavioural disturbance

Management

Elevated serum cortisol levels are found with absence of the normal diurnal rhythm (finding high, rather than expected low, midnight levels). A prolonged dexamethasone suppression test might be required to distinguish secondary causes (driven by ACTH, cortisol levels suppressible by dexamethasone) from primary causes (ACTH independent, not suppressible by dexamethasone). Computed tomography or MRI of the adrenal and pituitary glands might identify an adrenal tumour or pituitary adenoma. Treatment depends on the cause and might involve surgical resection and radiotherapy.

Adrenocortical insufficiency

Diminished production of adrenocortical hormones may be caused by primary or secondary adrenocortical insufficiency (see Table 7.5), or by congenital adrenal hyperplasia (CAH), which is an inherited inborn error of metabolism in biosynthesis of adrenal corticosteroids.

Clinical presentation

Clinical signs include:

- dizziness and postural hypotension
- abdominal pain, vomiting and diarrhoea/constipation
- hyperpigmentation (e.g., of the palmar creases)
- depression and psychosis

Intercurrent illness or trauma can trigger an adrenal/addisonian crisis (characterized by vomiting, dehydration and shock).

Management

Key investigations are to measure blood electrolytes and glucose.

Classically, there is hyponatraemia, hyperkalaemia and hypoglycaemia.

The short Synacthen test involves the administration of a synthetic version of ACTH and measuring the rise in plasma cortisol: if there is a rise after 30 minutes, primary adrenocortical deficiency (Addison disease) can be excluded. Treatment involves glucocorticoid (e.g., hydrocortisone) with or without mineralocorticoid (e.g., fludrocortisone) replacement.

HINTS AND TIPS

Steroid administration must not be stopped suddenly due to the risk of an addisonian crisis. If the child is sick, the steroid dose should be increased. All children should carry a steroid card with them which gives clear instructions on what to do in such a situation.

Congenital adrenal hyperplasia

CAH is a group of disorders caused by a defect in the pathway that synthesizes cortisol from cholesterol. The inheritance is autosomal recessive with the defective gene on chromosome 6. Prevalence is approximately 1 in 10,000. Approximately 90% of cases are caused by a deficiency in 21-hydroxylase and 5% to 7% are due to 11-hydroxylase deficiency; other defects occur rarely.

Clinical features
Clinical features are due to deficiency of cortisol and aldosterone, and excess of androgens:

- cortisol deficiency: hypoglycaemia, cardiovascular collapse
- aldosterone deficiency: salt-wasting crisis (this is less common with 11-hydroxylase deficiency) causing hyponatraemia, hyperkalaemia, volume depletion and shock
- virilization of female infants (ambiguous genitalia at birth, amenorrhoea later in life) and precocious puberty in males

It can be difficult to diagnose male infants with this disorder because they have few clinical manifestations at birth.

Investigations
Diagnosis rests on the demonstration of markedly elevated levels of 17α-hydroxyprogesterone in the serum and assessment of the urine steroid profile. In the 'salt-losing' form, the characteristic electrolyte disturbance of hyponatraemia, hypochloridaemia and hyperkalaemia provides a clue to the diagnosis.

Treatment
Initial management of a 'salt-losing' crisis involves volume replacement with normal saline and systemic steroids. Long-term treatment involves cortisol replacement with hydrocortisone and fludrocortisone to replace the deficient hormones and suppress ACTH and androgen overproduction. Parents are also taught to recognize early signs of illness and children should carry a steroid card to alert health professionals. Growth is used to monitor whether treatment is sufficient.

> **RED FLAG**
>
> Consider congenital adrenal hyperplasia as a differential for newborns with vomiting and dehydration – the salt-losing crisis is potentially lethal but easily treatable.

THYROID DISORDERS

Thyroid hormone is critical for normal growth and neurological development in infants and children; however, an excess can be dangerous in infancy and childhood. Worldwide, the most important condition affecting the thyroid gland is iodide deficiency, estimated to affect at least 800 million people.

Hypothyroidism

This might be present at birth (congenital hypothyroidism) or develop at any time during childhood or adolescence (acquired hypothyroidism).

Congenital hypothyroidism
This has an incidence of one in 4000 live births. The causes include:

- Developmental defects: thyroid agenesis or a failure of migration.
- Dyshormonogenesis: an autosomal recessive inborn error of thyroid hormone synthesis (accounts for 15%, a goitre usually occurs).
- Congenital pituitary lesions (rare).
- Transient congenital hypothyroidism in cases of maternal thyroid disease caused by transplacental passage of thyroid receptor antibodies or antithyroid medications.
- Maternal iodide deficiency: the most common cause worldwide.

Clinical features
Infants may appear clinically normal at birth. The clinical features that develop during infancy if untreated include:

- prolonged neonatal jaundice
- sleepiness
- feeding problems
- constipation
- umbilical hernia
- bradycardia and poor peripheral perfusion
- coarse facies, wide posterior fontanelle, large tongue
- hypotonia and learning difficulties
- goitre

Management
Testing for hypothyroidism is a part of the newborn blood spot screening in the UK and most infants are diagnosed this way. Most laboratories in the UK test for raised levels of TSH and some laboratories in the United States measure both TSH and thyroxine (T_4). In hypothyroidism secondary to a pituitary lesion, TSH will be normal or low. Early diagnosis and treatment with oral thyroxine can result in normal neurological function and intelligence.

Acquired hypothyroidism
Causes of acquired hypothyroidism include autoimmune disease (Hashimoto thyroiditis), iodide deficiency and iatrogenic (caused by thyroid surgery or medications).

Clinical presentation

Presentation in later childhood or adolescence is similar to adult hypothyroidism, and symptoms and signs may include the following:

- feeling cold
- weakness and fatigue
- low mood
- constipation
- menorrhagia (teenage girls)
- dry skin and coarse hair
- bradycardia and heart failure
- ataxia

Management

Thyroid function tests and thyroid autoantibodies should be measured. Radiographs of the left wrist and hand reveal bone age which is less than the chronological age. The mainstay of treatment is with oral thyroxine to normalize TSH.

Hyperthyroidism

As with hypothyroidism, hyperthyroidism can present at birth or later in childhood or adolescence.

Neonatal hyperthyroidism

Causes

Neonatal hyperthyroidism can occur in the infants of mothers with Graves disease (see below) or Hashimoto disease from the transplacental transfer of thyroid-stimulating immunoglobulins.

Clinical presentation

Antenatally, this may cause intrauterine growth restriction, tachycardia or foetal hydrops.

Neonatal presentations include:

- goitre
- increased appetite but faltering growth
- diarrhoea
- Central nervous system signs: irritability or jitteriness
- cardiovascular signs: tachycardia, arrhythmias, hypertension, heart failure

Management

This is usually self-limiting within 1 to 3 months but if severe, may require treatment with propranolol or carbimazole.

Acquired hyperthyroidism

This is most commonly caused by Graves disease, an autoimmune condition in which an antibody (human thyroid-stimulating immunoglobulin) mimics TSH by binding to and activating the TSH receptor. It usually presents during adolescence and is much more common in girls than boys. Less common causes include toxic multinodular goitre and rare monogenic activating mutations of the TSH receptor gene.

Clinical presentation

The clinical features are similar to those seen in adults:

- feeling hot
- diarrhoea
- increased appetite but weight loss
- tremor
- tachycardia, palpitations, cardiomyopathy
- Graves disease can cause eye signs including proptosis, chemosis, exposure keratitis and ophthalmoplegia

Additional features include deteriorating school performance, and puberty might be delayed or accelerated. Teenage girls may have amenorrhoea or oligomenorrhoea.

Management

On laboratory testing, serum levels of thyroxine (T_4) and triiodothyronine (T_3) are elevated and TSH levels are depressed. Thyroid autoantibodies are often detectable. Medical therapy with carbimazole is the first-line treatment. β-Blockers can be added for relief of severe symptoms but should be discontinued when thyroid function is controlled. Subtotal thyroidectomy or radioiodine treatments are options for relapse after medical treatment.

DIABETES MELLITUS

Diabetes mellitus is a heterogenous group of disorders of carbohydrate, fat and protein metabolism, caused by deficiency of or reduced efficacy of endogenous insulin. The prevalence of diabetes in children and young people is approximately 1/500 population.

Causes

- Over 95% of childhood-onset diabetes is type 1 diabetes, where there is T-cell-mediated autoimmune destruction of the β cells in the pancreatic islets of Langerhans, perhaps triggered by environmental factors (e.g., viruses) in people with a genetic predisposition. Associated with HLA-DR3/DR4.
- Type 2 diabetes involves reduced sensitivity to insulin. It is much more common in adulthood but its incidence is increasing in paediatric populations – risk factors include obesity, a positive family history, South Asian or African/Caribbean heritage, female sex.
- Maturity-onset diabetes of the young: an autosomal dominant form with a similar presentation to type 2 diabetes.

- Diabetes secondary to pancreatic destruction/failure: cystic fibrosis-associated diabetes, pancreatitis, pancreatic trauma or surgery.
- Associated with genetic syndromes (e.g., Down syndrome, Wolfram syndrome; DIDMOAD = diabetes insipidus, diabetes mellitus, optic atrophy and deafness).

Pathophysiology

The pathophysiological pathways of type 1 diabetes mellitus are described in Fig. 7.4. Key features include:

- Insulin deficiency becomes clinically significant when 90% of the β cells are destroyed.
- Osmotic diuresis ensues when blood glucose concentration exceeds renal threshold.
- Ketoacidosis develops when insulin deficiency is severe.

Clinical presentation

Type 1 diabetes most commonly presents with a several-week history which may include:

- polyuria: increased frequency of urination (possibly enuresis)
- polydipsia: increased thirst
- lethargy
- weight loss
- nausea, vomiting, abdominal pain

About 40% present in diabetic ketoacidosis (see Chapter 20: Emergencies).

HINTS AND TIPS

The 4Ts of diabetes were used in a public health campaign to raise awareness of the symptoms.

These are helpful to remember and can act as a prompt for history taking.

- Tired – are they feeling more tired than usual?
- Thirsty – are they unable to quench their thirst?
- Thinner – have they lost weight?
- Toilet – are they getting up at night and going to the toilet more frequently?

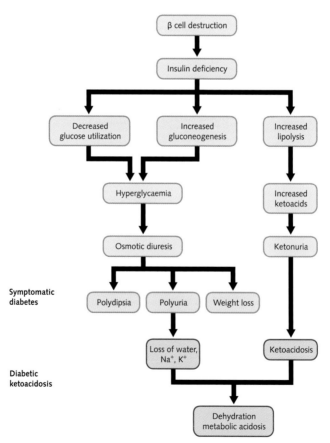

Fig. 7.4 Pathophysiology of diabetes mellitus.

Investigations

The World Health Organization (WHO) have defined criteria for diagnosis: a fasting plasma glucose >7 mmol/L or a random plasma glucose (or oral glucose tolerance test) of >11.1 mmol/L in the absence of other acute illnesses. If asymptomatic, these must be confirmed on a second occasion. The HbA1c indicates the average glucose level for the past 2 to 3 months but is not endorsed by the WHO or NICE in the diagnostic criteria. In children with type 1 diabetes, there may be raised levels of autoantibodies (antiglutamic acid decarboxylase antibodies or islet cell antibodies) and in type 2 diabetes, there will be raised C-peptide (a marker of endogenous insulin production); however, these are not recommended at presentation.

Management

The discovery of insulin in 1922 transformed type 1 diabetes mellitus from a fatal disease into a treatable one. Initial management depends on the child's clinical condition, and if they present in diabetic ketoacidosis, they will require hospital admission. Long-term management of this lifelong condition rests on:

- education and psychological support
- insulin replacement
- diet
- exercise
- monitoring
- management of acute complications: hypoglycaemia and diabetic ketoacidosis
- prevention of long-term complications

Education and psychological support

Children and their families require a comprehensive educational programme that covers:

- a basic understanding of diabetes
- the influence of diet and exercise on blood glucose levels
- practical aspects of insulin injection and blood glucose monitoring
- recognition and treatment of hypoglycaemia
- adjustments for intercurrent illness and the significance of ketonuria/ketonaemia
- the importance of good control in terms of long-term complications

Insulin replacement

National Institute for Health and Care Excellence (NICE) recommends the following regimens:

(1) Multiple daily injections 'basal-bolus regimen' – this involves using a long-acting or intermediate insulin before bedtime, and giving rapid-acting insulin boluses before meals, adjusted for the size of the meal. Injections are given subcutaneously and can be given in upper arms, outer thighs

or abdomen. The site must be rotated to avoid local complications such as fat atrophy.

(2) Continuous subcutaneous insulin infusion using a pump – a portable pump delivers rapid-acting insulin via a subcutaneous cannula (which should be changed every third day). This is particularly good for recurrent hypoglycaemia and unpredictable lifestyles/eating habits.

(3) Draft NICE Guidance (2023) has recommended a hybrid, closed-loop system—automatically balancing glucose levels through a glucose monitor that transmits data to a body-worn insulin pump—for patients who struggle to manage their diabetes.

- When a child is first started on insulin, there may be a 'honeymoon' or remission phase during which there are reduced insulin requirements due to residual islet cell function – this can last for weeks or months after presentation.
- During puberty, insulin requirements increase.
- Sick day rules: there may be an increased insulin requirement during illness.

Diet and exercise

Food intake needs to match the time course of insulin absorption and be adjusted depending on activity level. Dietary management therefore encompasses:

- High fibre, complex carbohydrates: this provides sustained release of glucose and avoids rapid swings in blood glucose generated by refined carbohydrates (e.g., sweets or ice cream).
- Food intake is divided between the three main meals and intervening snacks.
- Food intake is increased before or after heavy exercise to avoid hypoglycaemia.
- Working with the dietician in carbohydrate 'counting' to plan the number of grams of carbohydrates eaten and match the insulin dose accordingly.

Monitoring

Monitoring of blood glucose concentrations is necessary to evaluate the management and control. NICE recommends the following target ranges:

- fasting (on waking or premeals): 4–7 mmol/L
- post meals: 5–9 mmol/L

Previously this was by finger-prick samples recorded in a diary so changes to insulin regimens could be appropriately made. For children with type 1 diabetes, NICE Guidance now advises offering continuous glucose monitoring; either real-time continuous glucose monitoring (rtCGM) or for children over 4 years old intermittently scanned continuous glucose monitoring (isCGM – often called 'flash') if unable to use rtCGM or expressing a preference for isCGM. There is still a need for finger-prick samples as a backup and to occasionally check accuracy of CGM devices.

It is preferable to aim for the lower end of these ranges but without causing hypoglycaemia.

Urine or blood testing for ketones is important where ketoacidosis is suspected, for example, if the child is unwell or vomiting. The measurement of glycosylated haemoglobin (HbA1c) reflects glycaemic control over the past 6 to 8 weeks and allows long-term glucose control to be optimized. NICE recommends a target HbA1c level ≤48 mmol/L (≤6.5%).

Management of complications

These can be divided into immediate complications, which include hypoglycaemia and diabetic ketoacidosis, and late or long-term complications.

Hypoglycaemia

The concentration of glucose in the blood can fall when there is a mismatch between insulin dose, time of administration, carbohydrate intake and exercise. Hypoglycaemia can also occur in a nondiabetic child – causes and investigations are listed in the Boxes below.

Symptoms can occur at blood glucose levels below 4 mmol/L but more typically occur at ≤3 mmol/L. Initial symptoms reflect the compensatory sympathetic discharge and include feeling faint, dizzy or 'wobbly', sweating, tremulousness and hunger. More severe symptoms reflect glucose deprivation in the central nervous system and include lethargy, bizarre behaviour and—ultimately—coma or seizures. Many young children are not aware of hypoglycaemic episodes and repeated hypoglycaemic episodes increase this lack of awareness. Unlike adults and older children, in young children the behavioural and neuroglycopaenic symptoms predominate over autonomic symptoms.

Treatment of a 'hypo' is easily achieved at an early stage by administration of a sugary drink, glucose tablet or glucose polymer gel, which is well absorbed via the buccal mucosa, but this should be followed by a more complex form of carbohydrate. In severe hypoglycaemia, if consciousness is impaired or there is lack of cooperation, intravenous (IV) 10% dextrose or intramuscular glucagon (<8 years of age or <25 kg: give 500 µg, otherwise 1 mg) can be administered. Eating a snack just before exercising reduces the risk of exercise-induced hypoglycaemia.

CAUSES OF HYPOGLYCAEMIA		
Metabolic	**Hormonal**	**Hyperinsulinism**
Ketotic hypoglycaemia	Adrenocortical insufficiency	Islet cell adenoma
Liver disease	Panhypopituitarism	Exogenous insulin (in diabetes mellitus, otherwise as nonaccidental injury or self-harm in an adolescent)
Inborn errors of metabolism	Growth hormone deficiency	

Diabetic ketoacidosis (DKA)

This can occur at presentation or complicate established diabetes (e.g., if there is poor compliance or intercurrent illness). It is characterized by abdominal pain, vomiting, features of severe dehydration and ketoacidosis, and can have serious complications including cerebral oedema. It is considered in more detail in Chapter 20, Accidents and emergencies.

Late complications of diabetes

Good glycaemic control reduces the incidence of long-term complications of diabetes such as:

- cardiovascular disease
- retinopathy
- nephropathy
- neuropathy

Intensive control is associated with more hypoglycaemic episodes, hence may not be suitable for young children.

Type 2 diabetes mellitus

Although still uncommon, the incidence of T2DM in children is rising rapidly. 22.6% of reception-age children are overweight or obese, rising to 34.2% in Year 6. There is increasing consumption of sugar, saturated fats and salts and a reduction in physical activity.

Risk factors

- Obesity
- Family history of T2DM
- Black and Asian ethnic background
- Born to mothers with gestational diabetes
- Polycystic ovary syndrome

Presentation

It tends to present insidiously with few symptoms in adolescents. Generally, there are absent or mild symptoms of polyuria and polydipsia. There may be evidence of insulin resistance in the form of acanthosis nigricans. Children may also suffer with an increased frequency of infections. There is usually glycosuria but without ketonuria. Children with T2DM are far less likely to present in DKA.

Diagnosis

Diagnosis can be made based on fasting glucose, 2-hour glucose concentration during an oral glucose tolerance test (OGTT) or haemoglobin A1c (HbA1c). Diabetes autoantibody testing should be considered in all to rule out unusual presentations of T1DM.

Management

Lifestyle changes should be recommended at the time of diagnosis for all children. This includes strict dietary advice and the need for regular aerobic exercise. Initial pharmacologic treatment should include metformin or insulin, depending on degree of hyperglycaemia and metabolic disturbances, and presence or absence of ketosis/ketoacidosis.

At the time of diagnosis, it is important to assess for common comorbidities such as hypertension, dyslipidaemia and early renal impairment (elevated urine albumin/creatinine ratio). The overall risk of complications is higher than in T1DM and they tend to appear earlier.

Polydipsia

Polydipsia is an excessive thirst that leads to the consumption of larger than normal volumes of fluid. Children may have insatiable thirst and may even drink from taps and pet bowls.

Causes:

- Inadequate fluid intake.
- Excessive exercise; especially in hot environments.
- Psychogenic polydipsia/compulsive water drinking.
- Diabetes insipidus.
- Diabetes mellitus; hyperglycaemia secondary to undiagnosed or uncontrolled DM/DKA.
- Hypercalcaemia.
- Hyperthyroidism.

Investigations:

- Paired serum and urine osmolality.
- Serum and urinary glucose.
- Urinary ketones.
- Urea and electrolytes
- Calcium.
- Cortisol.
- Thyroid function test.

HINTS AND TIPS

It can be hard in clinical practice to differentiate fully between diabetes insipidus and psychogenic polydipsia. Investigations are key.

Diabetes insipidus (DI) – low urine osmolality and high plasma osmolality. Children pass large amounts of dilute urine. On water deprivation test, they are unable to concentrate their urine and the urine osmolality remains low. Administration of desmopressin will help differentiate between cranial and nephrogenic DI.

Psychogenic polydipsia – low urine osmolality but on water deprivation test, children are easily able to concentrate their urine resulting in a high urine osmolality.

Inborn errors of metabolism

This term is used to describe any of the inherited disorders that result in abnormal biochemical pathways. Several hundred of these conditions have been described. Individually they are rare,

Table 7.6 Inborn errors of metabolism

Category	Examples
Amino acid metabolism	Phenylketonuria
Organic acid metabolism	Maple syrup urine disease
Urea cycle disorders	Ornithine transcarbamylase deficiency
Carbohydrate metabolism	Galactosaemia Glycogen storage diseases
Mucopolysaccharidosis	Hurler syndrome Hunter syndrome

although certain ethnic groups are at increased risk of specific diseases. Inborn errors of metabolism are usually autosomal recessive, although some are X linked. The main categories are listed in Table 7.6.

Clinical features

The clinical effects are caused by accumulation of excess precursors, toxic metabolites or metabolic energy insufficiency. Clinical manifestations are nonspecific and often initially mistaken for sepsis. Metabolic stress often precipitates symptoms, for example, during the neonatal period, at weaning and with intercurrent infections. An inborn error of metabolism should always be a differential diagnosis for a sick neonate.

Features that may make it more likely include:

- parental consanguinity
- maternal HELLP (haemolysis, elevated liver enzymes, low platelet count) syndrome antenatally
- previous multiple miscarriages or stillbirths
- previous neonatal or sudden infant death
- encephalopathic episodes
- severe disease without a clear diagnosis

In older children, they should be considered as a potential cause of:

- faltering growth
- developmental delay
- progressive learning difficulties
- seizures
- coarse facies
- hepatosplenomegaly

Investigations

Initial screening investigations include:

- Blood acid–base status, anion gap, urea and electrolytes, liver function tests, glucose, lactate, ammonia levels, acylcarnitines and amino acids.

- Urine amino acids and organic acids: ketonuria is abnormal as neonates do not readily produce ketones in the urine.
- Cerebrospinal fluid lactate.

Common findings are of metabolic acidosis, hypoglycaemia or hyperammonaemia.

Treatment

The initial treatment is generic to all disorders and includes stopping feeds and administering IV dextrose to stop the metabolic load and further catabolism. Specific treatment for certain disorders is indicated and advice should be sought from a metabolic specialist. Correction of metabolic disturbances and ventilatory and renal support may be necessary. Although in some conditions the prognosis is poor, the diagnosis should be made so that prenatal diagnosis can be performed in future pregnancies.

Phenylketonuria

This is an autosomal recessive disorder with an incidence of 1/10,000 live births and a carrier rate of 1:50. In most cases, the defect lies in the enzyme phenylalanine hydroxylase, which normally converts phenylalanine to tyrosine. Hyperphenylalaninaemia occurs, with a build-up of toxic by-products, such as phenylacetic acid, which are excreted in the urine (hence phenylketonuria (PKU)).

Clinical presentation

Infants with PKU are clinically normal at birth. Symptoms and signs appear later in infancy and childhood if the disorder is undetected and untreated. These include:

- neurological manifestations: moderate to severe learning difficulty, hypertonicity, tremors, behaviour disorders and seizures
- faltering growth
- hypopigmentation: fair skin, light hair (due to the block in tyrosine formation that is required for melanin production)

Management

As PKU is relatively common and treatable, it is sought in the newborn bloodspot screening test. This is carried out at several days of age because it is necessary for the infant to have been fed milk, which contains phenylalanine. Treatment consists of dietary manipulation. The phenylalanine content of the diet is reduced.

Females with PKU must be on dietary restriction if planning a pregnancy, because maternal hyperphenylalaninaemia is associated with spontaneous abortion, microcephaly and congenital heart disease.

Galactosaemia

This causes neonatal liver dysfunction, coagulopathy and cataracts. It has an association with *Escherichia coli* sepsis. It is diagnosed by the presence of reducing substances in the urine and decreased or absent galactose-1-phosphate uridylyltransferase in red cells. A high suspicion of this disorder should be considered in all cases of severe neonatal jaundice. Treatment is by a lactose-free diet and it is an absolute contraindication to breastfeeding.

Glycogen storage diseases

This group of conditions is caused by defects in the enzymes involved in glycogen synthesis or breakdown. There is an abnormal accumulation of glycogen in tissues. The pattern of organ involvement depends on the enzyme defect and may include liver, heart, brain, skeletal muscle or other organs. There are at least six varieties, some of which have eponyms, for example, type 1A (von Gierke disease; glucose-6-phosphatase deficiency). Affected children have growth failure, hypoglycaemia and hepatomegaly. Treatment is by frequent feeds throughout day and night.

Mucopolysaccharidoses

Mucopolysaccharidoses (MPSs) are a group of disorders caused by defects in enzymes involved in the metabolism and storage of mucopolysaccharides. They are progressive multisystem disorders that can affect the central nervous system, eyes, heart and skeletal system. Characteristic features are:

- Developmental delay in the first year.
- Coarse facies: develop in most cases although children are normal at birth.

There are numerous types, many of which have eponymous designations, for example, MPS I (Hurler syndrome, which is autosomal recessive). Affected children develop coarse facial features, corneal opacities, hepatosplenomegaly, kyphosis and learning difficulties. Diagnosis is made by identifying the enzyme defect and identifying the excretion in the urine of the major storage substances, the glycosaminoglycans. Treatment is by bone marrow transplant if performed early.

Chapter Summary

- An understanding of the underlying physiology is important to understand endocrine pathologies.
- Short stature and delayed puberty are more likely to be pathological in girls, whereas precocious puberty is more likely pathological in boys.
- Endocrine causes of short stature are often associated with increased weight (e.g., hypothyroidism, Cushing syndrome, growth hormone deficiency).
- Consider congenital adrenal hyperplasia in infants with collapse, electrolyte disturbance and ambiguous genitalia. Diagnosis is based on elevated 17α-hydroxyprogesterone.
- Biochemical disturbance in hypoadrenalism/adrenal insufficiency includes hyperkalaemia, hyponatraemia and hypoglycaemia.
- The majority of cases of paediatric diabetes mellitus are type 1 – management is multidisciplinary with comprehensive patient and family education at its centre.
- Remember the 4Ts of tired, thirsty, toilet and thinner in history taking if diabetes is suspected.
- Always consider DKA as a cause of abdominal pain and/or tachypnoea.
- Consider endocrine and metabolic disorders in unwell neonates and children: always check a blood sugar and a blood gas if concerned.

UKMLA Conditions
Cushing's syndrome
Hypoglycaemia
Hypothyroidism
Thyrotoxicosis
Diabetes mellitus type 1 and 2
Diabetic ketoacidosis

UKMLA Presentations
Polydipsia (thirst)
Pubertal development

CHILDHOOD CANCER

Cancer in childhood is uncommon; affecting 1:600 children aged 1 to 15 years. Despite the dramatic increases in survival rate due to new treatments, it remains an important cause of death in childhood. The spectrum of cancer in childhood is very different from that in adults with leukaemia accounting for over one-third of cases (Fig. 8.1).

The aetiology, clinical features, investigation and management of malignant disease in childhood are considered in the following sections.

This chapter focuses on basics of paediatric oncology and haematology but **leukaemia** and **lymphomas** are covered in Chapter 9, Haematology.

Aetiology

Most childhood cancers are of uncertain cause and occur sporadically in otherwise healthy children. Risk factors include:

- Genetic predisposition: genetic factors are often more evident in childhood than in adult malignancy.
- Environmental factors.
- Infections.

Malignant cells proliferate and develop abnormally because they have escaped normal control mechanisms. In younger children, in particular, the malignant cells might be immature precursor cells that fail to mature into normal, differentiated functional cells.

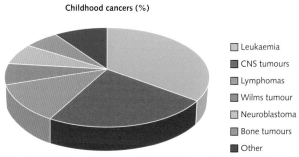

Childhood cancers (%)

- Leukaemia
- CNS tumours
- Lymphomas
- Wilms tumour
- Neuroblastoma
- Bone tumours
- Other

Fig. 8.1 Childhood cancer – clinical features at presentation. *CNS,* Central nervous system.

Genetic causes of childhood cancer

During periods of rapid proliferation, a normal cell may undergo a genetic alteration that transforms it into a malignant cell. Two important mechanisms of transformation are:

- activation of oncogenes
- loss of tumour suppressor genes

Some childhood cancers have an identifiable genetic aetiology. An important mutation associated with malignancy is that of *p53* (a tumour suppressor gene), but there are many others. Retinoblastoma is hereditary in approximately 40% of cases, whereby the child inherits a germline mutation of the tumour suppressor gene *RB1*. The determination of this pattern of inheritance played a key role in the understanding of cancer genetics.

There are also many genetic syndromes which are associated with increased risk of developing malignancy, including:

- Down syndrome
- Neurofibromatosis types 1 and 2
- Beckwith-Wiedemann syndrome
- Ataxia telangiectasia
- Li-Fraumeni
- WAGR
- Fanconi's anaemia
- Perlman syndrome

Infections

Two viruses are associated with malignancy:

- Epstein-Barr virus (EBV): present in the majority of Burkitt lymphoma. It produces a translocation disrupting the c-myc oncogene on chromosome 8 leading to malignant change, although the exact mechanism is poorly understood.
- Human immunodeficiency virus (HIV): HIV/acquired immune deficiency syndrome is associated with increased prevalence of malignancies (especially lymphoid).

Environmental

Carcinogens and toxins are less often a cause of cancer in children compared with that in adults, although importantly previous treatment of malignancy is a significant risk factor.

Clinical features

Cancer in childhood presents in a number of ways, some of which are nonspecific (Table 8.1).

Table 8.1 Childhood cancer – clinical features at presentation

Clinical feature	Type of cancer
Constitutional symptoms: fever, weight loss, night sweats	Leukaemia, lymphoma
A localized mass in: • Abdomen • Thorax • Soft tissue	See Table 8.3
Lymph node enlargement	Leukaemia, lymphoma
Bone marrow failure	Leukaemia
Bone pain	Leukaemia, bone tumours
Signs of raised intracranial pressure	Primary or metastatic central nervous system tumours

Investigations

Tumour histology provides a definitive diagnosis. This is provided by biopsy (although initial biopsy is not possible at some sites, e.g., brain tumours) or bone marrow aspiration.

Imaging is important and all modalities can be useful: ultrasound, X-ray, computed tomography (CT), magnetic resonance imaging (MRI) and nuclear imaging scans. Tumour markers are useful in certain tumours (e.g., α-fetoprotein in liver tumours and urinary catecholamines in neuroblastoma). Genome sequencing for all children with cancer is becoming part of routine care, enabling targeted treatments for each individual patient.

Management

The main therapeutic strategies available are:

- Surgery: including excisional biopsy and total or partial removal of solid tumours (debulking). This may be the sole management or come before or after other treatment modalities.
- Radiotherapy: often used in solid tumours.
- Chemotherapy: a number of highly effective antineoplastic agents have been developed in the last four decades and many children are enrolled in clinical trials on diagnosis.

Chemotherapy may be used as:

- primary therapy for disseminated malignancy (e.g., the leukaemias)
- to shrink bulky primary or metastatic disease before local treatment
- adjunctive treatment for micrometastases

Chimeric antigen receptor (CAR) T-cell therapy is an emerging therapy in paediatric haematology with relapsed/ refractory B-cell leukaemia/lymphomas. It is a promising treatment modality that seeks to replace or bridge progression to bone marrow

transplant. However, it isn't without potential serious side effects: Cytokine release syndrome (CRS) and immune effector cell-associated neurotoxicity syndrome (ICANS).

Bone marrow toxicity is the limiting factor for many therapeutic regimens. This can be circumvented by using bone marrow transplantation to 'rescue' patients after administering potentially lethal, but potentially curative, doses of chemotherapy or radiation.

Supportive care

Treatment produces many predictable and often severe side effects and supportive care is a vital part of cancer treatment. Pancytopenia may necessitate blood or platelet transfusions and close monitoring/treatment of infections at times of neutropaenia is vital. Antiemetics should be given preemptively to all children having chemotherapy and many will require nasogastric tube feeding or even total parenteral nutrition for short periods. Mucositis (drug induced, painful inflammation of any part of the gastrointestinal tract) can further complicate appetite and nutritional status and requires admission for feeding support and strong analgesia. Indwelling central venous catheters are inserted to allow pain-free blood sampling and injections, although these also carry an infection risk.

HINTS AND TIPS

Chemotherapy-related side effects are due to its action on rapidly dividing normal cells (e.g., those of the bone marrow, gastrointestinal tract and hair follicles). Whilst hair grows back, mucositis and sepsis resulting from febrile neutropaenia carry significant morbidity and mortality.

Cure may not always be possible for all children. Palliative treatment aims at reducing symptoms and maximizing quality of life. For survivors, regular follow-up is required to detect and manage long-term sequelae (see Box 8.1) and monitor for relapse.

COMMUNICATION

Psychosocial support is very important. Diagnosis of a potentially fatal illness provokes enormous anxiety, guilt, fear and sadness. Children and their siblings need an explanation of the illness tailored to their age. Help with practical difficulties such as transport and finances might be required and support from community nursing teams is very important.

BOX 8.1 SHORT- AND LONG-TERM SEQUELAE OF CANCER TREATMENT

Short term	Long term
Bone marrow suppression	Hearing loss (e.g., cisplatin)
Infection risk (bacteria, viral, fungal)	Peripheral neuropathy (e.g., vincristine)
Nausea and vomiting	Cardiac dysfunction (anthracycline related)
Mucositis (e.g., methotrexate)	Renal impairment (e.g., cisplatin)
Malnutrition	Cognitive impairment (e.g., methotrexate but also disrupted education)
Constipation (vincristine related)	Psychological effects
Hair loss	Reduced fertility
Colitis	Diabetes (abdominal radiotherapy)

BRAIN TUMOURS

Brain tumours are the most common solid tumour of childhood. Most are located infratentorially and present with signs and symptoms of raised intracranial pressure and cerebellar dysfunction. Metastasis is rare and diagnosis is often difficult and delayed.

Diagnosis

Brain tumours present in many different ways depending on the position of the tumour and the age of the child. Where a tumour is suspected clinically, an MRI scan is the preferred imaging modality.

RED FLAG

Brain tumours often present with nonspecific and common childhood complaints such as headache, vomiting and behavioural problems. They may also declare themselves with events such as seizures. A careful history and examination may reveal clues more specific to central nervous system pathology, such as:

- macrocephaly/hydrocephalus
- ataxia/cerebellar signs
- papilloedema
- focal neurological deficit (e.g., facial palsy, motor deficit)

For more information about paediatric brain tumours and their signs and symptoms as they vary by age, visit www.headsmart.org.uk.

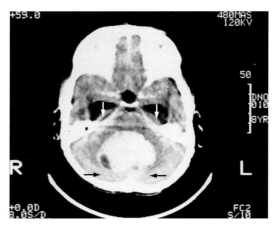

Fig. 8.2 Computed tomography of an enhancing posterior fossa tumour *(black arrows)* with hydrocephalus demonstrated by dilated temporal horns *(white arrows)*.

HINTS AND TIPS

Brain computed tomography (CT) scans are often more readily available in all hospitals. They are quick to perform and usually do not require sedation/anaesthesia of the patient. Despite this, magnetic resonance imaging (MRI) is gold standard as whilst a CT scan can detect large tumours and hydrocephalus (see Fig. 8.2), MRI is more sensitive for parenchymal lesions and the leptomeninges.

Whenever possible tumours of the CNS are biopsied. This is because the different types are classified by histology (see Table 8.2), some of which are described here.

Table 8.2 Histological classification of central nervous system (CNS) tumours seen in children

Types of central nervous system tumours	
Astrocytoma	Low-grade astrocytoma – for example, pilocytic astrocytoma, optic glioma High-grade supratentorial glioma – for example, glioblastoma multiforme Brainstem glioma –for example, diffuse intrinsic pontine glioma
Ependymoma	Subependymoma Ependymoma
Embryonal tumours	Medulloblastoma Craniopharyngioma Atypical teratoid rhabdoid tumour

Astrocytomas (40%)

This is a group of tumours that range from benign to highly malignant:

- Grade 1 – for example, pilocytic astrocytomas. Slow growing, unlikely to metastasize.
- Grade 2 – for example, diffuse astrocytoma. Slow growing but more difficult to resect due to poorly defined nature.
- Grade 3 – for example, anaplastic astrocytoma. Fast growing and often recur following treatment.
- Grade 4 – for example, glioblastoma multiforme. Fast growing and metastatic, associated with poor prognosis.

Clinical features

Cerebellar astrocytomas are usually low-grade cystic gliomas occurring between the ages of 6 and 9 years. Presenting features may include:

- Headache and vomiting: caused by obstructive hydrocephalus; papilloedema might be present.
- Cerebellar signs: ataxia, nystagmus and uncoordination.
- Diplopia, squint: sixth nerve palsy.

Supratentorial astrocytomas are less common and present with focal neurological signs and seizures.

Brainstem gliomas (6%) present with cranial nerve palsies, ataxia and pyramidal tract signs.

Diagnosis and management

This is usually based on clinical findings and MRI, as biopsy is hazardous. Whilst surgical resection is sometimes possible, prognosis is generally poor with median survival less than 1 year after diagnosis despite radiotherapy.

MEDULLOBLASTOMA (20%)

This is the most common malignant brain tumour of childhood, with a peak incidence between the ages of 2 and 6 years, and is more common in boys. They usually arise in the midline and

Table 8.3 Abdominal mass aetiology

Malignant	Wilms tumour, neuroblastoma, hepatoblastoma, leukaemia, lymphoma, rhabdomyosarcomas
Infective/inflammatory	Abscess, inflammatory mass with localized oedema
Gastrointestinal and hepatobiliary	Constipation, hepatomegaly, splenomegaly, splenic/hepatic cyst, cholecystitis, bowel obstruction
Genitourinary	Multicystic dysplastic kidney, ARPKD, hydronephrosis, ovarian cyst/tumour

invade the fourth ventricle and cerebellar hemispheres. Unlike other CNS tumours they seed through the CNS and up to 20% have spinal metastases at diagnosis.

Presentation is usually with headache, vomiting and ataxia.

Treatment is a combined modality approach with surgical removal, CNS radiotherapy and chemotherapy all playing a part. Prognosis is dependent on extent of metastasis and 5-year survival ranges from 20% to 80%.

HINTS AND TIPS

Radiotherapy is avoided in children under 3 years of age, as it can impair their continuing neurocognitive development. Proton beam radiotherapy is a modern technique which reduces damage to healthy surrounding tissue. Long-term complications of radiotherapy at any age include leukoencephalopathy, secondary malignancy and vasculopathy.

CRANIOPHARYNGIOMA (4%)

These arise from the squamous remnant of Rathke pouch and are locally invasive. They present with:

- visual field loss: due to compression of the optic chiasm
- pituitary dysfunction: growth failure, diabetes insipidus

Most are calcified and may be visible on skull radiographs; however, MRI is the investigation of choice. Treatment is by surgical excision with radiotherapy for residual or recurrent tumour. Prognosis is good but sequelae include visual impairment and pituitary/hypothalamic dysfunction.

NEUROBLASTOMA

Neuroblastoma is a malignancy of neural crest cells that normally give rise to the paraspinal sympathetic ganglia and the adrenal medulla. It is the second most common solid tumour of childhood, occurring predominantly in infants and preschool children with a median age at diagnosis of 2 years. It is unusual in that it can regress spontaneously in very young children (stage IV-S). They can occur anywhere in the sympathetic nervous system but are most commonly found in the adrenals or abdomen.

Clinical features

The clinical features depend on the location and may include:

- abdominal mass: a firm, nontender abdominal mass (common)
- systemic signs: pallor, weight loss, bone pain from disseminated disease

- hepatomegaly or lymph node enlargement
- unilateral proptosis: metastasis to the eye
- opsoclonus-myoclonus: 'dancing-eye' syndrome caused by an immune response.
- diarrhoea: due to secretion of vasoactive intestinal peptide
- respiratory distress: mediastinal mass (may also be incidentally detected on X-ray)

Diagnosis

Diagnosis may be suspected from characteristic clinical and radiological features (with calcium speckling of tumour). This is confirmed with:

- Biopsy demonstrating classical features on light microscopy with or without immunological staining.
- Raised urinary catecholamines (vanillylmandelic acid, homovanillic acid).
- Meta-iodobenzylguanidine, a radiolabelled tumour-specific agent, or other nuclear scan such as fludeoxyglucose positron emission tomography–CT is useful to measure disease extent.
- Bone marrow aspirates and trephines to detect infiltrative disease.

Treatment

Treatment of neuroblastoma includes:

- surgical resection
- chemotherapy
- radiotherapy (especially for high-grade tumours and complications, e.g., spinal cord compression)

Prognosis is worse for older children and those with metastatic disease. Overexpression of the N-myc oncogene in the tumour is associated with a poor prognosis.

WILMS TUMOUR (NEPHROBLASTOMA)

Wilms tumour arises from embryonal renal cells of the metanephros; there is cell proliferation without normal tubular and glomerular differentiation. It is predominantly a tumour of the first 5 years of life with a median age of presentation of 3 years of age. It can be sporadic, familial or syndromic. This is the most common childhood renal cancer, with other forms (e.g., clear cell tumours) being rare.

Clinical features

The most common clinical presentation is an asymptomatic abdominal mass that does not cross the midline. Other features may include:

- Abdominal pain: due to haemorrhage into the tumour.
- Haematuria.

- Hypertension: in 25% of cases. This can be caused by compression of the renal artery or renin production by tumour cells.

Genetics and aetiology

A Wilms tumour-susceptibility gene has been recognized on chromosome 11. There is an association with a number of syndromes including Beckwith-Wiedemann syndrome (with hemihypertrophy) and WAGR syndrome. Features of WAGR include:

- Wilms tumour
- aniridia
- genitourinary tract abnormalities
- learning disability (previously known as mental retardation)

Diagnosis

Diagnosis is normally made from the characteristic appearance on CT (Fig. 8.3), which shows an intrinsic renal mass with mixed solid and cystic densities, and from biopsy. A search for distant metastases, which are most common in lungs and liver, should be made.

Treatment

Treatment involves tailored chemotherapy with surgical resection of the primary tumour. Nephron-sparing surgery is attempted if disease is bilateral. Radiotherapy is used for more advanced disease. Overall, the prognosis is good, with a 90% chance of cure if there is no metastasis, although this falls to 30% to 40% with metastasis and unfavourable histology.

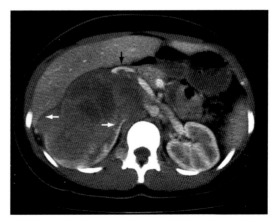

Fig. 8.3 Computed tomography scan of Wilms tumour. Mass arising out of right kidney *(white arrows)* displacing the inferior vena cava *(black arrow)*.

SOFT-TISSUE SARCOMAS

These arise from primitive mesenchyme. The most important is rhabdomyosarcoma, but even rarer forms include fibrosarcomas and liposarcomas. Rhabdomyosarcoma can occur anywhere in the body; however, head and neck tumours are common in younger children, whereas older children present with tumours in the extremities.

BONE TUMOURS

Primary malignant bone tumours account for 6% of childhood cancer. They are uncommon before puberty and are most common in adolescents with a preponderance in boys. The two main types are:

- osteosarcoma
- Ewing sarcoma

Osteosarcoma

This is a malignant tumour of the bone-producing mesenchyme usually found in older children and is twice as common in males as females.

Clinical features

The usual presenting feature is local pain and soft-tissue mass. Persistent bone pain precedes the detection of a mass. Half of all cases occur around the knee joint in the metaphysis of the distal femur or proximal tibia. Systemic symptoms are rare. Metastases are mainly to the lungs and are often asymptomatic.

Diagnosis

Bone X-ray shows destruction and a characteristic 'sunburst' appearance as the tumour breaks through the cortex and spicules of new bone are formed.

Treatment

Treatment involves surgery of primary and metastatic deposits. En bloc resection might allow amputation to be avoided. Aggressive neoadjuvant chemotherapy is important to treat micrometastatic disease. Survival has improved and is 60% to 80% for localized disease.

Ewing sarcoma

This is less common than osteogenic sarcoma and is more common in younger children. It is an undifferentiated sarcoma of uncertain tissue of origin that arises primarily in bone, but occasionally in soft tissues.

It mostly affects the long bones, especially the mid to proximal femur, but can also affect flat bones such as the pelvis.

Clinical features and diagnosis

Pain and localized swelling are the usual presenting complaints. X-ray demonstrates a destructive lesion with periosteal elevation or a soft-tissue mass (so-called onion-skin appearance). Metastases occur to the lungs and to other bones.

Treatment

Chemotherapy is usually the initial treatment followed by radiotherapy or definitive surgical resection. Prognosis depends mainly on the extent of disease at diagnosis.

RETINOBLASTOMA

This is a solid tumour affecting the eye and is bilateral in 40% of cases. It frequently presents with leukocoria (see Fig. 8.4) and is a cause of an absent red reflex in the neonate. It occurs when both copies of the *Rb* gene (tumour suppressor) on chromosome 13 are inactivated. It may be inherited (where one copy is already inactive) or be spontaneous. Early diagnosis and ophthalmology referral are vital to preserve visual development. Treatment includes systemic and intra-arterial chemotherapy, and sometimes enucleation. The 5-year survival rate is >90%.

LANGERHANS CELL HISTIOCYTOSIS

This encompasses a group of rare diseases characterized by the clonal proliferation of a myeloid dendritic cell with antigenic similarities to skin Langerhans cells. Langerhans cell histiocytosis (LCH) most often presents in children 1 to 3 years of age with bony lytic lesions, but is also highly

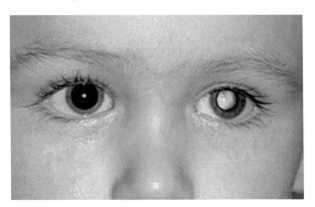

Fig. 8.4 Leukocoria of the left eye, which is a sign of potential retinoblastoma. (Republished with permission of McGraw-Hill Education from Richard P. Ustine, Mindy Ann Smith, Heidi S. Chumley, Camille Sabella, E.J. Mayeaux Jr., Elumalai Appach: *The Color Atlas of Pediatrics*.)

infiltrative. Diagnosis is confirmed with biopsy, preferably of a bony lesion. Other organs affected can include skin, lymph nodes, liver, spleen, oral mucosa, lung and CNS. Diabetes insipidus and neurodegeneration are typical of CNS infiltration of LCH. Whilst it is not currently considered a true malignancy, it is potentially an aggressive disease often requiring treatment with chemotherapy.

Chapter Summary

- Childhood cancer affects not only the child but also the surrounding family, so care needs not only to be holistic but also made in partnership with the patient and family.
- Supportive care embodies the biopsychosocial aspects of cancer care, thus allowing patients to receive the most benefit from their care.
- Brain tumours are the most common solid tumour in children. Presentation is variable and includes headache, vomiting and cerebellar signs.
- Cranial radiation is avoided in children under 3 years as it impairs neurodevelopment.
- Neuroblastoma commonly presents with an abdominal mass. Overexpression of N-myc oncogene is associated with a poor prognosis.

MLA Conditions
Raised intracranial pressure

UKMLA Presentations
Abdominal mass

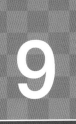

This chapter encompasses childhood haematological malignancy in addition to defects in the cellular elements of the blood or in those soluble elements involved in haemostasis. Normal developmental variations are important in the interpretation of changes in the blood in infancy and childhood.

THE LEUKAEMIAS

Leukaemia is the most common childhood malignancy (35% of all cases). They are characterized by proliferation of immature white cells. Acute leukaemia accounts for the majority (97%) of cases. Note that chronic myeloid leukaemia is rare and that chronic lymphocytic leukaemia is confined to adults. The malignant cells are termed 'blasts'.

The leukaemias are classified according to the white blood cell line involved:

- ALL: cells of lymphoid lineage
- acute myeloid leukaemia: cells of granulocytic or monocytic lineage

Prognosis has improved significantly with a 5-year overall survival rate of over 85%. It continues to improve with reductions in treatment-related mortality and matching of therapies to different prognostic groups.

Investigations

Peripheral blood may reveal:

- anaemia: normocytic, normochromic
- thrombocytopenia
- neutropenia (although the total white blood cell count might be low, normal or high)
- blast cells on film

Bone marrow examination reveals replacement of normal elements by leukaemic cells.

Acute lymphocytic leukaemia

ALL accounts for 80% of childhood leukaemia and has a peak incidence between age 2 and 5 years. It is slightly more common in boys than girls. Lymphoblasts in these children do not successfully complete the rearrangement of immunoglobulin and T-cell receptor genes necessary for full maturation. Coupled with genetic alterations which permit them to survive and proliferate, the lymphoblasts remain 'frozen' at an early stage of development.

ALL can be classified according to cell-surface antigens (immunophenotype) into:

- non-T-cell, non-B-cell (common) ALL: 80% are from B-cell precursor lineage
- T-cell ALL: 15%
- B-cell ALL: 1%

Clinical features

In most children with acute leukaemia, there is an insidious onset of symptoms and signs arising from infiltration of the bone marrow or other organs with leukaemic blast cells. Children will usually have one or more of the following:

- Pallor and malaise due to anaemia.
- Purpura, easy bruising or epistaxis due to thrombocytopenia.
- Infection due to neutropenia.
- Bone pain due to expansion of marrow cavity with or without periosteal involvement.
- Hepatosplenomegaly and lymphadenopathy due to reticuloendothelial cell infiltration.

T-cell ALL tends to occur in older children and teenagers, with a high peripheral white cell count and mediastinal mass.

Prognosis

The National Cancer Institute considers children aged >1 year to <10 years with a WCC $<50 \times 10^9$ g/L at diagnosis as standard risk with a 5-year event-free survival (EFS) of 90%. Some cytogenetics are favourable for prognosis including hyperdiploidy (95% EFS). There are several other factors that increase the risk classification which are outlined in Box 9.1.

Management

A typical treatment regimen can be divided into three phases:

1. Induction: an intensive regimen of between three and five drugs with the aim of reducing tumour load (90% achieve remission after induction).
2. Consolidation: short but continued intense therapy after remission.
3. Maintenance: total treatment is 3 years for boys and 2 years for girls.

Each stage will include central nervous system (CNS)-directed therapy. This is given to those with CNS-positive disease

BOX 9.1 POOR PROGNOSTIC GROUPS IN ACUTE LYMPHOBLASTIC LEUKAEMIA

High risk	Very high risk
White cell count >50 × 10⁹ g/L at diagnosis	Age <1 year
Age >10 years	Minimal residual disease positive at 28 days
Slow response to therapy	*MLL* rearrangements
Central nervous system positive	T-cell ALL
Testicular leukaemia	Philadelphia chromosome (t 9:22) positive

and as prophylaxis for CNS-negative patients in the form of intrathecal chemotherapy.

HINTS AND TIPS

When starting chemotherapy patients are at risk of tumour lysis syndrome, an oncological emergency. As the leukaemic cells are destroyed, they release potassium, phosphate and nucleic acid into the circulation. This results in dangerous hyperkalaemia and uric acid and calcium deposits within the kidney causing acute kidney injury. Treatment is aimed at prevention with hyperhydration and allopurinol.

Relapses may occur in the bone marrow, CNS or more rarely testes or lymph nodes. The prognosis is less good in these cases; they are treated with intensified chemotherapy and may be candidates for bone marrow transplant once remission is achieved. For those with Philadelphia translocation, monoclonal antibody therapy (imatinib) is showing some promise.

Acute myeloid leukaemia

This is classified into subtypes depending on cytogenetic abnormality. Prognosis is worse than for ALL – around 85% achieve remission with chemotherapy, but relapse is common and recurrence-free survival ranges from 30% to 45%. Treatment approach is similar. Allogeneic bone marrow transplant has been shown to improve survival and may be offered depending on risk stratification and where a suitable donor is found.

LYMPHOMAS

These can be classified into:

- Non-Hodgkin lymphoma (NHL): more common in young children.
- Hodgkin disease: more common in adolescents and young adults.

Non-Hodgkin lymphoma

NHL is a heterogeneous group of lymphomas with different characteristics and cells of origin. The most common types being Burkitt lymphoma, diffuse large B-cell lymphoma, T-cell lymphoblastic lymphoma and anaplastic large cell lymphoma. It accounts for 7% of all childhood cancer. They can develop in immunocompromised children; for example, those with HIV, severe combined immunodeficiency or other severe inherited immunodeficiencies.

Clinical features

Symptoms of NHL develop over weeks, most commonly presenting with rapidly enlarging, nontender lymphadenopathy. The disease tends to be aggressive and can also present acutely with:

- respiratory distress (mediastinal masses can compress the trachea, oesophagus and major vessels such as the superior vena cava)
- acute abdominal pain (intussusception from gastrointestinal lymph node mass)
- tumour lysis syndrome (spontaneous onset)

Management

Chemotherapy is the mainstay of treatment but surgical debulking might be required for abdominal tumours. Localized disease has a 90% survival at 5 years.

Hodgkin lymphoma

This is another malignant lymphoma which is characterized histologically by the Reed-Sternberg cell. Up to 50% of cases are associated with EBV infection. It usually presents in adolescence or young adulthood, with a slight predominance in females.

Clinical features

The usual presentation is with painless cervical or supraclavicular lymphadenopathy. Systemic symptoms are uncommon. Metastatic disease occurs in the lungs, liver and bone marrow.

Diagnosis

Diagnosis is confirmed by histological examination of a lymph node biopsy. Classification based on histopathology identifies four subtypes of different prognosis:

1. lymphocyte predominance: best prognosis
2. mixed cellularity
3. nodular sclerosing: most common in children and adolescents
4. lymphocyte depletion: least common, worst prognosis

Management

The disease is staged using imaging of chest, mediastinum and abdomen. Treatment is chemotherapy and field radiotherapy which is risk adapted. In advanced or recurrent disease, bone marrow transplant may be of benefit. The overall prognosis is good and 80% to 90% of patients are cured overall.

HAEMATOPOIESIS

Early prenatal haematopoiesis occurs in the liver, spleen and lymph nodes. It commences in the bone marrow at about the fourth or fifth month of gestation. At birth, haematopoietic activity is present in most of the bones, especially long bones.

Cells in the peripheral blood have a relatively short lifespan. Continuous replenishment in massive amounts from the bone marrow is required to maintain adequate blood counts.

> **HINTS AND TIPS**
>
> Lifespan of peripheral blood cells:
> - red cells: 120 days
> - platelets: 10 days
> - neutrophils: 6 to 7 hours

Normal developmental changes in haemoglobin

The haemoglobin (Hb) concentration and haematocrit are relatively high in the term newborn infant because of the low oxygen tension in utero. The wide range encountered, 14 to 20 g/dL, is accounted for by:

- variation in umbilical cord clamping
- the infant's position after delivery

If cord clamping is delayed and the baby is lower than its placenta, Hb and blood volume are both increased by a placental transfusion. These values subsequently decline, reaching a nadir at around 7 weeks in preterm infants and 2 to 3 months in term infants.

The lower limit of normal for this 'physiological' anaemia is 9.0 g/dL. During this period, there is erythroid hypoplasia of the marrow and a change from foetal to adult Hb. Foetal haemoglobin (HbF) constitutes around 60% to 80% of total Hb in the newborn; values decline postnatally to 2% of total Hb at 6 to 12 months.

ANAEMIA

Anaemia is defined as a decrease of the Hb concentration in the blood to below normal or reduction in red blood cell (RBC) mass. Dietary iron deficiency is the most common cause but there are many others. Anaemia can be classified initially according to:

- colour intensity of RBCs (normochromic/hypochromic)
- size of RBCs (microcytic/normocytic/macrocytic)

Important causes based on this classification are shown in Box 9.2.

BOX 9.2 CLASSIFICATION AND CAUSES OF ANAEMIA

Microcytic, hypochromic anaemia
Defects of haem synthesis
- Iron deficiency
- Chronic inflammation

Defects of globin synthesis
- Thalassaemia

Normocytic, normochromic anaemia
Haemolytic anaemias
- Intrinsic red cell defects

Membrane defects: spherocytosis
Haemoglobinopathies: sickle cell disease
Enzymopathies: glucose-6-phosphate dehydrogenase deficiency
- Extrinsic disorders

Immune mediated: Rh incompatibility
Microangiopathy
Hypersplenism
Haemorrhage (acute or chronic)
- Hookworm infestation
- Meckel diverticulum
- Iatrogenic (excessive venesection)
- Menorrhagia

Hypoproduction disorders
- Red cell aplasia (e.g., renal disease)
- Pancytopaenia (e.g., marrow aplasia, leukaemia)

Macrocytic anaemia
Bone marrow megaloblastic
- Vitamin B12 deficiency
- Folic acid deficiency

Bone marrow not megaloblastic
- Hypothyroidism
- Fanconi anaemia

The history and physical examination will often provide a good idea of the likely cause; however, few symptoms will occur with Hb above 7 to 8 g/dL, except in acute blood loss. It is easy to miss mild anaemia, especially in patients with pigmented skin.

History

When anaemia is suspected, the history should include enquiry about:

- the presence of chronic diseases (especially renal) or prematurity
- gastrointestinal symptoms
- dietary history: adequate iron intake?
- family history: relatives with haematological disorders
- place of birth: sickle cell screening has been part of the Newborn Blood spot test in the UK since 2002
- ethnicity:
  - Afro-Caribbean: sickle cell disease
  - Mediterranean and Asian: thalassaemia

Examination

Physical examination may narrow down the differential causes, and key observations include:

- Pallor: best observed in the conjunctiva and palmar creases.
- Jaundice: suggests acute haemolysis.
- Petechiae or bruising: suggests marrow failure.
- Splenomegaly: suggests haemolysis, haemoglobinopathy or marrow failure.

RED FLAG

Peripheral vasoconstriction also causes pallor (e.g., in hypovolaemic shock) and tachycardia may be present in both conditions. A patient in shock will be cool peripherally with a prolonged capillary refill time. This would not be the case in anaemic patients, unless hypovolaemic shock was a result of acute blood loss.

Investigations

The most important initial investigation is a full blood count (FBC) to confirm reduced Hb concentration and document red cell indices (Box 9.3). Additional valuable information from the FBC includes:

- Reticulocytes: an increase suggests haemolytic anaemia; a decrease suggests marrow aplasia.
- Pancytopaenia: a reduction in all cell types suggests marrow failure or hypersplenism.

BOX 9.3 RED CELL INDICES AND BLOOD FILM

Mean corpuscular volume:
- low: microcytic (e.g., iron deficiency, thalassaemia)
- high: macrocytic (e.g., folate or vitamin B12 deficiency (rare), normal in neonates)

Mean corpuscular haemoglobin concentration:
- low: hypochromic (e.g., iron deficiency, thalassaemia)
- high: hyperchromic (e.g., spherocytosis)

Red cell distribution width:
- normal: aplastic anaemia, chronic disease
- high: iron, vitamin B12 or folate deficiency, sickle cell disease

Blood film may reveal:
- sickle cells – sickle cell disease
- spherocytes – hereditary spherocytosis
- blast cells – malignancy

Depending on the initial results, further investigations to clarify the cause might include:

- iron studies: ferritin (If required, serum iron and total iron-binding capacity)
- direct antiglobulin test (Coombs test): this is positive in immune-mediated haemolysis
- red cell folate, vitamin B12
- Hb electrophoresis
- Red cell enzymes: glucose-6-phosphate dehydrogenase (G6PD), pyruvate kinase
- Bone marrow aspiration

Iron-deficiency anaemia

Iron-deficiency anaemia is a microcytic, hypochromic anaemia and the commonest cause of anaemia in childhood. Unlike in adults, it usually results from inadequate dietary intake rather than loss of iron through haemorrhage.

Iron requirements

The foetus absorbs iron from the mother across the placenta:

- Term infants have adequate reserves for the first 4 months of life.
- Preterm infants have limited stores and higher demands. Their rapid growth rate means they utilize all their reserves by 8 weeks.

Both breast milk and unmodified cow's milk are low in iron concentration (0.05–0.10 mg/100 mL). However, 50% of the iron in breast milk is absorbed, compared with just 10% from cow's milk. Most formula milks are fortified with iron and contain 10 times the concentration in breast milk (1.0 mg/100 mL); however, only 4% is absorbed.

Dietary sources of iron include red meat, fortified breakfast cereals, dark green vegetables and bread. About 10% to 15% of dietary iron is absorbed. Absorption is enhanced by ascorbic acid (vitamin C) and reduced by tannin in tea.

Whilst in adults most iron supplies (95%) come from the recycling of broken-down RBCs, infants require 30% of iron to come from dietary sources to match their rapid growth rate. Iron requirements increase during adolescence, especially for girls who lose iron through menstruation.

Causes of iron deficiency

Nutritional deficiency is common in certain at-risk groups (Box 9.4). Blood loss is a less common cause but might occur with:

- menstruation
- hookworm infestation
- repeated venesection in babies
- Meckel diverticulum
- recurrent epistaxis
- inflammatory bowel disease
- coeliac disease

Clinical features

Mild iron deficiency is asymptomatic. As it becomes more severe there might be:

- lethargy
- fatigue
- anorexia

On examination, the only signs might be pallor of mucous membranes. If severe there may also be a flow murmur due to a hyperdynamic circulation.

Iron deficiency in infancy and early childhood causes developmental delay and poor growth, which is reversible by long-term oral iron treatment. Severe anaemia can cause cardiac failure.

Diagnosis

Diagnosis is confirmed by the FBC, blood film and iron studies:

- FBC: low Hb, low mean corpuscular Hb
- blood film: microcytic, hypochromic RBCs

BOX 9.4 HIGH-RISK GROUPS FOR IRON-DEFICIENCY ANAEMIA

- Premature infants
- Early introduction of unmodified cow's milk (before 1 year)
- Delay in weaning (beyond 6 months)
- Poor diet (associated with low socioeconomic status, strict vegetarian/vegan diet, etc.)
- Malabsorption

- iron studies:
  - ◦ low serum ferritin (reflecting iron stores)
  - ◦ low serum iron (iron circulating in blood)
  - ◦ high total iron binding capacity (proteins available in the blood to bind to iron, e.g., transferrin)

COMMUNICATION

It is important to take a detailed dietary history. You must ask specifically what type of milk and how much is consumed in a day. It is also important to advise parents about appropriate diet and give information regarding iron-containing foods.

Management

Primary prevention in infants can be achieved by:

- Avoidance of unmodified cow's milk until 12 months.
- Iron supplementation in vulnerable infants (e.g., preterm).

Mild to moderate anaemia is treated with dietary counselling and oral iron supplements. A referral to a dietician may also be required. Replacement should be continued for 3 months after correction of anaemia to allow replenishment of iron stores.

Severe anaemia with cardiac compromise might require transfusion. Investigation for occult gastrointestinal tract bleeding is indicated if there is a failure of response to treatment or recurrence despite an adequate intake.

Thalassaemias

The thalassaemias are a group of hereditary anaemias caused by defects of globin chain synthesis.

HINTS AND TIPS

Haemoglobin is a tetramer. Normal foetal haemoglobin is made up of one pair of α-globin chains and one pair of γ-globin chains. Normal adult haemoglobin (HbA) is made up of one pair of α-globin chains and one pair of β-globin chains. Disease occurs when the normal balance of globin chains is disrupted.

Thalassaemia is classified as:

- α-thalassaemia: reduced synthesis of α-globin chains
- β-thalassaemia: reduced synthesis of β-globin chains

Mutations in the globin genes lead to a reduction or absence of the corresponding globin chains. Excess unpaired globin chains produce insoluble tetramers that precipitate causing membrane damage and either:

- Cell death within the bone marrow (ineffective erythropoiesis).

Or

- Premature removal by the spleen (resulting in haemolytic anaemia).

β-Thalassaemia

This occurs most frequently in people from the Mediterranean countries and the Middle East. There are two main types:

1. β-thalassaemia major (homozygous)
2. β-thalassaemia trait (heterozygous)

β-Thalassaemia major. There is usually a complete absence of β-globin chain production (genotype $β^0/β^0$), although some mutations allow partial synthesis (genotype $β^+/β^+$); HbA cannot be synthesized.

Clinical features. Affected infants usually present after 6 months, as HbF levels decline, with severe haemolytic anaemia, jaundice, failure to thrive, lethargy and hepatosplenomegaly. If untreated, bone marrow hyperplasia occurs with development of the classical facies:

- maxillary hypertrophy
- skull bossing

Diagnosis FBC will reveal a severe microcytic hypochromic anaemia and blood film will show abnormal RBC morphology with inclusion bodies termed 'Heinz bodies', which represent α-globin chain precipitates. Diagnosis is confirmed on Hb electrophoresis (see Table 9.1).

HINTS AND TIPS

Both iron-deficiency anaemia and thalassaemia present with a microcytic hypochromic picture. It is important to distinguish these so that iron supplements are not given to patients with thalassaemia who are already at risk of iron overload. A high red cell distribution width (anisocytosis on blood film) distinguishes true iron-deficiency anaemia.

Treatment. The mainstay of treatment is regular blood transfusion, aiming to maintain the Hb concentration above 10 g/dL. Unfortunately, chronic transfusion therapy is complicated by accumulation of iron in parenchymal organs including the heart, liver, pancreas, gonads and skin. Iron-associated cardiomyopathy is a major cause of mortality in the second and third decades. Iron chelation is therefore vital using either oral or subcutaneous agents but does not eradicate the problem completely.

Table 9.1 β-Thalassaemia genotypic profiles and haemoglobin electrophoresis

Type	Genotype	Haemoglobin (Hb) electrophoresis
Minor (heterozygous)	$β/β^0$ or $β/β^+$	Normal or high HbA_2
Intermediate (homozygous)	$β^+/β^+$	Normal or high foetal haemoglobin (HbF)
Major (homozygous)	$β^0/β^0$	Absent adult haemoglobin (HbA; only HbF and HbA_2)

Splenectomy is useful in selected patients, and bone marrow transplantation is potentially curative. Gene therapy (betibeglogene autotemcel), harvesting stem cells to which functional genes are added by a viral vector, has been approved in the United States by the medicines regulator; but the manufacturer has withdrawn operations in Europe, including the UK.

β-Thalassaemia trait. The only abnormality is a mild, hypochromic, microcytic anaemia. Most are asymptomatic. β-Thalassaemia trait can be misdiagnosed as iron-deficiency anaemia. The important diagnostic feature is the raised HbA_2 and about 50% have a mild elevation of HbF (1%–3%) on electrophoresis.

α-Thalassaemia

This is caused by absence or reduced synthesis of α-globin genes. Most result from gene deletions. The manifestations and severity depend on the number of genes deleted (Table 9.2).

Table 9.2 Clinical manifestations of α-thalassaemia variants

Variant	Number of genes deleted	Haemoglobin (Hb) pattern	Clinical features
α-Thalassaemia major	Four $--/--$	γ4 (Hb Bart)	Hydrops fetalis/death in utero
Haemoglobin H disease	Three $α-/--$	β4 (Hb H; beyond early infancy)	Severe anaemia persists through life
α-Thalassaemia minor	Two $αα/--$ or $α-/α-$	Normal	Mild anaemia
Silent carrier	One $αα/α-$	Normal	No anaemia Normal red blood cell indices

General principles of management include regular check-ups and full blood count monitoring. Folic acid supplements are required due to increased erythropoiesis. Genetic counselling is important in all haemoglobinopathies.

HAEMOLYTIC ANAEMIA

Haemolytic anaemia occurs when the lifespan of the RBC is shorter than the normal 120 days. Haemolytic anaemia can be caused by:

- intrinsic red cell defects
- membrane defects
- haemoglobinopathies
- red cell enzyme defects
- extrinsic defects (e.g., rhesus (Rh) or ABO incompatibility (see Chapter 15), microangiopathy and hypersplenism)
  It is characterized by:
- anaemia
- reticulocytosis
- increased erythropoiesis in the bone marrow
- unconjugated hyperbilirubinaemia

Hereditary spherocytosis

This is an autosomal dominant disorder caused by abnormalities in spectrin, a major supporting component of the RBC membrane. About 25% of cases are sporadic and are due to new mutations. As the name suggests, the red cell shape is spherical and the lifespan is reduced by early destruction in the spleen.

Clinical features

The clinical features are highly variable and include:

- mild anaemia: Hb 9 to 11 g/dL
- jaundice
- splenomegaly: mild to moderate

May be complicated by:

- Aplastic crises: triggered by parvovirus B19 infection.
- Gallstones: caused by increased bilirubin excretion.

Diagnosis

Spherocytes are seen on peripheral blood film. Diagnosis is confirmed by the osmotic fragility test (spherocytes already have maximum surface area-to-volume ratio and rupture more easily than biconcave red cells in hypotonic solutions). Other tests exist including gel electrophoresis to identify the protein defect or molecular genetic studies.

Management

Mild disease requires no treatment other than folic acid to meet the increased demands of the marrow.

Splenectomy is indicated for more severe disease, but should be deferred until school age because of the increased risk of overwhelming infection. The child should receive:

- *Haemophilus influenzae* type B (Hib), meningococcal and pneumococcal vaccines before splenectomy.
- Prophylactic penicillin for life afterwards.
- This is due to the risk of invasive infection from encapsulated bacteria such as *Streptococcus pneumoniae, H. influenzae* and *Neisseria meningitides.*

Sickle cell disease

This is a chronic condition characterized by sickling of RBCs, which results in haemolysis, anaemia and vaso-occlusion. It occurs in patients homozygous for a single base mutation in the β-globin gene where valine is substituted for glutamine, resulting in HbS production. In the deoxygenated state, HbS aggregates into long polymers that distort the red cells into a sickle shape.

The heterozygous state (sickle cell trait) confers some protection against falciparum malaria; this 'heterozygote advantage' explains the high incidence of the mutation in populations originating in malaria endemic areas such as tropical Africa, the Mediterranean, the Middle East and parts of India. Regardless of sickle cell status, everyone should be advised to take antimalarial precautions.

Clinical features

The synthesis of HbF during the first few months affords protection until the age of 4 to 6 months. Progressive anaemia with jaundice and splenomegaly then develops. Infants typically present with dactylitis (painful swelling of the digits) or severe infection. The subsequent course of the disease is punctuated by crises, of which 'vaso-occlusive' crises are by far the most common.

Vaso-occlusive crises

These episodes are due to the sickled RBCs becoming trapped in the microcirculation causing painful ischaemia. They are often precipitated by infection, hypoxia, dehydration, cold weather or vascular stasis. The clinical features depend on the tissue involved but episodes most commonly manifest as a 'painful' crisis, with pain in the long bones or spine. Priapism can also occur.

Table 9.3 Life-threatening crises in sickle cell disease

Type	Symptoms	Signs	Management principles
Acute chest crisis (pulmonary ischaemia)	Fever Chest pain Shortness of breath Cough	Tachypnoea Respiratory distress Hypoxia Wheeze Chest X-ray changes	• High-flow oxygen • Pain relief • Adequate hydration • Antibiotics • Top-up transfusion (aim for haemoglobln (Hb) 10 g/dL) • Exchange transfusion[a]
Stoke (cerebral ischaemia)	Headache Weakness Speech difficulties Visual disturbances Collapse Seizures	Dysarthria/aphasia Motor deficit Confusion Cerebellar signs Reduced Glasgow Coma Scale	• The airway, breathing, circulation approach including airway protection • High-flow oxygen • Pain relief • Adequate hydration • Top-up transfusion[b] • Exchange transfusion[a]
Girdle syndrome (bowel ischaemia)	Abdominal pain Vomiting Constipation	Tachycardia Tender, tense abdomen (peritonitis) Absent bowel sounds	• High-flow oxygen • Pain relief • Adequate hydration • Exchange transfusion[a] • Surgical review (may require resection of ischaemic bowel)
Acute splenic sequestration	Lethargy Abdominal distension	Pallor Splenomegaly Hypovolaemic shock	• High-flow oxygen • Pain relief • Fluid resuscitation • Top-up transfusion[a] • Splenectomy if recurrent

[a]*Aim for HbS less than 30%.*
[b]*Top-up transfusion: aim for patients' baseline Hb to avoid causing hyperviscosity.*

Less commonly but more serious vaso-occlusive crises include cerebral infarctions (stroke), pulmonary infarctions (acute chest crisis) or bowel ischaemia (Girdle syndrome). See Table 9.3 for clinical features and management.

Repeated vaso-occlusive episodes lead to infarction, fibrosis and scarring of the spleen. These patients are, therefore, at risk of overwhelming infection with encapsulated organisms such as *H. influenzae* and *S. pneumoniae* due to functional hyposplenism. There is also an increased risk of osteomyelitis due to *Salmonella* and other organisms. All forms of crises have a low threshold for antibiotics if febrile.

The long-term consequences of sickle cell disease include:

• myocardial damage and heart failure
• aseptic necrosis of long bones
• leg ulcers
• gallstones
• renal papillary necrosis
• retinopathy
• psychological implications of chronic disease

Management

Antenatal and neonatal screening is available and this allows initiation of antibiotic prophylaxis early in life. Sickle cell screening has been part of the Newborn Blood spot test since 1995. Prophylactic penicillin should be taken to prevent pneumococcal infection. Daily folic acid supplements help to meet the demands of increased red cell breakdown. It is important that all children are vaccinated against pneumococcus, meningococcus and *H. influenzae* B according to the routine vaccination schedule. They should also receive the seasonal influenza vaccine. Hydroxyurea reduces crises in several ways, including an increase in HbF and is useful for those experiencing frequent painful crises or severe anaemia.

HINTS AND TIPS

In sickle cell disease:

• Splenomegaly is present in early life, but splenic infarction subsequently reduces the spleen in size.
• A sudden increase in the size of the spleen suggests a sequestration crisis and parents are taught how to check for this at home.

The general treatment of a vaso-occlusive crisis includes:

- analgesia: opioids for severe pain
- oxygenation
- maintaining good hydration with intravenous fluids if necessary

Exchange transfusion, designed to reduce the proportion of sickle cells, is indicated for brain or lung infarction and priapism. Vaso-occlusive crises can result in loss of function of the limb or organ if not treated early. It is important to give adequate information to parents about its symptoms and advise them to seek medical advice early in such an event.

Serial transcranial Doppler ultrasound can identify those most at risk of stroke and allow commencement of transfusion programme or hydroxyurea treatment. Retinopathy is also a risk and regular ophthalmology review is recommended. Children should be reviewed annually by a paediatric haematologist who will coordinate their care.

Sickle cell trait

The heterozygote with sickle cell trait (HbAS) is asymptomatic unless subjected to hypoxic stress (e.g., general anaesthesia). Sickle cells are not seen on peripheral smear and diagnosis is by Hb electrophoresis. The trait is worth detecting to allow genetic counselling and precautions to be taken against hypoxaemia during flying and general anaesthesia.

Red cell enzyme deficiencies

These include G6PD deficiency and the much rarer pyruvate kinase deficiency.

G6PD deficiency

This is an X-linked recessive disorder with variable clinical severity. Over 400 million people are affected worldwide, particularly in the Mediterranean, Middle Eastern, Oriental and Afro-Caribbean populations. G6PD-deficient red cells do not generate enough glutathione to protect the cell from oxidant agents. Males are more severely affected but females can manifest the phenotype.

Clinical features

G6PD deficiency is characterized by episodes of acute rather than chronic haemolysis. It can manifest with:

- Neonatal jaundice.
- Haemolytic episode: induced by infection, oxidant drugs and fava beans. Fever, malaise, jaundice and the passage of dark urine (haemoglobinuria) may occur.

Management

The mainstay of management is educating patients to avoid precipitating factors. Examples of oxidant drugs include nonsteroidal antiinflammatories (NSAID), sulphonamides, antimalarials and nitrofurantoin. When haemolysis does occur, it is usually self-limiting and does not require transfusion. Neonatal jaundice requires monitoring and may need treatment with phototherapy or, if severe, exchange transfusion.

Pyruvate kinase deficiency

This is an autosomal recessive condition caused by deficiency of the enzyme pyruvate kinase. Infection (e.g., parvovirus) may precipitate severe haemolysis; however, due to a right shift on the oxygen dissociation curve, patients can tolerate very low Hb concentrations. Management includes folic acid, occasional blood transfusions and splenectomy in severe cases.

SPLENOMEGALY

In neonates and very thin children, the tip of the spleen is often palpable. The spleen can enlarge during acute infections and in various haematological diseases. Hepatosplenomegaly suggests a different aetiology from that associated with isolated splenomegaly (Figs. 9.1 and 9.2).

HINTS AND TIPS

The spleen in sickle cell disease:

- In infancy, there is splenomegaly.
- Recurrent infarction and 'autosplenectomy' cause the spleen to regress and become impalpable after 5 years.
- Splenic hypofunction renders patients susceptible to infections with encapsulated organisms.

History

- Systems review: this might elicit symptoms related to the many infective causes.
- Family history: inherited anaemias, storage disorders (e.g., Gaucher disease).

Examination

Note coexistent lymphadenopathy, hepatomegaly, pallor, fever or rash.

Investigations

- haematological: FBC, blood film, reticulocyte count
- infections: serology (e.g., Epstein-Barr virus), blood cultures, film for malaria parasites
- malignancy: bone marrow aspiration
- liver disease: liver function tests, hepatitis serology
- abdominal ultrasound scan

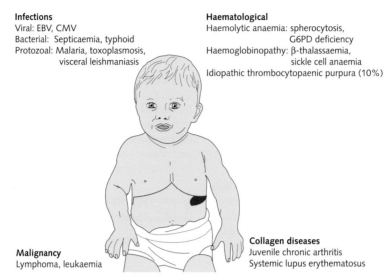

Infections
Viral: EBV, CMV
Bacterial: Septicaemia, typhoid
Protozoal: Malaria, toxoplasmosis,
　　　　　　visceral leishmaniasis

Haematological
Haemolytic anaemia: spherocytosis,
　　　　　　　　　　　G6PD deficiency
Haemoglobinopathy: β-thalassaemia,
　　　　　　　　　　　sickle cell anaemia
Idiopathic thrombocytopaenic purpura (10%)

Collagen diseases
Juvenile chronic arthritis
Systemic lupus erythematosus

Malignancy
Lymphoma, leukaemia

Fig. 9.1 Causes of splenomegaly. *CMV,* Cytomegalovirus; *EBV,* Epstein-Barr virus; *G6PD,* glucose-6-phosphate dehydrogenase.

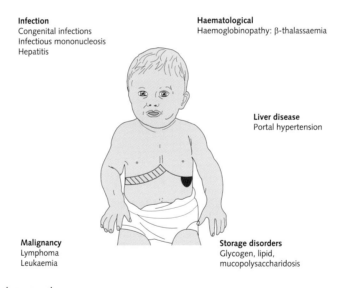

Infection
Congenital infections
Infectious mononucleosis
Hepatitis

Haematological
Haemoglobinopathy: β-thalassaemia

Liver disease
Portal hypertension

Malignancy
Lymphoma
Leukaemia

Storage disorders
Glycogen, lipid,
mucopolysaccharidosis

Fig. 9.2 Causes of hepatosplenomegaly.

BLEEDING DISORDERS

Normal haemostasis requires a complex interaction between three factors:

- blood vessels
- platelets
- coagulation factors

A bleeding diathesis can result from a deficiency or disorder of any of these elements. Clinical presentation of a generalized bleeding diathesis might include:

- Bleeding into the skin:
- Petechiae: small red spots <3 mm.
- Purpura: confluent petechiae up to 1 cm.
- Ecchymosis: large area of extravasated blood >1 cm (synonym for bruise).

- Haematoma: extravasated blood that has infiltrated subcutaneous tissue or muscle to cause a deformity.
- Haemarthrosis: bleeding into joints.
- Prolonged bleeding after dental extraction, surgery or trauma.

Test small lesions on the skin using a transparent glass to see if they blanch. Failure to blanch indicates extravasated blood.

> **RED FLAG**
>
> When assessing a child with bruising, it is important to know what is normal and what is abnormal. Mobile toddlers commonly have multiple bruises on bony prominences (e.g., forehead/nose, knees). Bruises in nonmobile infants, over soft areas of the body or in hidden areas of the body, suggest possible nonaccidental injury.

Disorders of blood vessels

Injury to blood vessels provokes two responses that limit bleeding:

- vasoconstriction
- activation of platelets and coagulation factors by subendothelial collagen

Rare inherited disorders include Ehlers-Danlos syndrome associated with excessive capillary fragility and hereditary haemorrhagic telangiectasia.

Acquired disorders include vitamin C deficiency (scurvy) and Henoch-Schönlein purpura.

Henoch-Schönlein purpura

Henoch-Schönlein purpura (HSP) is the commonest vasculitis in children. It is a multisystem vasculitis involving the small blood vessels. It typically follows an upper respiratory tract infection or exposure to a drug or allergen, and is immune-mediated with IgA suspected to play a major role.

It is more common in boys and 75% of affected children are under 10 years.

Clinical features

The condition affects skin, joints, gastrointestinal tract and kidneys (see Table 9.4).

Diagnosis and management

Diagnosis is clinical. Normal platelet count and coagulation studies exclude other causes of purpura.

HSP is usually self-limiting and prognosis is excellent. Treatment is supportive with rest and pain relief. Steroids are of benefit in severe gastrointestinal disease and renal involvement.

Table 9.4 Clinical features of Henoch-Schönlein Purpura

Body system	Clinical feature
Skin	Purpuric rash (typically legs and buttocks)
Gastrointestinal (GI) tract	Diffuse abdominal pain GI bleeding Intussusception
Joints	Arthralgia Swelling of large joints (e.g., knees and ankles)
Kidneys	Glomerulonephritis (hypertension, microscopic haematuria and/or proteinuria)

BOX 9.5 CAUSES OF THROMBOCYTOPAENIA

Decreased production
Bone marrow failure
- Aplastic anaemia
- Leukaemia

Wiskott-Aldrich syndrome
Thrombocytopaenia with absent radii (TAR) syndrome

Reduced survival
Immune-mediated thrombocytopaenia
- Idiopathic thrombocytopaenic purpura (most common)
- Secondary to viral infection, drugs

Hypersplenism
Kasabach-Merritt syndrome
Disseminated intravascular coagulation

Most children recover within 4 to 6 weeks, although, rarely, chronic renal disease can develop and follow-up monitoring for hypertension and proteinuria should be arranged.

Disorders of platelets

These might be quantitative or qualitative, with the former (thrombocytopaenia) being most common.

Thrombocytopaenia

A decreased number of platelets (from the normal count of 150–450×10^9/L) is the most common cause of abnormal bleeding. Purpura usually occurs when the count is below 20×10^9/L. The cause might be decreased platelet production or reduced platelet survival (Box 9.5).

Idiopathic thrombocytopaenic purpura

Idiopathic thrombocytopaenic purpura (ITP) is the most common cause of thrombocytopaenia in childhood and refers to an immune-mediated thrombocytopaenia for which an exogenous cause is not apparent. The platelets are destroyed within the reticuloendothelial system, mainly in the spleen.

Clinical features

There may be a history of recent viral illness. ITP mainly affects children between 2 and 10 years of age. Presentation is with purpura and minor bleeding, for example, from mucosal surfaces (e.g., epistaxis). The spleen is palpable in a minority of cases.

Diagnosis

The differential diagnosis includes:

- acute leukaemia
- nonaccidental injury
- Henoch-Schönlein purpura

An FBC reveals thrombocytopaenia but no pancytopaenia. Bone marrow aspiration is unnecessary in typical ITP, but should be performed where there is doubt over the diagnosis or in those who develop chronic disease. An increase in megakaryocytes (platelet precursors) is characteristic.

Treatment

In most children, the disease is acute, benign and self-limiting, and no therapy is required. However, chronic thrombocytopaenia can occur in up to 20% of cases. Serious bleeding is extremely rare and platelet levels as low as $<10 \times 10^9$ are tolerated as the platelets function more efficiently. Platelet infusions are rapidly destroyed and are only useful in life-threatening emergencies. Advice regarding lifestyle (e.g., avoid contact sports) should be given.

Pharmacological intervention remains widely debated. Both immunoglobulin infusions and corticosteroids cause a rise in the platelet count; however, this has not been shown to change the risk of serious or intracranial bleeding. Current recommendations suggest treatment in:

- life-threatening bleeding
- increased risk of bleeding (e.g., haemophilia)
- prior to invasive procedures

Teenage girls have a higher risk of chronic disease (>1 year), treatment is primarily with thrombopoietin receptor agonists (eltrombopag, or romiplostim) splenectomy is very rarely indicated in childhood ITP.

COAGULATION DISORDERS

An understanding of the clotting cascade (Fig. 9.3) and how to interpret clotting studies (discussed in Chapter 2) are helpful in understanding the following conditions.

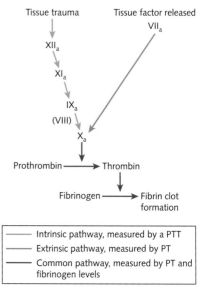

Fig. 9.3 Clotting cascade and coagulation studies. *PT,* Prothrombin time; *PTT,* partial thromboplastin time.

Haemophilia A and B and von Willebrand disease account for the majority of inherited coagulation disorders.

Haemophilia A (factor VIII deficiency)

This is an X-linked recessive disorder due to reduced or absent factor VIII. The incidence is 1 in 5000 to 10,000 males. It is the result of a new mutation in one-third of cases. The factor VIII molecule is a complex of two proteins:

- VIII:C – small molecular weight protein, antihaemophilic factor
- VIII:R – large molecular weight protein, von Willebrand factor

Clinical features

Haemophilia A results from deficiency of VIII:C. Clinical severity varies greatly and depends on factor VIII levels (Table 9.5). The characteristic clinical feature is spontaneous or traumatic bleeding, which can be:

- subcutaneous
- intramuscular
- intraarticular

Mild haemophilia might remain undetected until excessive bleeding occurs (e.g., after dental extraction). Even severely affected boys often have few problems in the first year of life (unless circumcision is performed), but early bruising and

Table 9.5 Factor VIII levels in haemophilia A

Severity	Factor VIII levels	Typical presentation
Mild	5%–25% of normal	Bleeding following surgery or major trauma
Moderate	1%–4% of normal	Bleeding following minor injury, minor spontaneous bleeds
Severe	<1% detectable activity	Spontaneous bleeding or following trivial injury

abnormal bleeding are noted from the time they begin to walk and fall over.

In later life, recurrent soft tissue, muscle and joint bleeding are the main problems. Haemarthrosis cause pain and swelling of the affected joint(s) and repeated haemorrhage might result in chronic joint disease. Life-threatening internal haemorrhage (e.g., intracranial) can follow trauma.

Diagnosis

Diagnostic evaluation reveals a prolonged activated partial thromboplastin time (APTT) with normal prothrombin time (PT). Factor VIII assay confirms the diagnosis.

HINTS AND TIPS

Bleeding into skin and mucous membranes: platelet or vascular disorder.
Bleeding into muscle or joints: coagulation disorder.

Genetic testing is useful for other family members and prenatal diagnosis is possible.

Management

Bleeding is treated by replacement of the missing clotting factor with intravenous infusion of factor VIII concentrate. The amount required depends on the site and severity of the bleed. Prompt and adequate therapy is important to avoid chronic arthropathy; home therapy can avoid delay and minimize inconvenience.

Recombinant DNA technology is now used to produce factor VIII that is safer than the blood products previously used. Antibodies to factor VIII can develop.

Mild haemophilia can be managed with infusion of desmopressin that releases factor VIII from tissue stores.

Haemophilia B (factor IX deficiency, Christmas disease)

This is an X-linked recessive disorder caused by deficiency of factor IX. It is clinically similar to haemophilia A, but much less common. Investigation reveals a prolonged APTT and reduced factor IX activity (although presentation is heterogeneous with very variable factor IX levels). Treatment is with prothrombin complex concentrate.

von Willebrand disease

This is due to a deficiency of von Willebrand factor (VIII:R), which has two major roles:

- Acts as carrier protein for factor VIII:C (preventing it from breakdown).
- Facilitates platelet adhesion.

Around 1% of the population is known to be affected. Inheritance is usually autosomal dominant with variable penetrance. The clinical hallmark is bleeding into the skin and mucous membranes (gums and nose).

Disseminated intravascular coagulation

Intravascular activation of the coagulation cascade may be secondary to various disease processes:

- damage to vascular endothelium: sepsis, renal disease
- thromboplastic substances in the circulation (e.g., in acute leukaemia)
- impaired clearance of activated clotting factors (e.g., in liver disease)

In disseminated intravascular coagulation (DIC) there is fibrin deposition in small blood vessels with tissue ischaemia, consumption of labile clotting factors and activation of the fibrinolytic system.

Clinical features

Clinical features are:

- a diffuse bleeding diathesis, with oozing from venepuncture sites
- pulmonary haemorrhage
- gastrointestinal haemorrhage

Diagnosis and management

Investigations reveal:

- prolonged PT, APTT and thrombin time
- thrombocytopaenia and microangiopathic red cell morphology
- hypofibrinogenaemia
- elevated fibrinogen degradation products

Management is supportive with treatment of the underlying cause and replacement of platelets and clotting factors (with fresh frozen plasma).

RED FLAG

A petechial or purpuric rash in a febrile child should always be treated as meningococcal sepsis until proven otherwise.

THROMBOTIC DISORDERS IN CHILDHOOD

Recognition of thrombotic disorders in children is increasing. Although thrombosis is usually rare in children, certain genetic conditions predispose to it:

- Factor V Leiden: caused by an abnormal factor V protein that is resistant to activated protein C.
- Protein C deficiency: protein C inactivates the activated forms of factor V and VIII and stimulates fibrinolysis.
- Protein S deficiency: protein S is a cofactor to protein C.
- Antithrombin III deficiency.

In addition to genetic predispositions, some conditions are associated with prothrombotic states such as nephrotic syndrome and malignancy. Low-molecular-weight heparin is commonly used in children; however, specific therapies like protein C replacement are available.

Chapter Summary

- Acute leukaemia accounts for over a third of malignancy in children and prognostic indicators exist which determine risk stratification and chemotherapy treatment regime.
- Anaemia is classified by both colour intensity of red blood cells (RBCs; normochromic/hypochromic) and size of RBCs (microcytic/normocytic/macrocytic).
- Iron deficiency is the commonest cause of anaemia in children. It is microcytic and hypochromic and is managed by either dietary advice or iron supplementation.
- Thalassemia and sickle cell disease are examples of haemoglobinopathies that cause haemolytic anaemia and are chronic conditions that require a multidisciplinary team approach.
- Bleeding disorders occur due to abnormal blood vessels, deficient clotting factors or thrombocytopaenia. They can usually be distinguished by the bleeding pattern, which may range from petechiae to recurrent haemarthrosis.

UKMLA Conditions
Anaemia
Henoch- Schonlein purpura
Hyposplenism/splenectomy
Leukaemia
Lymphoma
Pancytopenia
Sickle cell disease

UKMLA Presentations
Bruising
Pallor

Despite the achievements of public health measures and immunization programmes, infectious disease remains a major cause of mortality and morbidity in childhood. Worldwide, millions of children die from preventable infections such as gastroenteritis, pneumonia, measles and malaria per year. Diseases such as measles have had a resurgence in the UK following adverse media reports on the safety of immunization.

FEVER

Fever is a common presenting symptom in children and can be a major challenge to healthcare professionals. Fever is defined as a central temperature greater than 38°C. Electronic tympanic membrane thermometers correlate moderately well with rectal temperature and are adequate for most practical purposes. Most fevers are due to benign, self-limiting viral infections but skill is needed to distinguish these from potentially serious bacterial infections. The latter have the potential to deteriorate rapidly so it is essential to identify and treat them as early as possible.

History

- Duration of fever – prolonged fever ≥5 days will require further investigations.
- Are there any localizing symptoms? (Fig. 10.1)
- Any unwell contacts or foreign travel?

> **HINTS AND TIPS**
>
> Vomiting in children is not a specific sign for gastritis/gastroenteritis – it can be a sign of any infection including urinary tract infection and central nervous system infection.

> **COMMON PITFALLS**
>
> Younger children (<2 years of age) might not localize symptoms and therefore fever might be the only presentation of serious infection.

Examination

- Is the child systemically unwell? An active, playing and communicative child is unlikely to have sepsis. However, any febrile child should be examined to look for a source.
- Look for localizing signs (Fig. 10.1) – tonsillitis, otitis media, pneumonia, meningitis and septic arthritis may all be revealed on examination.
- Assess for signs of serious sepsis.
- A set of observations is an important part of your observation (Table 10.1). Tachycardia is an important clinical sign (>160 bpm in <1 year, >150 bpm in 1–2 years, >140 in 2–5 years).

> **HINTS AND TIPS**
>
> Assume sepsis in all febrile infants aged <3 months until proven otherwise.

> **RED FLAG**
>
> For serious bacterial sepsis
> - Children <3 months
> - Bulging fontanelle
> - White cell count >20 × 10⁹/L or <4 × 10⁹/L, or high C-reactive protein >100 mg/L
> - Shock
> - Decreased consciousness or lethargy
> - Irritability
> - Persistent tachycardia (tachycardia in the absence of fever)
> - Cold extremities
> - Poor capillary refill time
> - Apnoea
> - Nonblanching rash (particularly spreading petechiae or purpura)

Investigations

In a well child in whom a confident clinical diagnosis of a viral infection has been possible, no investigation is required. In

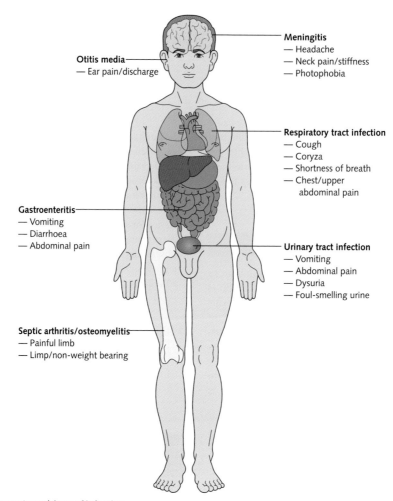

Meningitis
— Headache
— Neck pain/stiffness
— Photophobia

Otitis media
— Ear pain/discharge

Respiratory tract infection
— Cough
— Coryza
— Shortness of breath
— Chest/upper
abdominal pain

Gastroenteritis
— Vomiting
— Diarrhoea
— Abdominal pain

Urinary tract infection
— Vomiting
— Abdominal pain
— Dysuria
— Foul-smelling urine

Septic arthritis/osteomyelitis
— Painful limb
— Limp/non-weight bearing

Fig. 10.1 Localizing symptoms/signs of infection.

children <3 months or in older children with a fever who are clinically unwell without clear localizing signs, a septic screen should be performed:

- a full blood count
- C-reactive protein (CRP)
- blood culture
- urine dipstick + culture
- chest X-ray (if respiratory signs)
- stool culture (if diarrhoea)

A throat swab may be helpful. A lumbar puncture should be performed if there is a fever in a child under 1 month, a child aged 1 to 3 months who looks unwell or has a white cell count $<5 \times 10^9$/L or $>15 \times 10^9$/L.

COMMON PITFALLS

While a raised white cell count and C-reactive protein are useful if there is uncertainty in diagnosis or for serial measurement of a septic child, normal values cannot rule out serious infection.

Management

If a benign viral infection is suspected, then only symptomatic therapy is needed. In the very young, or those who are very unwell, broad-spectrum intravenous (IV) antibiotics are started before the

Table 10.1 Traffic light system for identifying risk of serious illness in under 5s

	Green – low risk	Amber – intermediate risk	Red – high risk
Colour (of skin, lips or tongue)	• Normal colour	• Pallor reported by parent/carer	• Pale/mottled/ashen/blue
Activity	• Responds normally to social cues • Content/smiles • Stays awake or awakens quickly • Strong normal cry/not crying	• Not responding normally to social cues • No smile • Wakes only with prolonged stimulation • Decreased activity	• No response to social cues • Appears ill to a healthcare professional • Does not wake or if roused does not stay awake • Weak, high-pitched or continuous cry

Respiratory		• Nasal flaring
		• Tachypnoea:
		  - RR >50 breaths/minute, age 6–12 months
		  - RR >40 breaths/minute, age >12 months
		• Oxygen saturation ≤95% in air
		• Crackles in the chest
			• Grunting
			• Tachypnoea: RR >60 breaths/minute
			• Moderate or severe chest indrawing

Circulation and hydration	• Normal skin and eyes
	• Moist mucous membranes
		• Tachycardia:
		  - >160 beats/minute, age <12 months
		  - >150 beats/minute, age 12–24 months
		  - >140 beats/minute, age 2–5 years
		• CRT ≥3 seconds
		• Dry mucous membranes
		• Poor feeding in infants
		• Reduced urine output
			• Reduced skin turgor

Other	• None of the amber or red symptoms or signs	• Age 3–6 months, temperature ≥39°C • Fever for ≥5 days • Rigors • Swelling of a limb or joint • Non-weight bearing limb/not using an extremity	• Age <3 months, temperature ≥38°C* • Non-blanching rash • Bulging fontanelle • Neck stiffness • Status epilepticus • Focal neurological signs • Focal seizures

CRT, capillary refill time; RR, respiratory rate
*Some vaccinations have been found to induce fever in children aged under 3 months.
This traffic light table should be used in conjunction with the recommendations in the NICE guideline on fever in under 5s.

results of diagnostic testing are available because quickly ruling out serious infection is often impossible; treatment can be tailored when the results are back. Antipyretics can be used as needed.

The child with fever and a petechial rash

The most important differential diagnosis in this common scenario is serious sepsis, especially meningococcal disease which requires immediate treatment. The majority of children presenting with fever and petechiae do not have serious sepsis; however, National Institute for Health and Care Excellence (NICE) advises performing blood tests including a blood culture and treating with IV ceftriaxone or cefotaxime if there is a raised CRP or white cell count.

HINTS AND TIPS

Nonblanching or rapidly spreading rash should be treated as meningococcal sepsis until proven otherwise.

Meningococcal sepsis

Principles of management are:

The sepsis six:

1) measure serum lactate
2) measure urine output
3) take blood cultures
4) give high-flow oxygen
5) give IV fluid resuscitation
6) give IV third-generation cephalosporin, ceftriaxone 80 mg/kg or cefotaxime 50 mg/kg

Other investigations: full blood count, CRP, coagulation screen, meningococcal polymerase chain reaction (PCR), blood gas, glucose, renal function, liver function and throat swab. A lumbar puncture should be performed for suspected meningitis or meningococcal disease unless there are signs of raised intracranial pressure, extensive purpuric rash, clotting abnormalities, shock or seizures.

Pyrexia of unknown origin

The designation pyrexia of unknown origin should be reserved for a child with a documented protracted fever (>7 days) and no diagnosis despite initial investigation. It is frequently misapplied to any child presenting with a fever of which the cause is not immediately obvious. Most are infectious and 40% to 60% will resolve without diagnosis. Particular patterns of fever and response to treatment can be helpful in making important diagnosis (e.g., Kawasaki disease, juvenile idiopathic arthritis; Table 10.2).

Table 10.2 Causes of pyrexia of unknown origin

Infection	Pyelonephritis
	Osteomyelitis
	Abscess
	Endocarditis
	Tuberculosis
	Typhoid
	Cytomegalovirus
	Human immunodeficiency virus
	Hepatitis
	Malaria
Inflammation	Kawasaki disease
	PIMS-TS
	Rheumatoid arthritis
	Inflammatory bowel disease
Malignancy	Leukaemia
	Lymphoma
Factitious	By parent or child/young person

Kawasaki disease

Kawasaki disease is an uncommon systemic vasculitis affecting the small and medium vessels which can include the coronary arteries leading to aneurysm formation.

Incidence

Kawasaki disease typically affects children between the age of 6 months and 4 years (peak at 1 year). It is much more common in children of Asian origin. In the UK the incidence is 8 cases per 100,000.

Clinical features

The clinical criteria for diagnosis are a fever for 5 days or more, with four of the following features:

- bilateral nonpurulent conjunctivitis
- polymorphous maculopapular rash
- oral changes: red, cracked lips or a strawberry tongue
- changes to the extremities: reddening or oedema of the hands and feet, or peeling of the skin (classically a late sign)
- cervical lymph nodes >1.5 cm

The signs may emerge sequentially and not be present all at once. Characteristically, the child is extremely miserable. Coronary aneurysms will occur in 30% of untreated cases and typically develop within the first 4 to 6 weeks of the illness.

> **RED FLAG**
>
> In any child with a fever of ≥5 days, consider Kawasaki disease. Early recognition and treatment are vital to reduce the risk of potentially life-threatening cardiac complications. Kawasaki disease has replaced rheumatic fever as the most common cause of acquired heart disease in children.

Investigations

The differential diagnosis includes measles, scarlet fever, rubella, roseola and fifth disease. The following investigations are undertaken if Kawasaki is suspected:

- Full blood count – thrombocytosis is common but often a late feature.
- CRP and erythrocyte sedimentation rate – raised.
- Urea and electrolytes and liver function tests – bilirubin and AST may be raised.
- Throat swab and antistreptolysin O titre – scarlet fever is an important differential.
- Blood cultures and viral titres.
- Echocardiography – the most important investigation which must be done to look for coronary aneurysms.
- Electrocardiogram (ECG).

Management

The most effective treatment involves a single dose of IV immunoglobulin (IVIG; 2 g/kg). This reduces both the incidence and severity of coronary artery aneurysm formation if given within the first 10 days. Aspirin is given concurrently to reduce the risk of thrombosis at a high dose initially (7.5–12.5mg/kg 4 times/day) for 2 weeks or until afebrile, followed by a lower dose (5 mg/kg once daily) continued for 6 to 8 weeks; if there is no evidence of coronary aneurysms, it is discontinued.

> **COMMUNICATION**
>
> Immunoglobulin is a blood product and parents should be informed of the potential benefits (reduction in chance of aneurysm formation) and adverse effects (which can include anaphylaxis and infection).

VIRAL INFECTIONS

Viral exanthems

The term 'exanthem' is applied to diseases in which a rash is a prominent manifestation. Classically, six exanthems with similar rashes were described. They are numbered in the order in which they were described (Table 10.3). Note that the second exanthem, scarlet fever, is an actual consequence of bacterial infection (see later in this chapter), and fourth disease is no longer recognized as an entity.

Table 10.3 Viral exanthems

Exanthem	Disease	Causative agent
First	Measles	Paramyxovirus
Second	Scarlet fever	Group A β-haemolytic streptococcus (*Streptococcus pyogenes*)
Third	Rubella	Togavirus
Fourth (historical – not used in clinical practice)	–	–
Fifth	Erythema infectiosum	Parvovirus B19
Sixth	Roseola infantum	Human herpes virus 6 and 7

Measles

Measles is caused by a highly infectious single-stranded RNA paramyxovirus virus which spreads by droplets with an incubation of about 10 days. Patients remain infectious until about 5 days after the rash disappears. After the introduction of the vaccination, rates fell considerably; however, outbreaks have been seen as a consequence of reduced uptake rates – secondary to public concerns about the safety of the measles, mumps and rubella (MMR) vaccine.

> **COMMUNICATION**
>
> In February 1998, a paper authored by Dr Andrew Wakefield was published in *The Lancet* claiming links between measles, mumps and rubella (MMR) and autism. Further publications by Dr Wakefield ensued, criticizing the MMR vaccine, and as a result there was an unprecedented collapse in public confidence. In January 2010, Dr Wakefield was found guilty of three dozen charges and removed from the medical register. *The Lancet* also fully retracted the paper. Parents must therefore be strongly reassured that there is no link between the MMR vaccine and autism, and reminded of the benefits of vaccination.

Clinical features

There is several-day prodrome with fever, a dry cough, coryza and lymphadenopathy. In this stage, conjunctivitis and pathognomonic white Koplik spots on the buccal mucosa (see Fig. 10.2) may be seen. This is followed after 3 to 5 days by an erythematous maculopapular rash which starts on the face and spreads down the body, becoming confluent. The rash tends to desquamate during the second week of illness.

Complications

Complications include otitis media, pneumonia, diarrhoea and convulsions. Rarer complications include encephalitis (1–4/1000–2000 measles cases) and subacute sclerosing pan encephalitis (SSPE). The mortality varies with age; high in children under one, lower in children aged 1 to 9 years and again higher in teenagers and adults. SSPE is a very rare (1/25,000 measles cases) immune-mediated neurodegenerative disease that can occur 7 to 10 years after measles. Measles is particularly dangerous to immunocompromised children. Worldwide, malnutrition and vitamin A deficiency are major contributors.

Management

Diagnosis can be made following a buccal swab analysis. Measles can also be confirmed by the detection of specific IgM in serum

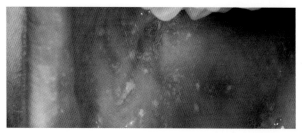

Fig. 10.2 Koplik spots on buccal mucosa as seen in measles. (Photo under license from TT Nyhetsbyrå, Stockholm.)

samples ideally taken from 3 days after the appearance of the rash. The disease is notifiable. Treatment is supportive only.

Rubella

This mild childhood disease is caused by infection with the rubella togavirus which has an incubation period of 2 to 3 weeks. Its importance lies in the devastating effect of maternal infection in early gestation on the developing foetus.

Clinical features

Infection is subclinical in up to half of infected individuals. In those who are symptomatic, a low-grade fever is followed by an erythematous maculopapular rash, which starts on the face and spreads rapidly over the entire body (see Fig. 10.3). The rash is fleeting and might have gone entirely by the third day. Generalized lymphadenopathy, particularly affecting the suboccipital and postauricular nodes, is a prominent feature.

Complications

Complications are unusual in childhood but include arthritis (typically affecting the small joints of the hand), purpura and very rarely encephalitis.

Management

Diagnosis is clinical and differentiation from other viral exanthems is often difficult. In circumstances in which it is important, detection of rubella-specific IgM in the saliva or serum is necessary to confirm the diagnosis. The live, attenuated rubella vaccine is given as the MMR – vaccine failure is rare.

Congenital rubella

The risk and extent of foetal damage are mainly determined by the gestational age at the onset of maternal infection. Maternal infection at up to 10 weeks' gestation confers a 90% risk of some degree of damage that is often severe and includes deafness,

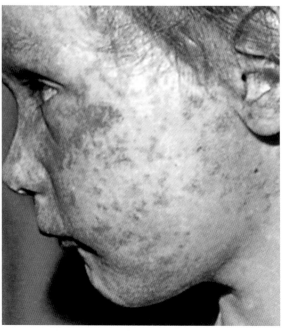

Fig 10.3 Facial exanthem as seen in rubella. (From Kliegman RM et al. *Nelson Textbook of Pediatrics*. 19th ed. Philadelphia, PA: Saunders; 2011.)

congenital heart disease and cataracts. Transmission rapidly declines after 13 weeks gestation, damage is typically limited to sensorineural hearing loss. After 16 weeks gestation damage is unlikely.

Clinical features of congenital rubella include:

- intrauterine growth restriction
- hepatosplenomegaly
- eye (glaucoma, cataract, retinopathy)
- congenital heart disease (pulmonary stenosis, patent ductus arteriosus)
- sensorineural hearing loss

Erythema infectiosum or slapped cheek disease (fifth disease)

This is caused by infection with parvovirus B19, a small DNA virus which is the only parvovirus pathogenic to humans. Transmission can occur via respiratory secretions, from mother to foetus, and by transmission of contaminated blood products.

Clinical features

Asymptomatic infection is common. Erythema infectiosum describes the most common disease pattern of fever followed

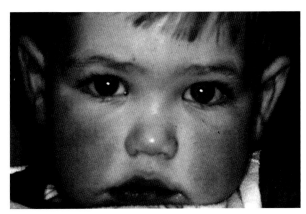

Fig 10.4 Slapped cheek appearance as seen in erythema infectiosum (parvovirus B19). (From Baren JM, Rothrock SG, Brennan J, et al. *Pediatric Emergency Medicine*. 1st ed. Philadelphia, PA: Saunders; 2007.)

a week later by a characteristic rash (see Fig. 10.4). This starts with malar erythema (hence the name 'slapped-cheek disease') and progresses to a symmetrical lacy rash on the limbs and trunk.

Complications

The virus suppresses erythropoiesis for up to 7 days. In children with haemolytic anaemia, such as sickle cell disease or hereditary spherocytosis, parvovirus infection can cause an aplastic crisis. Maternal infection during pregnancy can be transmitted to the foetus and causes hydrops fetalis (due to foetal anaemia and myocarditis), foetal death or spontaneous abortion.

Management

Diagnosis is clinical, but if confirmation is important (e.g., in pregnancy), specific IgM can be detected 2 weeks after exposure. Management is symptomatic.

Roseola infantum (sixth disease)

Roseola infantum is caused by infection with human herpesvirus (HHV)-6 or HHV-7. Most children acquire the infection between the age of 3 months and 4 years; population-based studies show that 40% are seropositive by 1 year of age, 77% by age 2.

Clinical features

There is sudden onset of a high fever (>39°C) with irritability lasting for about 3 to 5 days. The fever then falls abruptly and a widespread rose-pink maculopapular rash appears on the face, neck and trunk. Other common features include cervical lymphadenopathy, cough and coryza.

Complications

During the febrile period, febrile convulsions can occur. Up to one-third of febrile convulsions in children <2 years of age are caused by HHV-6. Rare complications include aseptic meningitis, encephalitis, hepatitis and massive lymphadenopathy.

Management

Diagnosis is clinical. Management is supportive, antipyretics for discomfort with fever and fluid rehydration.

Herpes infections

There are eight HHVs. They cause a number of common and important diseases in children. The hallmark of these viruses is their capacity to become latent with subsequent recurrence, causing, for example, shingles (varicella zoster) and cold sores [herpes simplex virus 1 (HSV-1)].

The HHVs and their corresponding diseases are shown in Table 10.4. Note, HHV-6/7 are discussed in the 'Viral exanthems' section.

Table 10.4 Human herpesviruses

Human herpesviruses (HHVs)	Virus	Disease
HHV-1	Herpes simplex virus 1	Oral infection, encephalitis
HHV-2	Herpes simplex virus 2	Genital infection, neonatal infection
HHV-3	Varicella zoster	Chickenpox Shingles
HHV-4	Epstein-Barr virus	Glandular fever
HHV-5	Cytomegalovirus	Congenital infection Infection in immunosuppression
HHV-6/7	HHV-6/7	Roseola infantum

Herpes simplex virus 1 (HSV-1; HHV-1)

Most primary infections with HSV-1 are asymptomatic. The most common clinical manifestation in childhood is gingivostomatitis. The child (usually a toddler) presents with high fever and vesicular lesions on the lips, gums, tongue and hard palate, which might progress to painful, extensive ulceration. The illness can last as long as 2 weeks.

Less commonly, infection can involve the:

- eye: causing dendritic ulcers on the cornea
- skin: causing eczema herpeticum-particularly severe in children with eczema
- fingers: causing a herpetic whitlow
- brain: causing herpes simplex encephalitis

Management

Occasionally, IV fluids will be required for gingivostomatitis, but in this condition oral aciclovir has only a marginal effect. High-dose IV aciclovir is used in herpes simplex encephalitis. The virus becomes latent in the dorsal root ganglion supplying the trigeminal nerve where subsequent reactivation (by UV light, stress or menstruation) can cause labial herpes (cold sores) in later life.

Herpes simplex virus 2 (HSV-2; HHV-2)

Transmission of herpes simplex virus 2 (HSV-2) from the genital tract of a mother who is often asymptomatic can result in neonatal herpes infection. Neonatal HSV-2 has high mortality and morbidity. It causes a generalized infection with pneumonia, hepatitis and encephalitis, with onset usually in the first week of life. Treatment is high-dose IV aciclovir and supportive care. Elective caesarean section is indicated when a mother with active genital herpes goes into labour as this mode of delivery offers neonatal protection.

Varicella zoster virus (VZV; HHV-3)

Chickenpox is a common childhood disease caused by primary infection with the varicella zoster virus. It is highly infectious with transmission occurring by droplet infection, direct contact or contact with soiled materials. The average incubation period is 2 weeks. The period of infectivity is from 2 days before eruption of the rash until all the lesions have crusted over.

Clinical features

A brief coryzal period is followed by the eruption of an itchy rash which progresses from macules to papules to vesicles before crusting over. This starts on the scalp or trunk and spreads centrifugally; mucous membranes may be involved. Typically, new crops develop over 3 to 5 days.

Complications

Complications are unusual in immunocompetent children but can include secondary bacterial infection of the skin with staphylococci or streptococci and encephalitis (often affecting the cerebellum), which appears 3 to 6 days after onset of the rash. Chickenpox can, however, be more serious in adults, particularly pregnant women and those who smoke. In children, severe disease can occur in the immunosuppressed child and in the newborn infant if the mother develops chickenpox just before delivery; before antiviral treatments were introduced, fatality rates were high (7% and 30%, respectively). Persisting fever after the typical chickenpox rash has erupted should prompt evaluation for secondary infection.

Management

Diagnosis is clinical but virus isolated from vesicular fluid can be identified by electron microscopy or culture. Treatment is generally symptomatic; however, aciclovir can be given for severe chickenpox or clinical infection in an infant or immunosuppressed child. Varicella zoster immune globulin (VZIG) provides passive immunity and should be given to an immunosuppressed child exposed to the virus or to newborn babies if the mother develops chickenpox or shingles in the 7 days before or after birth – its release is authorized by a consultant virologist. A live, attenuated vaccine does exist but is not currently given routinely in the UK – reserved either for nonimmune healthcare workers, or healthy, nonimmune contacts of immunosuppressed patients (where close contact is unavoidable; siblings of a child being treated for leukaemia, or a child of a parent being treated with chemotherapy).

Congenital varicella

Maternal chickenpox during the 20 weeks of pregnancy (particularly 13–20 weeks), can result in congenital varicella syndrome in 2% of those infected. This can cause pigmented skin scarring, cortical atrophy and microcephaly, as well as limb hypoplasia. Infected mothers should be treated with aciclovir.

Herpes zoster (shingles)

This is due to reactivation of latent varicella zoster and is uncommon in childhood. A vesicular eruption occurs in the distribution of a sensory dermatome, mainly in the cervical and sacral regions. In adults they tend to be thoracic and lumbar. In addition, unlike adults, postherpetic neuralgia and malignant association are rare. Treatment with antivirals is not routinely indicated.

Epstein-Barr virus (EBV; HHV-4)

The Epstein-Barr virus (EBV) has a particular tropism for the epithelial cells of the oropharynx and nasopharynx, and for B lymphocytes. It is the major cause of infectious mononucleosis (glandular fever) and is also involved in the pathogenesis of Burkitt lymphoma and nasopharyngeal carcinoma. Transmission occurs by droplet transmission or directly via saliva (colloquially it is also known as 'kissing disease'). The incubation period is 4 to 5 weeks.

Clinical features

Most people are infected asymptomatically in childhood. Symptomatic infection (infectious mononucleosis or glandular fever) is most common in adolescents. Glandular fever is characterized by fever, malaise, pharyngitis (tonsils may be grossly enlarged with a membranous exudate) and cervical lymphadenopathy. Petechiae might be seen on the palate and a fine maculopapular rash might occur but rapidly disappears. There can also be transient bilateral upper eyelid oedema. Splenomegaly is present in 50% of cases and hepatomegaly with hepatitis (usually anicteric) in 10%. The infection can persist for up to 3 months.

Management

Diagnosis is usually clinical. The blood shows atypical lymphocytes (T cells) with a blue-rimmed cytoplasm, and in the majority, heterophile antibodies are formed which can be tested with agglutination tests such as the monospot and Paul-Bunnell tests. The latter appear only in the second week and might not be produced in young children. Specific EBV serology (IgM to viral capsid antigen) is more reliable. The differential diagnosis is from other causes of infectious mononucleosis [cytomegalovirus (CMV), toxoplasmosis] and other causes of pharyngitis. Management is symptomatic. Rarely, massive pharyngeal swelling can compromise the airway. This is helped by corticosteroid treatment.

COMMON PITFALLS

If amoxicillin is given to a patient with Epstein-Barr virus infection (e.g., if they are wrongly thought to have a streptococcal throat infection), they may develop a widespread maculopapular rash.

COMMUNICATION

A teenager with Epstein-Barr virus should be warned to avoid contact sports as there is a risk of splenic rupture with splenomegaly.

Cytomegalovirus (CMV; HHV-5)

In the UK, about half of all pregnant women are susceptible to CMV and about 1% of these will have a primary CMV infection during pregnancy. In almost half of these mothers, the infant will be infected, making CMV the most common congenital infection with an incidence of 3/1000 live births.

Severe congenital infection causes:

- Intrauterine growth restriction.
- Hepatosplenomegaly, jaundice and thrombocytopaenia.
- Microcephaly, intracranial calcification and chorioretinitis.
- Long-term sequelae include cerebral palsy, epilepsy, learning disability and sensorineural hearing loss. Hearing loss might develop later in life without signs of infection in the newborn period.

However, many infants with congenital CMV are asymptomatic and develop normally.

To confirm congenital infection, specimens for viral isolation must be taken within 3 weeks of birth. Newborns can be treated with ganciclovir.

Human papillomavirus

Human papillomavirus (HPV) infects the squamous epithelium (skin and mucosa). There are 100 types of HPV – 40 of which infect the genital tract. Genital HPV is transmitted by sexual contact, most infections are transient with no clinical consequence, but persistent infection with a high-risk HPV type (types 16 and 18 conferring the greatest risk) is the most important factor for developing cervical cancer. HPV infection is also associated with anal and oropharyngeal cancers. Studies show vaccination confers an 89% reduction in the risk of cervical cancer, or cancerous change (found on cervical screening). Vaccination is recommended from 11 years of age, but eligibility extends up to the age of 25 years for those who have missed out. In the UK, Gardasil 9 is the vaccine of choice. It protects against 9 HPV variants including 16 and 18 – the variants linked to most HPV-related cancers.

Other viruses

Mumps

Mumps is caused by infection with an RNA paramyxovirus. Routine MMR vaccination has markedly reduced the incidence. Transmission is by droplet spread and the incubation period is 2 to 3 weeks. Patients are infectious from 7 days before the onset of parotid swelling to up to 3 days after the enlargement subsides.

Clinical features

The clinical manifestations include fever, malaise and parotitis. Pain and swelling of the parotid gland might initially be unilateral. Parotid gland enlargement is more easily seen than felt, between the angle of the mandible and sternomastoid – extending beneath the ear lobe, which is pushed upwards and outwards. The swelling usually subsides within 7 to 10 days.

Complications

Complications include central nervous system (CNS) involvement: up to 50% of patients have cerebrospinal fluid lymphocytosis and 10% have signs of a meningoencephalitis. This usually resolves within a few days. Other complications include sensorineural hearing loss, epididymo-orchitis (usually in postpubertal boys), pancreatitis, hepatitis, arthritis and myocarditis. Infection in the first trimester of pregnancy can cause miscarriage.

Management

Diagnosis is usually clinical; treatment is symptomatic.

Enteroviruses

The human enteroviruses include:
- coxsackie virus A and B
- echoviruses
- poliovirus

Coxsackie viruses can cause aseptic meningitis, myocarditis, pericarditis, Bornholm disease (pleurodynia) and hand, foot and mouth disease.

Hand, foot and mouth disease

Hand, foot and mouth disease is a mild viral illness caused by coxsackie virus A16 or enterovirus 71. It causes mild fever, sore throat, cough and coryza with a vesicular rash on the palms, soles and mouth which heal without crusting. Very rare complications include myocarditis and encephalitis.

Polio

Poliovirus is an enterovirus with antigenic types 1, 2 and 3. Immunization has rendered poliovirus infection uncommon in countries with widespread uptake of the vaccination but it remains endemic in parts of Africa and India. Transmission is by the faecal–oral route with an incubation period of 7 to 21 days.

The clinical features vary:
- Over 90% of cases are asymptomatic.
- 5% have a 'minor illness' – fever, headache, malaise.
- 2% progress to CNS involvement – aseptic meningitis.

- In under 2%, 'paralytic polio' occurs due to the virus attacking the anterior horn cells of the spinal cord.

Viral hepatitis

Viral hepatitis can be caused by:
- hepatitis virus A, B, C, D, E or G
- generalized infections: CMV, EBV, Arbovirus (yellow fever)

Hepatitis A virus

This is an RNA virus spread by faecal–oral transmission. The incubation period is 2 to 6 weeks. It is the most common cause of viral hepatitis worldwide, particularly in Africa, South America and South-East Asia.

Clinical features

In infants and young children, many infections are asymptomatic or present as a nonspecific febrile illness without jaundice. Older children (and adults) are more likely to be symptomatic and develop fever, malaise, anorexia, abdominal pain (due to tender hepatomegaly), nausea/vomiting and diarrhoea. If a cholestatic jaundice occurs, it is usually a week after symptom onset; it may be preceded by dark urine (due to urobilinogen).

Investigations

Diagnosis is often made on the combination of clinical features and history of exposure, but might be confirmed by measurement of IgM anti-HAV antibody which remains elevated for up to 6 months after acute infection. Serum transaminases and bilirubin levels are elevated.

Treatment

There is no specific treatment. The majority of children have a mild, self-limiting illness and recover within 2 to 4 weeks. The most serious but rare complication is fulminant hepatic failure.

Active immunization is available and is mostly used for frequent travellers or those at high risk. Postexposure prophylaxis for those at high risk of severe disease (immunosuppression, chronic liver disease)is with intramuscular human normal immunoglobulin (HNIG). Prevention methods involve improved sanitation and hand hygiene.

Hepatitis B virus

This is a DNA virus of the *Hepadnavirus* genus. It is a double-shelled particle with an inner core antigen (HBcAg) and an outer lipoprotein coat comprising the hepatitis B surface antigen (HBsAg). Hepatitis e antigen (HBeAg) is the extracellular form of HBcAg, formed by self-cleavage and its presence is a marker of active viral replication. Transmission is parenteral via blood and other body fluids. In infants, the most important source of infection is vertical perinatal transmission from infected mothers. Most transmission occurs during or just after birth from exposure to maternal blood. In adolescents, sexual transmission is important to consider. The average incubation period is 20 days. Childhood hepatitis B is relatively rare in the UK, but it is endemic in many parts of the world including parts of Africa, South America, Asia and the Middle East.

Clinical features
In most children, the initial infection is asymptomatic, although features of acute hepatitis might occur. Like with hepatitis A, young children are much less likely to become jaundiced compared with older children and adults. Fulminant hepatic failure occurs in 1% of cases. The most important consequence of infection is the risk of becoming a carrier with subsequent development of cirrhosis or hepatocellular carcinoma. The risk of developing carrier status rises with infection at a young age (reaching 90% in those infected perinatally). Between 30% and 50% of carrier children will develop chronic hepatitis B virus (HBV) liver disease.

Investigations
Diagnosis is dependent on serological testing for antibodies and antigens related to HBV (Table 10.5). Acute HBV infection is associated with the presence of HBsAg and IgM antibodies to HBc antigen. Carrier status is defined as HBsAg persisting for more than 6 months. The presence of HBeAg correlates with high infectivity, whereas the presence of antibodies to HBeAg indicates low infectivity.

Management
Hepatitis B vaccination now forms part of the routine childhood immunization programme in the UK. It is also recommended:

- after perinatal exposure
- for individuals at risk (e.g., healthcare professionals)
- postexposure (e.g., needlestick injury)

The NICE guidelines suggest active treatment for chronic hepatitis B in children if significant fibrosis or persistently abnormal alanine aminotransferase is present. First-line treatment is a 6 to 12-month course of pegylated interferon α-2a, a significant undertaking with potential adverse effects.

Perinatal exposure
All pregnant women should have antenatal screening for the HBsAg. All babies born to women known to be HBsAg positive should commence a course of hepatitis B vaccine within 24 hours of birth (in addition to the standard immunization schedule). Unless the mother is known to be anti-HBe positive, the baby should also receive hepatitis B-specific Ig.

Non-A–E hepatitis
Acute non-A–E hepatitis are not as common as the above; hence early identification of the aetiology can take time. In children, there are numerous (uncommon and rare) causes of hepatitis and acute liver failure. Having an appreciation of the causes will help you choose what investigations are pertinent to perform.

- Infections – HSV, adenovirus, CMV, EBV and parvovirus, septic shock
- Autoimmune – autoimmune hepatitis, haemophagocytic lymphohistiocytosis (HLH)
- Drugs/toxins – paracetamol overdose, isoniazid, sodium valproate
- Vascular – Budd-Chiari syndrome
- Metabolic – galactosaemia, iron storage disorders, fatty acid oxidation disorder, Wilsons disease

Management, like investigations is directed at the cause, however, in cases of acute liver failure, it is wise to check and correct (if necessary) clotting derangement, and promptly treat for sepsis if clinical concerns are present for that.

Table 10.5 Serological markers of hepatitis B virus (HBV) infection

	Hepatitis B surface antigen (HBsAg)	Anti-HbS	Anti-HBc immunoglobulin M (IgM)	Anti-HBc IgG
Acute HBV infection	+	−	+	+
HBV carrier	+	−	+ or −	+
Immune – previous infection	−	+ or −	−	+
Immune – immunization	−	+	−	−

Coronavirus-induced severe acute respiratory syndrome (SARS); COVID-19

SARS-CoV-2, also called coronavirus disease 2019 (COVID-19), is aptly named due to first appearing in 2019 before spreading around the globe. Like most viruses, COVID-19 has several common and very contagious variants such as alpha, delta and omicron. Each of them has slightly different symptoms and signs. The virus, which is similar to Middle East respiratory virus (MERS) but less deadly, predominantly affects the respiratory system. It can be mild and may present with cold and flu-like symptoms or may progress to respiratory distress syndrome and respiratory failure requiring intubation. Transmission is via bioaerosol inhalation or direct self-inoculation with contaminated hands. As with adults, certain comorbidities made children more prone to having more severe infection, those being: genetic conditions, cardiac conditions, obesity, diabetes mellitus, being immunosuppressed, neurological conditions or metabolic conditions.

The clinical manifestation of COVID-19 varies but presented with one or more of these symptoms and signs: fever, respiratory symptoms (cough, shortness of breath), ENT symptoms (rhinorrhoea, sore throat), neurological (headache, loss of smell or taste), musculoskeletal (myalgia) and abdominal (nausea and vomiting, abdominal pain, diarrhoea). In children less than 12 months presentations of poor feeding, fever of unknown origin and apnoeas can be seen.

One of the further and later complications of having COVID-19 in children was the phenomenon of paediatric multisystem inflammatory syndrome temporally associated with COVID-19 (PIMS-TS or PIMS).

Another complication that has been observed is 'long COVID', which is characterized by persistence of symptoms (≥12 weeks) following COVID-19 infection. The symptoms are (but not limited to): weakness, fatigue, disturbed sleep, myalgia, loss of sense of smell/taste and respiratory issues.

Investigation of COVID-19 would be appropriate for children being admitted to hospital due to the severity of their disease. Point of care testing is used to isolate/cohort cases; investigations to consider (alongside confirming COVID-19 via antigen testing) would be renal and liver function, clotting profiles, bone profiles, D-dimer, inflammatory markers, troponin and pro-NT-BNP. Investigation of the respiratory distress can be monitored via blood gases. Chest X-rays can be performed to rule out any alternate pathologies, such as pneumothorax or secondary bacterial infection.

Management of COVID is largely supportive in nature and is dependent on the severity of the illness. Supportive measures range from – oxygen, and dexamethasone for those requiring a certain proportion of oxygen to biologics. Intravenous fluids versus nasogastric feeds should be considered dependent on the severity of the respiratory distress seen.

Table 10.6 Clinical and biochemical features of PIMS-TS

Clinical features	Biochemical features
Persistent Fever	Raised CRP/ESR, ferritin, fibrinogen
Single/multi-organ involvement/injury	Neutropaenia/ lymphopaenia
Respiratory – cough, sore throat, oxygen requirement, patchy infiltrates, pleural effusion	Recent or currently positive for SARS-CoV-2 by PCR, serology or antigen test
Abdominal – pain, diarrhoea +/- vomiting	Hypoalbuminaemia, renal dysfunction, hyponatraemia
Neurological – headache, lethargy, confusion, irritability	Raised D-dimer
Cardiovascular – hypotension/shock, coronary artery abnormalities, myocardial dysfunction	Elevated troponin/ pro-NT-BNP
Dermatological – rash, periorbital swelling/ erythema, swollen hands/ feet, conjunctivitis, mucus membrane changes	

https://www.osmosis.org/learn/Measles_virus

PIMS-TS

PIMS-TS has similarities in presentation to Kawasaki disease, sepsis and toxic shock syndrome. The diagnostic features of PIMS-TS (WHO definition) are seen in Table 10.6.

Prompt recognition of PIMS-TS is needed because it has a high rate of mortality.

PIMS-TS can be treated with a few different medications dependent on the clinical and biochemical features. These treatments would involve one of, or a combination of the following: Corticosteroids, intravenous immunoglobulins (IVIG), anticlotting medications (low-molecular-weight heparin and aspirin), proton pump inhibitors/histamine receptor antagonists (reduce development of gastritis or ulcers) or biologics (anakinra or tocilizumab – if IVIG and corticosteroids prove ineffective).

BACTERIAL INFECTIONS

Streptococcal infections

Streptococci are gram-positive cocci. They can be divided based on their pattern of haemolysis on a blood agar plate into alpha-haemolytic (incomplete haemolysis) and beta-haemolytic (complete haemolysis) streptococci.

Alpha-haemolytic streptococci

The viridans group of alpha-haemolytic streptococci are normal upper respiratory tract flora but are an important cause of dental caries and infective endocarditis. *Streptococcus pneumoniae* (pneumococcus) is an encapsulated bacterium which means it is a particular risk to patients who lack a spleen, for example, children with sickle cell disease. It is the most important cause of community-acquired pneumonia, and can also cause otitis media, meningitis and sepsis.

Beta-haemolytic streptococci

The beta-haemolytic streptococci are further into the Lancefield groups based on the carbohydrate antigens in their cell walls. The most important pathogens affecting paediatric patients are group A and group B. Group B streptococci are the main cause of neonatal sepsis and are covered in Chapter 15.

Group A beta-haemolytic *Streptococcus pyogenes* (GAS) is responsible for a number of common and important paediatric diseases, from noninvasive infections to life-threatening invasive disease (iGAS) that can be caused by:

- direct infection
- toxins
- postinfectious immune-mediated mechanisms (acute glomerulonephritis, rheumatic fever)

iGAS infections are notifiable, household contacts developing GAS symptoms or high-risk contacts (including neonates, recent chickenpox or influenza infection) should be treated with antibiotic prophylaxis.

Infections caused by streptococci are shown in Table 10.7. Most of these are described elsewhere: tonsillitis (see Chapter 4), pneumonia (Chapter 4), meningitis (Chapter 13), glomerulonephritis (Chapter 6) and rheumatic fever (Chapter 3).

Scarlet fever

This occurs in children who have streptococcal pharyngitis. The organism produces a toxin, which causes a characteristic rash.

The clinical features include:

- Tonsillitis.
- Fever.
- Strawberry tongue.
- Palatal petechiae.
- Rash: a widespread, erythematous rash starting on the trunk that becomes punctate and desquamates on resolution after 7 to 10 days (flushing of the face is often associated with circumoral pallor).

Diagnosis is clinical, but can be confirmed by isolation of the streptococcus from a throat swab, and by elevated antistreptolysin O titres. Treatment is with penicillin (or erythromycin/clarithromycin if the patient has penicillin allergy).

Table 10.7 Infections caused by streptococci

Organism	Disease caused
Group A streptococcus	Pharyngitis/tonsillitis Cellulitis Osteomyelitis Septicaemia Toxin mediated: • scarlet fever • erysipelas • toxic shock syndrome
Streptococcus pneumoniae	Otitis media Pneumonia Meningitis Septicaemia
Group B streptococcus	Neonatal infection (e.g., pneumonia, meningitis or septicaemia)

Erysipelas

This intradermal infection is caused by toxin-producing *S. pyogenes*. The face or leg is the usual area affected. The skin is dusky and vesicles or bullae might develop. Skin swabs and blood cultures might be negative; treatment is with parenteral antibiotics.

Staphylococcal infections

The coagulase-positive bacterium *Staphylococcus aureus* is the main pathogen but coagulase-negative bacteria (e.g., *Staphylococcus epidermidis*) are a major problem in intensive care units, and children with central lines (for cancer treatments or parenteral nutrition). Methicillin-resistant *S. aureus*, which lives harmlessly in the nose and skin of about one-third of people, can cause infection in vulnerable individuals.

S. epidermidis is part of the normal skin flora and *S. aureus* is found in the nares and skin in up to 50% of children. Infections occur when defences are compromised. Many infections are therefore caused by the body's own bacteria, but transmission between individuals occurs with close contact.

S. aureus most commonly causes superficial infections such as boils and impetigo, and occasionally deeper infections (e.g., of the bones, joints or lungs; Table 10.8) Toxin-producing *S. aureus* causes scalded skin syndrome and toxic shock syndrome.

Impetigo

This highly contagious skin infection commonly occurs on the face in infants and young children – especially if there is preexisting skin disease (e.g., eczema). Erythematous macules develop

Table 10.8 Infections caused by *Staphylococcus aureus*

Direct infection	Toxin mediated
Impetigo	Toxic shock syndrome
Folliculitis/boils	Scalded skin syndrome
Wound infections	Food poisoning
Abscess	
Pneumonia	
Osteomyelitis	
Septic arthritis	

into characteristic honey-coloured crusted lesions. Some cases are due to streptococcal infection. Topical antibiotics can be used for mild cases (e.g., mupirocin) but more severe infections require systemic antibiotics (e.g., flucloxacillin). Nasal carriage is an important source of reinfection and can be eradicated by nasal cream containing chlorhexidine and neomycin.

Boils and abscesses

A boil (or furuncle) is an infection of a hair follicle or sweat gland and is usually caused by *S. aureus*. A painful, red, raised, hot lesion develops and usually discharges a purulent exudate heralding spontaneous resolution. Treatment is with systemic antibiotics. Deeper infection can lead to abscess formation in which case incision and drainage are usually required.

Staphylococcal scalded skin syndrome

Staphylococcal scalded skin syndrome (SSSS) is a potentially life-threatening, toxin-mediated manifestation of localized skin infection. SSSS results from the effect of epidermolytic toxins produced by certain phage types. They cause blistering by disrupting the epidermal granular cell layer. The lesions look like scalds. Management requires attention to fluid balance and treatment with IV flucloxacillin.

Gram-negative infections

Typhoid and paratyphoid fever

Typhoid fever is caused by *Salmonella Typhi* and paratyphoid by *Salmonella Paratyphi*. Both occur worldwide, but mostly in the developing world and the main reservoir is humans; they are invasive, systemic infections. Salmonellosis occurs after infection with *Salmonella enteritidis* or *Salmonella typhimurium,* which usually causes gastroenteritis (food poisoning) and is more common in the UK than typhoid fever – animals constitute the main reservoir for these strains and nearly half the human infections are transmitted by poultry products. Salmonellae are gram-negative bacilli. Transmission of typhoid fever, by contrast, is by ingestion of food or water contaminated by faeces or urine from an infected person. The incubation period is 1 to 3 weeks.

Clinical features

The clinical presentation is similar in each case, but paratyphoid fever is milder. Typhoid (enteric) fever is characterized by slow onset of fever, malaise, headache and tachypnoea. Signs include splenomegaly, and a characteristic rash of 'rose spots' on the trunk. Unlike adults, children do not usually develop a relative bradycardia. Paratyphoid is a milder illness, but diarrhoea is more common.

Diagnosis

Diagnosis is made by culture of organisms from the blood (early in the disease) or from stool and urine (after the first week).

Management

If the child is systemically unwell, then a course of antibiotics is indicated for usually 14 days. *Salmonella* antibiotic resistance is a global concern that includes multidrug-resistant strains. Traditional first-line antibiotic medications include ampicillin, amoxicillin or cotrimoxazole. If resistance is suspected or proven, ceftriaxone, ciprofloxacin or azithromycin are used. Family and close contacts should be screened with stool cultures. Three consecutive negative stools signify clearance of infection. Long-term symptomless carriage can occur with a reservoir of infection in the gall bladder and excretion in the faeces.

Orbital and preseptal cellulitis

Preseptal and orbital cellulitis are presentations that are more commonly seen in children compared to adults.

Preseptal cellulitis (also known as periorbital cellulitis) is an infection that occurs anterior to the orbital septum. It is common in children, following sinusitis or localized infections, cuts/trauma. In children, compared to adults, this can progress to orbital cellulitis if not recognized and treated early.

Orbital cellulitis is an ophthalmic emergency that can cause impairment/loss of sight and if not treated, cause death. The causes of this can be linked to: untreated preseptal cellulitis, inoculation from trauma or surgery to the orbit, haematogenous spread from bacteria elsewhere.

The causative agents are mostly *Streptococcus* and *Staphylococcus* spp. but *Haemophilus influenzae* can be seen in children.

On presentation, these conditions can appear similar but there are discrete differences. Both preseptal and orbital cellulitis causes eyelid oedema, but orbital oedema can cause restriction of gaze, blurred/double vision, pain on eye movement, proptosis and may have an associated fever.

Investigations of preseptal and orbital cellulitis are aimed at finding the cause. In children it is prudent to order a CT of the sinuses and orbit to look for any collections or cavernous sinus thrombosis.

Management of children with presumed preseptal or orbital cellulitis would be admission to hospital for ophthalmology assessment and commencement of intravenous antibiotics. If orbital cellulitis is the main differential, then referral to ENT is prudent for joint management with ophthalmology.

Tuberculosis

Tuberculosis (TB) remains a major global health problem, particularly in patients with human immunodeficiency virus (HIV). New multidrug-resistant (MDR-TB) strains have emerged, causing increasing challenges to treatment.

The incidence of TB steadily declined last century until the 1980s when it increased until 2011, since when it has again been in decline. This pattern illustrates the change in disease epidemiology – from being endemic in the whole population, now shifting to specific high-risk groups; in the context of deteriorating TB control globally. TB was declared a global public health emergency in 1993 by the WHO. TB is more common in areas of socioeconomic deprivation, especially in urban areas as well as in those who are immunocompromised. It occurs in all racial groups, but high rates are seen in children whose families have come from endemic areas such as:

- The Indian subcontinent (India, Pakistan and Bangladesh).
- Sub-Saharan Africa.

Pathophysiology

TB is caused by infection with the acid-fast, slow-growing bacillus *Mycobacterium tuberculosis*. Children are usually infected by inhalation of infected droplet nuclei from an adult who is a regular or household contact. Children with the disease (even with active pulmonary disease) are almost always noninfectious. Therefore, once a child is identified as having TB, notification to public health is essential to identify the index case and contact trace.

Clinical features

The clinical features of TB reflect the wide variation in outcomes that follow inhalation of the tubercle bacillus or primary infection. Children under 4 years are at particularly high risk of disseminated disease (e.g., TB meningitis; Fig. 10.5).

Tuberculous infection: asymptomatic infection

This is most common. A local inflammatory reaction limits disease progression and the disease becomes latent. Reactivation can occur subsequently.

Tuberculous disease: symptomatic infection

Multiplication within macrophages occurs at the peripheral alveolar site (the primary or Ghon focus) and the bacilli spread to the regional lymph nodes causing hilar lymphadenopathy. The peripheral lung lesion and nodes comprise the 'primary or Ghon complex'. Systemic symptoms can then develop, including fever, anorexia, weight loss and cough.

The pulmonary pathology can evolve in several different ways. Bronchial obstruction by enlarged lymph nodes might cause segmental collapse and consolidation. Rarer outcomes include development of a pleural effusion or progressive primary pulmonary TB with cavity formation (in adolescents and adults). Spread into the lymphoid system can result in cervical, supraclavicular or axillary lymphadenopathy.

Haematogenous dissemination

In addition to the aforementioned intrathoracic events, haematogenous spread probably occurs in most children, although dormant lesions rather than disease occur in these distant sites. Tubercle bacilli might spread to the bones (especially the vertebral column), joints, kidneys and meninges. Miliary TB is the most severe result of haematogenous spread. It occurs particularly in small infants or immunosuppressed individuals – lesions are found throughout the lungs, liver, spleen and bone marrow.

Diagnosis

This can be difficult and requires a high index of clinical suspicion. A history of close contact to an adult with smear-positive TB, symptoms (weight loss, night sweats, cough), clinical signs, tuberculin testing, chest X-ray and examination of appropriate specimens by microscopy ('smear') and culture (induced sputum, early morning gastric aspirates or NPA) can diagnose the infection.

Tuberculin skin testing

The Mantoux test quantifies the skin reaction to an intradermal injection of tubercular purified protein derivative – in the UK the first dose is 2 units, normally made on the flexor aspect of the forearm. The site is read after 48 to 72 hours by measuring the transverse diameter of induration in millimetres. A 5-mm diameter reaction is considered positive, especially if risk factors are present. When previous bacille Calmette-Guérin (BCG) immunization has been carried out, a reaction of >10 mm is indicative of infection.

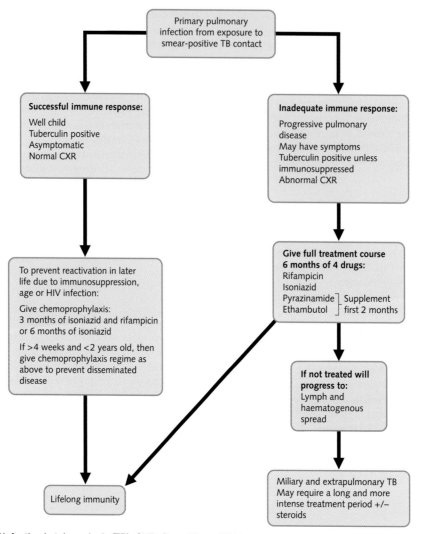

Fig. 10.5 Course of infection in tuberculosis (TB). *CXR,* Chest X-ray; *HIV,* human immunodeficiency virus.

Interferon-gamma release assay (IGRA)

This blood test exposes white blood cells in a sample to tuberculous antigens. If infection is present, the white cells will secrete interferon-gamma. The amount secreted is measured to give the result. This test (commercially either QuantiFERON or T-Spot-TB) can be used in individuals with equivocal tuberculin results or those who have received BCG immunization for greater diagnostic accuracy.

Culture and histology

Isolation of *M. tuberculosis* by culture is the 'gold standard' but positive cultures are obtained in a minority (40%) of children.

Sputum, or in younger children who can't produce sputum, early-morning gastric aspirates on 3 successive days are the best specimens. It takes 6 to 8 weeks for the bacillus to grow. Microscopy is often negative but histological examination of a lymph node biopsy may reveal caseating granulomata and acid-fast bacilli.

Polymerase chain reaction

PCR (Xpert MTB/RIF) can be used in real time (results within 2 hours) to detect the presence of *M. tuberculosis* and rifampicin sensitivity (suggesting MDR-TB). Although it is less sensitive than culture in children, it is very specific – overall detecting

30% to 70% of samples that are smear negative, but culture positive.

Radiology
TB is suggested by hilar or mediastinal lymphadenopathy, especially if it is unilateral, or in combination with a 'wedge' of collapse or consolidation. Calcification also suggests TB.

Treatment and prevention
A 6-month regimen consisting of four drugs, isoniazid, rifampicin, pyrazinamide and ethambutol for 2 months, followed by isoniazid and rifampicin for a further 4 months is used in most instances except in tuberculous meningitis, where a 12-month regimen is appropriate. All children diagnosed with TB should be offered an HIV test. The most important preventive measures are prompt and complete treatment of infectious cases and thorough contact tracing.

The BCG vaccine has been used in the UK since the 1950s to protect against TB, especially TB meningitis. Routine BCG immunization of all schoolchildren has been replaced by a more targeted approach since 2005. Currently in the UK, BCG is given to neonates in areas of high incidence or to neonates and children likely to be exposed to contacts.

COMMUNICATION

It is important to stress the importance of treatment – these children often become symptom free after the first few weeks and the medication may be unpleasant. Compliance can be poor thereafter, which can lead to clinical infection later on. Parents should be made aware of the risks of inadequate treatment, including emergence of drug resistance. Some children require supervised treatment, either daily (preferred) or three times weekly (if daily supervision is not available).

PARASITIC INFECTIONS

Malaria

Malaria is a major global health problem causing millions of deaths annually. In 2021, the WHO recommended routine use of the RTS,S malaria vaccine in sub-Saharan Africa and other areas with moderate-high *Plasmodium falciparum* malaria transmission. Imported cases are seen in the UK (most commonly from returned travellers visiting friends and relatives in West Africa). Malaria is caused by infection with any of the five species of the protozoan parasite *Plasmodium*. On average 1500 cases of malaria are reported annually in the UK; most (75%) are due to *P. falciparum*, and children under 16 account for 10% of cases. Most cases did not take chemoprophylaxis.

HINTS AND TIPS

Fever in a child who has been to a malaria endemic area within the last year is malaria until proven otherwise.

Pathophysiology
Transmission is vector borne via the female anopheles mosquito. The onset is usually 7 to 10 days after inoculation but might be delayed by months or even years. The feeding female mosquito injects sporozoites, which pass to the liver via the bloodstream. After asexual multiplication in hepatocytes, these emerge as merozoites, which invade, multiply in and destroy the host's red blood cells. Some of the merozoites form gametocytes, which are sucked up by a feeding mosquito; the sexual phase of the life cycle then takes place in the mosquito with the formation of a new generation of sporozoites.

Clinical features
Malaria presents with fever, and nonspecific symptoms include headache, rigors, abdominal and muscle pains, cough, diarrhoea and vomiting. Common misdiagnoses include viral influenza, gastroenteritis or hepatitis. Apart from the fever, which is rarely periodic, there are no consistent clinical signs. Splenomegaly, anaemia and jaundice can all occur and a number of signs characterize the severe complication of algid malaria (shock), cerebral malaria (coma, seizures) or blackwater fever (haemoglobinuria and renal failure).

Diagnosis
Diagnosis is made by the examination of thick and thin blood films; rapid detection tests (based on the detection of antigen) are used in addition, but do not replace thick and thin blood films. The former allows rapid scanning of a larger volume of blood per microscopic field. At least three films should be taken, as one negative film does not exclude malaria. If falciparum or knowlesi malaria is diagnosed, the percentage of parasitaemia should be determined; parasitaemia >2% indicates an increased chance of developing severe disease, even if the patient appears well; 10% parasitaemia represents severe disease.

Management
Children with confirmed or suspected falciparum malaria require hospitalization and treatment with an artemisinin

combination therapy. This is given orally in uncomplicated disease or intravenously if the parasite count is high or complications are present. In addition, in severe infection, broad-spectrum antibiotics are recommended until bacterial infection is excluded. In vivax infection, 2 to 3 weeks of primaquine is needed to clear dormant hypnozoite hepatic infection; falciparum does not have a dormant life cycle. Travellers to endemic areas should seek advice about the most appropriate treatment for the area they plan to visit. Treatment is taken from 1 week before to 4 weeks after travel. Even with chemoprophylaxis, efforts should be made to avoid mosquito bites by the use of nets and repellent.

Toxocariasis

Human toxocariasis is mainly caused by infection with *Toxocara canis,* a common gut parasite of dogs. *Toxocara* eggs are ingested when a child eats soil, play-pit sand or unwashed vegetables contaminated with infective dog or cat faeces.

Clinical features

There are two distinct forms of disease:

- Visceral larva migrans: characterized by fever, hepatomegaly, wheezing and eosinophilia.
- Ocular larva migrans: a granulomatous reaction in the retina causing a squint or reduced visual acuity.

Management

Treatment is with antiparasitic drugs such as albendazole or mebendazole for visceral larva migrans. Steroids may be tried for ocular disease. *Toxocara* infection could be prevented by the regular deworming of cats and dogs and by not allowing animals to defecate in public places, including sandpits.

IMMUNODEFICIENCY

Immunodeficiency can be classified into:

- Primary: in which there is an inherited, intrinsic defect in the immune system.
- Secondary: in which a defect in the immune system has been acquired, as occurs in malnutrition, infections (e.g., HIV), immunosuppressive therapy (e.g., steroids, cytotoxic drugs), hyposplenism (e.g., sickle cell disease).

  Primary immunodeficiency occurs in 1/5000 live births and should be suspected in the following circumstances:

- recurrent or persistent infections of unusual severity – often respiratory tract, cutaneous or soft-tissue infections
- infection with unusual organisms (Table 10.9)
- faltering growth

- chronic diarrhoea
- incomplete response to antibiotics
- complications of live vaccines
- noninfectious manifestations of primary immunodeficiency include severe eczema, autoimmune and lymphoproliferative disease

Primary immunodeficiencies

These can be inherited as X-linked (affecting boys only) or autosomal recessive disorders. About 40% are diagnosed in first year of life. The most important are combined (T-cell & antibody) deficiencies, major antibody deficiencies and major neutrophil disorders.

Combined (T-cell and antibody) deficiency disorders

- Severe combined immunodeficiency (SCID)
- Wiskott-Aldrich syndrome
- Ataxia telangiectasia
- SCID defines a heterogeneous group of disorders with profoundly defective cellular and humoral immunity (hence the name 'combined'). It presents in the first 6 months of life with faltering growth, diarrhoea, persistent candidiasis and recurrent, severe infections. A full blood count often shows lymphopaenia. Bone marrow transplantation can be curative.

Table 10.9 Immune defects and clinical presentation

Type of primary immunodeficiency	Presentation
T-cell deficiency	Pneumonitis, chronic diarrhoea and growth faltering, persistent thrush
Antibody deficiency	Encapsulated bacterial infections - commonly Sino-pulmonary infections, pneumonia, otitis media, tonsillitis - less commonly meningitis, chronic diarrhoea
Combined (T-cell and antibody) deficiency	Features of both T-cell and antibody deficiency
Neutropaenia	Sepsis, lymphadenopathy
Phagocyte disorders	Superficial boils, abscesses, poor wound healing
Asplenism (surgical, functional and congenital)	Encapsulated bacterial infections - sepsis
Complement deficiency	Encapsulated bacterial infections - sepsis, meningitis

Major antibody deficiency

X-linked agammaglobulinaemia (XLA)

XLA (Bruton's disease) is the commonest primary antibody deficiency. There is a failure of B-cell development and Ig production. It presents with severe bacterial infections, often from around 3–6 months as prior to this the baby is protected by transplacental maternal IgG antibodies.

Common variable immunodeficiency disorders (CVID)

CVID encompasses a heterogeneous group of patients who have low levels of serum IgG and IgA. It usually presents in late childhood with recurrent bacterial infection of the sinuses or lungs. In addition, these patients have a high rate of autoimmune disease.

Other antibody deficiencies tend to be asymptomatic; selective Ig A deficiency is common, particularly amongst Caucasian people, affecting up to 1/300. The majority are asymptomatic but it can be associated with respiratory and gastrointestinal infections, as well as an increased risk of coeliac disease.

Major neutrophil disorders

- Chronic granulomatous disease (CGD)
- Leucocyte adhesion deficiency (LAD)
- Severe congenital neutropaenia (SCN)

CGD is an inherited disorder, usually X linked, in which phagocytic cells fail to produce the oxidative burst required for the intracellular killing of pathogens. It presents with repeated bacterial and fungal infections involving the skin, lymph nodes, lungs, liver and bones. Granulomas and abscesses form in these sites. Diagnosis is confirmed by failure to reduce nitro blue tetrazolium (NBT test).

Management

The key steps in the management of primary immunodeficiency include:

- Antibiotic prophylaxis (e.g., cotrimoxazole for pneumocystis pneumonia).
- Aggressive treatment of infections with IV antibiotics.
- IVIG for severe antibody deficiency.
- Bone marrow transplant can be curative but has a high mortality rate.
- Gene therapy: this has been used for adenosine deaminase deficiency caused by SCID.

HINTS AND TIPS

Live vaccines are contraindicated in severe immunodeficiency (see Chapter 19).

Secondary immunodeficiency

Immunosuppressive therapy

Cytotoxic chemotherapy for malignancy (e.g., acute leukaemia) causes immunosuppression due to marrow suppression and neutropaenia. Febrile children with neutrophil counts less than 0.5×10^9/L are at risk of serious and potentially fatal bacterial and fungal infection.

Children on high-dose corticosteroids (e.g., for nephrotic syndrome) are particularly at risk for disseminated chickenpox infection. Children with organ transplants are prone to infection with CMV.

Human immunodeficiency virus

Worldwide, the most important infection which causes immunodeficiency is the human immunodeficiency virus (HIV), a retrovirus. This is the virus that causes acquired immunodeficiency syndrome (AIDS) through the destruction of CD4+ lymphocytes.

According to the Joint United Nations Programme on HIV/AIDS (UNAIDS), there were 38.4 million people worldwide with HIV/AIDS and approximately 150,000 new paediatric infections each year – most would be preventable through integrated antenatal services providing HIV testing and treatment. In the UK 489 children were being treated in paediatric HIV services in 2021, approximately half of whom were born abroad. There is increasing access to antiretroviral treatment on a worldwide basis, and access to treatment in the UK has turned a previously fatal illness into a manageable, chronic condition.

Transmission

The main route of transmission to children is vertically from mother to child: intrauterine, intrapartum or via breastfeeding. Transmission rates vary with geographical area: lower in Europe and higher in Africa. With optimal management, the risk of vertical transmission can be reduced to <1%. Sexual transmission is an important source of infection for the adolescent population.

Clinical features

At primary infection, some people become transiently unwell with fever, malaise, a rash or generalized lymphadenopathy but this often goes unnoticed. Once the CD4 count falls, the child may present with chronic diarrhoea, faltering growth, widespread candidiasis and severe, opportunistic infections such as pneumocystis pneumonia. AIDS-defining malignancies such as Kaposi sarcoma are rare in the paediatric population.

Diagnosis

All newborns born to HIV-infected women will have circulating maternal HIV antibodies but only a proportion of these are infected with the virus. Passively acquired antibody disappears at 15 to 18 months of age, so this is not a reliable test for infection under 18 months. HIV PCR is the usual test for infection in the infant.

Management

Antiretroviral therapy (ART) is extremely effective and is recommended from the point of diagnosis, irrespective of age, CD4 count or viral load. Infants born to HIV mothers require urgent diagnosis and treatment. The key issue is adherence, particularly during adolescence, as there can be adverse effects associated with ART. Coordinated psychological and social support for the whole family is a vital aspect of managing an HIV-infected child. Issues include:

- telling children the diagnosis
- retaining confidentiality
- social or cultural isolation
- stigma of diagnosis

COMMUNICATION

Children need to learn about their human immunodeficiency virus diagnosis at a time appropriate to them. Guidelines suggest this should be during their primary school years, usually by age 9.

Prevention

All pregnant women should be tested for HIV. Antiretroviral therapy during pregnancy for the mother and for the baby after birth greatly reduces the risk of vertical transmission. Formula feeding rather than breastfeeding the infant plays a vital role in prevention in the developed world.

Chapter Summary

- In an unwell child with fever, the most important differential is meningococcal sepsis which requires rapid treatment with a third-generation IV cephalosporin.
- In the child who has travelled abroad who has a fever, a key differential is malaria.
- Poor compliance is a big issue in the treatment of infections such as TB, which requires many months of treatment, and HIV, which needs lifelong treatment.
- Consider immunodeficiency in the child with chronic diarrhoea, faltering growth and recurrent infections.

UKMLA Conditions
Candidiasis
Cellulitis
Conjunctivitis
Hepatitis
Herpes simplex virus
Human immunodeficiency virus
Human papilloma virus infection
Impetigo
Influenza
Lower respiratory tract infection
Kawasaki disease
Malaria
Measles
Meningitis
Mumps
Periorbital and orbital cellulitis
Rubella
Tonsillitis
Toxic shock syndrome
Tuberculosis
Upper respiratory tract infection
Viral exanthema

UKMLA Presentations
Fever

Allergy and anaphylaxis

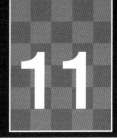

11

Allergy is a hypersensitivity reaction of the immune system to an external stimulus (allergen). Atopy describes a genetic predisposition to mount a type 1 hypersensitivity reaction to environmental allergens. The 'atopic triad' describes asthma, eczema (atopic dermatitis) and hay fever (allergic rhinitis). There is also an increased likelihood of developing allergic conjunctivitis, food allergies and anaphylaxis. This chapter will cover mainly food allergy and anaphylaxis, as the others are discussed elsewhere.

EPIDEMIOLOGY

There is a greatly increasing prevalence of childhood allergy which has led to an increased need for specialized services dealing in childhood allergy. Approximately 6% to 8% of all children experience food allergy and 6% of all asthmatics have food-induced wheeze. In atopic eczema, approximately 60% will have a reaction to certain foods. Different types of allergy tend to occur in different age groups (Fig. 11.1):

- gastrointestinal (e.g., diarrhoea): in infancy, for example, cow's milk protein allergy (CMPA)
- atopic dermatitis: peak incidence around 1 year
- wheeze: increasingly common through toddler years
- allergic rhinitis: from middle childhood

PATHOPHYSIOLOGY

Allergic reactions may be divided into immunoglobulin E (IgE)- and non-IgE-mediated forms. Acute allergic reactions, anaphylaxis, asthma and allergic rhinitis/conjunctivitis are usually IgE mediated. Atopic dermatitis (eczema) and CMPA manifest by delayed symptoms (within 24–48 hours of ingestion, developing flare of eczema, vomiting or diarrhoea) are typically non-IgE mediated.

IgE-mediated allergy

IgE-mediated allergy involves an initial sensitization to an allergen where T helper 2 (Th2) cells stimulate B cells to produce IgE to the allergen; the IgE then binds to binding sites on mast cells and basophils. On re-exposure to that allergen, it causes cross-linking of the IgE which leads to degranulation of the mast cells and basophils with release of inflammatory mediators (Fig. 11.2). IgE reactions classically produce a biphasic response with an early and late component (Fig. 11.2).

Non-IgE-mediated allergy

The mechanism for non-IgE-mediated allergy is less well understood but is thought to be T-cell mediated and often causes more subacute reactions.

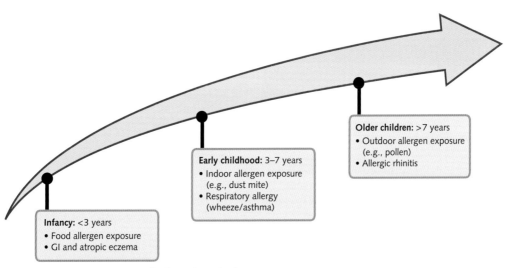

Older children: >7 years
- Outdoor allergen exposure (e.g., pollen)
- Allergic rhinitis

Early childhood: 3–7 years
- Indoor allergen exposure (e.g., dust mite)
- Respiratory allergy (wheeze/asthma)

Infancy: <3 years
- Food allergen exposure
- GI and atropic eczema

Fig. 11.1 The allergic march of childhood. *GI,* Gastrointestinal.

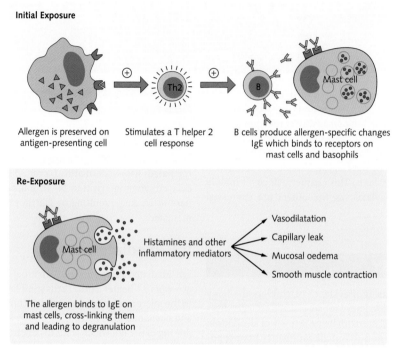

Initial Exposure

Allergen is preserved on antigen-presenting cell → Stimulates a T helper 2 cell response → B cells produce allergen-specific changes IgE which binds to receptors on mast cells and basophils

Re-Exposure

Mast cell → Histamines and other inflammatory mediators →
- Vasodilatation
- Capillary leak
- Mucosal oedema
- Smooth muscle contraction

The allergen binds to IgE on mast cells, cross-linking them and leading to degranulation

Fig. 11.2 The pathophysiology of immunoglobulin E (IgE)-mediated allergy.

Cross-reactivity

It is important to note that children sensitized to one allergen can develop reactions to another even though previous exposure has not occurred. This is due to molecular mimicry between allergens. Examples are:

- peanuts: soya beans, lentils, grass
- banana: kiwi fruit, latex
- cow's milk: soya

AETIOLOGY

Although part of the increase in cases of allergy stems from greater awareness and reporting, population-based studies have shown a significant rise in atopy and allergic diseases. There are several hypotheses for this increase; however, there is no definitive evidence for any one theory:

- Hygiene hypothesis: excessive cleanliness and improved standard of living leads to less early exposure to infectious pathogens which may prevent switching of the immune system from a predominantly Th2-cytokine-based system at birth to a predominantly Th1-cytokine system. This predisposes to hypersensitivity.
- Delayed introduction of foods: there is some evidence that late weaning and delay in exposure of the gut to allergens may increase likelihood of a reaction.

- Food processing: change in type of food to more highly processed forms may change the way antigens are presented from the gut.

Other theories include reduced antioxidants in the diet, change in types of fats ingested, vitamin D deficiency and a possible role for *Staphylococcus aureus*-derived enterotoxins.

CLINICAL ASPECTS OF ALLERGY

History

Investigations for allergy can be difficult to interpret. The history is critical to their interpretation and diagnosis. The aim is to distinguish true allergy from more common nonallergic reactions (e.g., 90% of cases of reported reactions to penicillin are nonallergic). It should also try to distinguish IgE-mediated from non-IgE-mediated allergy.

The history should include:

- age of onset
- symptoms: skin, gastrointestinal, respiratory, anaphylaxis (see Table 11.1)
- severity of previous reactions – did they need hospital admission?
- suspected causative agent
- temporal relationship: length of time between ingestion and symptom onset, duration of reaction

Table 11.1 Clinical features of allergy

	Immunoglobulin E (IgE) mediated	Non-IgE mediated
Skin	Pruritis	Pruritis
	Erythema	Erythema
	Acute urticaria	Atopic eczema
	Acute angioedema	
Gastrointestinal system	Angioedema lips/tongue/palate	Gastro-oesophageal reflux
	Oral pruritis	Infantile colic
	Nausea/vomiting	Abdominal pain
	Colicky abdominal pain	Constipation
	Diarrhoea	Loose/frequent stools
		Blood/mucus in stools
		Food refusal/aversion
		Perianal redness
		Pallor/tiredness
		Faltering growth (in conjunction with at least one of the aforementioned symptoms)
Respiratory system	Rhinorrhoea or nasal congestion	
	Cough	
	Wheeze	
	Shortness of breath	
	Chest tightness	

- frequency and reproducibility of reaction
- feeding history: if breastfed, consider maternal diet
- any foods eliminated–reintroduced and impact on symptoms
- personal or family history of atopic disease

HINTS AND TIPS

When taking a history of a drug allergy it is important to identify the type of reaction as a true allergy is uncommon. You should ask about the timing between drug ingestion and the reaction, and whether the reaction was witnessed.

Examination

Examination of the child should focus on eliciting signs of allergy (see Table 11.1), comorbid atopic features (e.g., asthma, allergic rhinitis) and growth/nutritional status.

Investigations

Allergy testing is indicated where there is suspicion of an IgE-mediated reaction and evidence from the history of the potential allergen. So-called 'fishing expeditions', using tests to multiple possible allergens with no correlation in the history, are not helpful. The main options for IgE-mediated allergies are skin-prick testing or specific serum IgE assays. There is no equivalent test available at present for non-IgE-mediated allergy and the only option is a trial of elimination (for 2–6 weeks) and reintroduction.

Skin-prick testing

This is the most common test because it is cheap, quick and has a good safety profile. Small amounts of allergen are injected subcutaneously (along with saline and histamine controls) and the amount of wheal and flare observed. A wheal ≥3 mm than the negative control is a positive result. Reactions must be interpreted with a good clinical history because a positive test gives only a 50% to 60% chance that the child will react to the allergen; however, a negative test has a >95% chance the child is not allergic to the allergen. If there is a strong history of food reaction and a positive skin-prick test, then a food challenge is not needed to confirm the allergen responsible for symptoms. Skin-prick testing should only be performed in places equipped to deal with anaphylaxis.

Serum-specific IgE

This may take the form of radioallergosorbent testing (RAST), although other assays are increasingly used. They measure levels of IgE that are food specific and are useful where skin-prick testing is unsuitable (e.g., active eczema or patients on steroids or antihistamines where the drug cannot be stopped) or unavailable. Like skin-prick tests, a negative result is good for ruling out allergens, but a positive result is useful only in the context of a positive history.

HINTS AND TIPS

Size of skin-prick reaction and immunoglobulin E levels are poor predictors of severity of reaction.

Food challenge

A blinded food challenge following a period of elimination is the gold standard and is used where there is diagnostic uncertainty, particularly where non-IgE mechanisms are suspected. This is the only investigation that can predict the severity of reaction following allergen exposure. It is rare to have IgE-mediated reactions to more than three foods and allergy testing results that show cross-reaction should be confirmed by food challenge.

HINTS AND TIPS

Allergen challenging is useful but can cause anaphylaxis. It should only be done in the hospital setting, and informed consent must be taken from parents.

Management

Children with suspected allergy should be assessed by a paediatrician with expertise in allergy and with support from a dietician. The education of both family and school plays an important part. A major consideration in management is the anxiety that affects both child and carers. Avoidance of the allergen might be difficult. It is often hard for parents to identify suitable foods; the help of a dietician is thus essential. Inhaled allergen avoidance is extremely difficult and the effectiveness of allergen avoidance in these cases is controversial. Asthma and eczema should be treated as outlined in the relevant chapters. An adrenaline auto-injector should be given (see the 'Anaphylaxis' section). Antihistamines can be useful. Immunotherapy usage (either sublingual or subcutaneous) is increasing in children with severe hay fever or house dust mite allergy – refractory to other treatments.

COMMUNICATION

Parents often want to know the likely outcome of food allergy – the majority of children outgrow milk and egg allergies in their toddler years, but peanut allergy is often lifelong.

ANAPHYLAXIS

Anaphylaxis is a severe, life-threatening, generalized hypersensitivity reaction that manifests as affecting the airway and/or breathing and/or circulation. As with other forms of allergy the prevalence is increasing. It causes approximately 20 deaths annually in the UK.

Pathophysiology

It is caused by rapid degranulation of mast cells and basophils, with systemic release of inflammatory mediators leading to vasodilatation, capillary leak, mucosal oedema and smooth muscle contraction. Bronchospasm and airway oedema cause acute airway obstruction; vasodilatation and capillary dilatation cause shock.

Causes

In children the most common cause of anaphylaxis is food; in adults this is superseded by drugs.

- Foods – peanuts are the most common food triggering anaphylaxis, followed by tree nuts, cow's milk and shellfish.
- Insect venom – anaphylaxis to venom is rare in children but it is associated with the greatest anxiety.
- Latex – anaphylaxis to latex is rare in children and is usually found in those who have had numerous surgical procedures. Note cross-reaction with banana.
- Drugs – vaccines and penicillins account for the majority of reactions, but are rare. Parents can be concerned about giving vaccinations in children with egg allergy. The measles, mumps and rubella (MMR) vaccination no longer contains any egg as it is grown on chick fibroblasts. It can be safely given to children with egg allergy. Where there has been a previous severe anaphylactic reaction to egg, discussion with an expert is advised about location of immunization (e.g., in hospital). Influenza and yellow fever vaccines should not be given to children with egg allergy.

COMMUNICATION

It important to advise latex-allergic adolescents of the potential reaction from latex condoms.

Clinical presentation

Early recognition and treatment of anaphylaxis are life-saving. The diagnosis is highly likely when there is a combination of mucosal involvement (angioedema of the lips, tongue and face, pruritis) and/or widespread urticarial rash with one or more of the following:

- respiratory compromise (dyspnoea, wheeze, stridor, hypoxia)
- cardiovascular compromise (hypotension, tachycardia, syncope)
- gastrointestinal involvement (crampy abdominal pain, diarrhoea, vomiting)

Respiratory difficulty is more common than cardiovascular collapse. Initial symptoms can be subtle and progression rapid. The patient may also experience a feeling of impending doom.

> **RED FLAG**
>
> Signs of life-threatening anaphylaxis:
> - airway: swelling, hoarseness, stridor
> - breathing: tachypnoea, wheeze, cyanosis, hypoxia, fatigue, confusion
> - circulation: pale, clammy, hypotensive, faint, drowsiness/coma

Management

Anaphylaxis is an emergency which must be treated promptly with an airway, breathing, circulation (ABC) approach (Table 11.2). The mainstay of drug treatment is adrenaline which both acts as a bronchodilator and supports the cardiovascular system through inotropic effects and peripheral vasoconstriction:

- Remove allergen where possible.
- Intramuscular adrenaline – out of hospital an adrenaline autoinjector should be used. (Table 11.2).
- If no response after 5 minutes repeat IM adrenaline and administer an IV fluid bolus (10 mL/kg).
- In cases where two appropriate doses of IM adrenaline have been administered and respiratory or cardiovascular symptoms have not improved, this is now refractory anaphylaxis and warrants critical care support early. Management of this is covered in (Table 11.3).

- Adrenaline and salbutamol nebulizers for upper airway obstruction and bronchospasm can be useful adjuncts to IM adrenaline, respectively.
- Antihistamines and corticosteroids are not recommended for the emergency treatment of anaphylaxis; they may be considered only following stabilization of the child, and should not be given preferentially to adrenaline.
- Blood should be taken for mast cell tryptase – if the cause is thought to be venom related, drug related or idiopathic (two samples, one as soon as possible after emergency treatment given, the second within 4 hours).
- All under 16-year-olds who have had emergency treatment for anaphylaxis need to be admitted for observation.

Prevention

Allergen avoidance is the only preventive measure and all children with suspected anaphylaxis should be referred to a specialist allergy service for allergen testing. The use of an adrenaline (epinephrine) autoinjector (the three main types are EpiPen, Jext or Emerade) which allows intramuscular administration of adrenaline (epinephrine) can be life-saving but it is essential that carers are trained in its use. Ongoing management should also include:

- identifying causes
- education on allergen avoidance
- individualized treatment plan
- training of carers and school
- annual reinforcement

> **COMMUNICATION**
>
> How to use an adrenaline autoinjector (EpiPen, Jext or Emerade).
> - Remove cap and check expiry date.
> - Form a fist around the pen – do not put your finger over the end.
> - Hold alongside outer thigh with injecting side facing towards body.
> - Inject firmly into outer thigh.
> - Do not inject into buttocks as this may be ineffective.
> - Attend hospital immediately after injection.

Table 11.2 Emergency treatment of anaphylaxis

Age	Adrenaline 1/1000 intramuscularly (IM)	IV fluid challenge (crystalloids)
<6 months	0.1–0.15 mL = 100–150 µg	10 mL/Kg for all ages
6 months to 6 years	0.15 mL = 150 µg	↓
6–12 years	0.3 mL = 300 µg	↓
>12 years (adult dosing)	0.5 mL = 500 µg	↓

Table 11.3 Emergency treatment of refractory anaphylaxis

Establish IV/IO access for sole use of adrenaline infusion	**Seek expert help early**	**Airway:** Partial airway obstruction: nebulized adrenaline Total airway obstruction: expert help needed – follow difficult airway algorithm
Give IM adrenaline every 5 minutes until adrenaline infusion has been started	**Start adrenaline infusion** (on its own line) + **Give rapid IV fluid bolus** (0.9% sodium chloride/ alternative crystalloid)	**Breathing:** Oxygenation = more important than intubation If apnoeic: + Bag-mask ventilation + Consider tracheal intubation Severe/ persistent bronchospasm: + nebulized salbutamol with ipratropium + oxygen Consider IV bolus +/– salbutamol infusion/aminophylline + inhalational anaesthesia
Give high-flow oxygen (aim SATS 94%–98%)	Continue adrenaline infusion and treat ABC symptoms Titrate according to clinical response	**Circulation:** Give further boluses + titrate to response: Child = 10 mL/kg
Monitor HR, BP, SATS and ECG for cardiac arrythmia Bloods for mast cell tryptase, urea and electrolytes and capillary or arterial blood gas		**Cardiac arrest** – follow APLS algorithm - Adrenaline dosing different for both anaphylaxis and cardiac arrest protocol

Hereditary angioedema (C1-esterase inhibitor deficiency)

This is an autosomal dominant disease caused by either a lack/ deficiency or dysfunctional C1-inhibitor protein. Triggers (trauma, infections and stress) cause angioedema to the upper airway, skin and gastrointestinal tract. In distinction to allergic anaphylaxis (histamine-mediated angioedema), itching/pruritis is rare, urticaria does not occur and the progression of attacks tends to be slower over hours – but lasts longer (2–5 days). It is uncommon (1/50,000) but presents in the first two decades of life and is an important differential consideration in anaphylaxis since the treatments used in allergic angioedema: adrenaline, steroid and antihistamines are ineffective. Treatment is by administering C1-esterase inhibitor; either in fresh frozen plasma or a partially purified form. Preventative/prophylactic medications are used to prevent attacks.

● Chapter Summary

- The 'atopic triad' describes asthma, eczema (atopic dermatitis) and hay fever (allergic rhinitis).
- The most severe form of allergy is anaphylaxis which can be life-threatening; those at risk should have an adrenaline autoinjector for use at any time.
- A careful history is key to determining the type of allergic reaction, in particular the nature of symptoms and the time course of the reaction.
- Adrenaline (appropriate dose and timing), fluid resuscitation and oxygenation are the most key points in treating anaphylaxis effectively.

UKMLA Condition
Anaphylaxis

UKMLA Presentation
Allergies

THE CHILD WITH A RASH

A rash is a very common childhood presentation. The majority are harmless and they can occur with any underlying viral illness; however, occasionally they are caused by a major systemic infection or an underlying dermatological condition. Careful clinical history and examination are essential and investigation is occasionally needed.

Causes

Causes of a rash include the following:

- infection (viral, bacterial, toxin associated)
- infestation (e.g., scabies)
- dermatitis (eczema, psoriasis)
- allergy
- vasculitis and bleeding disorders (rare)

History

Key questions to ask about the rash include:

- Duration, site of onset, evolution and spread.
- Does it come and go (e.g., urticaria)?
- Does the rash itch (e.g., eczema, scabies)?
- Has there been any recent drug ingestion or exposure to potentially provocative agents (e.g., sunlight, food, allergens, detergents)?
- Are there any other associated symptoms (e.g., sore throat, upper respiratory tract infection, malaise)?
- Are any other family members or contacts affected (e.g., viral exanthems, infestations)?
- Is there any family history (e.g., atopy, psoriasis)?

Examination

Assess for systemic features including:

- fever
- lymphadenopathy
- splenomegaly
- arthropathy

Examine all of the skin, including the mucous membranes, nails and hair. Describe the rash systematically.

Site and distribution

- generalized (e.g., to flexor surfaces – eczema, or to extensor surfaces – Henoch-Schönlein purpura) or localized

- number of lesions
- pattern of lesions: discrete, grouped, confluent

Morphology

- Describe the size, shape and colour of lesions:
  - macules: flat, nonpalpable, pigmented
  - papules: palpable, raised <5 mm diameter
  - nodules: palpable, raised >5 mm diameter
  - vesicles: fluid filled (serous), palpable, raised <5 mm
  - bullae: fluid filled (serous), palpable, raised >5 mm
  - pustule: pus filled, palpable, raised
  - petechiae: pinhead-sized lesion of extravasated blood; do not blanch
  - purpura: larger (2–10 mm) lesion of extravasated blood; do not blanch
  - ecchymosis: largest lesion (>10 mm) of extravasated blood; do not blanch
- Describe the surrounding skin.
- Palpate the rash for scale, thickness, texture and temperature.

HINTS AND TIPS

It is often helpful to draw a diagram of a rash in the clinical notes, in order for colleagues to later assess whether it has changed.

COMMUNICATION

With petechial rashes or cellulitis, it is key to know whether they spread, therefore it is very helpful to draw around them on the child's skin. Explain this to the child and their parents before doing so.

Investigations

Investigations are rarely required but might include skin scrapings for fungi or scabies. If the skin looks infected, a swab of any discharge can be helpful. If there are signs of systemic illness, other investigations including blood tests or cultures might be needed, or a full septic screen (see Chapter 10). See Table 12.1.

Table 12.1 Types of rash

Type of rash	Description	Examples
Maculopapular	Flat, non-palpable, pigmented rash/vesicular: fluid-filled, palpable, raised lesions	Viral exanthems (see Chapter 10), for example, measles, rubella, roseola infantum, any viral infection Scarlet fever Kawasaki disease
Vesicular rash		Chickenpox Eczema herpeticum
Haemorrhagic rash	Caused by extravasation of blood, therefore no blanching on pressure. From smallest to largest: petechiae, purpura, ecchymoses	Meningococcal sepsis Acute leukaemia Idiopathic thrombocytopenic purpura Henoch-Schönlein purpura: distribution is usually on the legs and buttocks. Arthralgia and abdominal pain might be present. Bleeding disorders: haemophilia, von Willebrand disease
Urticarial rash	Transient, itchy rash characterized by raised weals. Appears rapidly and fades	Food allergy (e.g., shellfish, eggs) Drug allergy (e.g., penicillin) Contact allergy (e.g., grass, animal fur) Hereditary Angioedema (e.g., C1 esterase deficiency)

HINTS AND TIPS

Take care to consider suspected nonaccidental injury in cases of traumatic or nontraumatic bruising.

RED FLAG

Nonblanching or rapidly spreading rash should be treated as meningococcal sepsis until proven otherwise.

ACUTE RASHES

Viral exanthems

These rashes are widespread that is normally associated with systemic symptoms (fever, headache and malaise). In children they are very common and largely caused by viruses but can occasionally have alternate aetiologies which are important to consider in the absence of viral symptomatology.

There are classical viral exanthems that have been labelled as first to sixth disease in the order they were found, and these are described in Chapter 10 with associated pictures.

Other causes of exanthems

Pityriasis rosea

This common, acute, benign and self-limiting condition is thought to be of viral origin. It begins with a 'herald patch', an oval or round, scaly, erythematous macule on the trunk, neck or proximal part of limbs. This is followed within 1 to 3 days by a shower of smaller dull pink macules on the trunk in a so-called Christmas tree pattern following the lines of the ribs. Spontaneous resolution occurs within 6 to 8 weeks. No treatment is required.

Erythema multiforme

A distinctive, symmetrical rash characterized by annular target (iris) lesions and various other lesions including macules, papules and bullae (Fig. 12.1). The severe form with mucous membrane involvement is Stevens-Johnson syndrome. Causes include

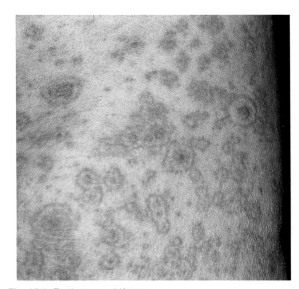

Fig. 12.1 Erythema multiforme.

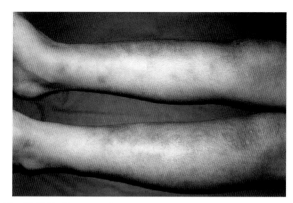
Fig. 12.2 Erythema nodosum.

infections (most commonly herpes simplex, mycoplasma or Epstein-Barr virus) and drugs. Mostly it is idiopathic and self-limiting.

Erythema nodosum

Red, tender, nodular lesions usually occur on the shins. Important causes include inflammatory bowel disease, streptococcal infections and tuberculosis (Fig. 12.2).

Napkin dermatitis

Rashes in the nappy area are common and can be due to:

- an irritant contact dermatitis (nappy rash)
- candidiasis
- seborrhoeic dermatitis
- candidiasis

Nappy rash

Ordinary nappy rash is due to the prolonged contact of urine and faeces with skin. Particular causes include skin wetness and ammonia from the breakdown of urine by faecal enzymes. The skin is red, moist and might ulcerate. The inguinal folds are spared. Nappy rash can be prevented by frequent nappy changes and barrier creams. Exposure to air can hasten recovery.

Candidiasis

Candidiasis is also common and is distinguished by bright red skin with satellite lesions and involvement of the skin folds. Candidal infection can be treated with a topical and oral antifungals such as nystatin.

Acne vulgaris

This is the most common skin disease amongst adolescents. The aetiology is multifactorial, with circulating androgens during puberty causing increased sebum production and proliferation of the bacterium *Propionibacterium acnes*.

Clinical features

A variety of lesions occur, chiefly on the face and upper trunk. Characteristically, comedones occur: plugs of keratin and sebum within the dilated orifice of a hair follicle. These can be open (blackheads) or closed (whiteheads). They progress to papules and pustules (bacterial superinfection) and in severe cases to cystic and nodular lesions, which can cause scarring.

Management

Treatment options include:

- Topical treatment with keratolytic agents (e.g., benzoyl peroxide).
- Topical antibiotics (e.g., clindamycin or low-dose oral antibiotics (e.g., doxycycline or erythromycin)).
- Vitamin A analogues, 13-*cis*-retinoic acid: can be given topically or orally (for severe acne only; prescribed by specialists only).

COMMUNICATION

Having a skin condition such as acne can be extremely difficult psychologically, and it is important to explore the impact that it is having on the patient's life – are they comfortable going to school or socializing with friends?

HINTS AND TIPS

Oral isotretinoin (roaccutane) is teratogenic – it is important to counsel teenage girls about this before it is prescribed.

Chronic rashes

Eczema

Eczema is a chronic inflammatory skin condition that usually starts in childhood. Three main varieties occur in infants and children:

- atopic eczema
- infantile seborrhoeic eczema
- napkin dermatitis

Atopic eczema

Atopic eczema is very common and affects 10% to 20% of children. There is often a family history of atopic disorders (eczema, asthma and allergic rhinitis), reflecting a genetic predisposition that confers an abnormal immune response to environmental allergens. Eczema is often the first manifestation of the 'allergic march' that may continue with allergic rhinitis and asthma.

Clinical features

It is usually an episodic condition though may be continuous in severe cases. A dry, red itchy rash occurs that usually starts on the extensor surfaces and face in infants and young children, and the flexures (the antecubital and popliteal fossae) in older children (Fig. 12.3). The skin appearance can vary from an acute, weeping papulovesicular eruption to the chronic, dry, scaly, thickened (lichenified) skin that develops in older children (Fig. 12.4). Itching is often the most problematic symptom.

Investigations

The diagnosis is clinical although total immunoglobulin E is likely to be raised. Food and environmental allergens play a role and identifying these using exclusion diets or radioallergosorbent testing and skin prick tests may be helpful.

Management

The mainstay of treatment is the regular use of emollients even when the eczema is under control. In addition to this a stepwise approach should be used, applying topical steroids of appropriate potency to affected areas. If treatment with emollients and topical steroids alone is not sufficient, topical therapies such as tacrolimus and pimecrolimus may be used (topical calcineurin inhibitors). Systemic therapy with immunosuppressive agents is required for a small number of children with severe eczema. Having a child with severe eczema can be quite distressing to parents. Parents should be armed with an individual management plan detailing how to respond to flares and step treatment up and down as appropriate. Education is essential and community nurses play a valuable role in demonstrating the use of the topical therapies and monitoring response. Many children grow out of their eczema by their teens.

> ### HINTS AND TIPS
>
> Remember the increasing potency of topical steroids with this mnemonic:
>
> #### Help every budding dermatologist
> - *h*ydrocortisone (least potent)
> - *e*umovate
> - *b*etnovate
> - *d*ermovate (most potent)

Complications

The most important is secondary infection with either viruses or bacteria. Infection with herpes simplex (eczema herpeticum; see Fig. 12.5) is potentially serious and should be treated with aciclovir.

Bacterial superinfection is most commonly by staphylococci and requires antibiotic treatment.

Infantile seborrhoeic eczema

This mild condition presents most commonly in the first 2 months of life with a scaly, nonitchy rash initially on the scalp (cradle cap); this might spread to involve the face, flexures and nappy area (Fig. 12.6). Treatment is with emollients and mild topical steroids.

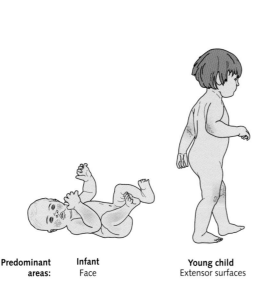
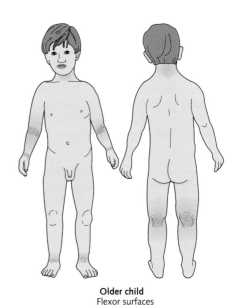

| Predominant areas: | Infant Face | Young child Extensor surfaces | Older child Flexor surfaces |

Fig. 12.3 Distribution of atopic eczema.

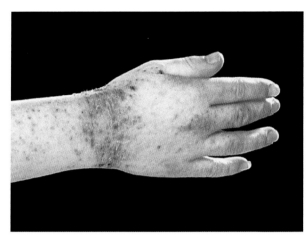

Fig. 12.4 Atopic eczema.

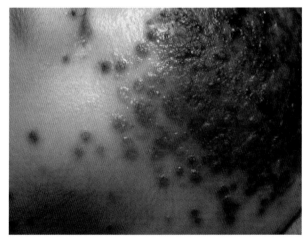

Fig. 12.5 Eczema herpeticum.

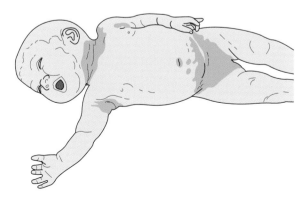

Fig. 12.6 Distribution of infantile seborrhoeic eczema.

Bacterial skin infections

Bacterial infections of the skin in children include common and important entities such as:

- impetigo
- boils and furuncles
- staphylococcal scalded skin syndrome
- erysipelas

These are considered in Chapter 10.

Viral skin infection

Viral warts

The human papillomavirus causes viral warts. Two types are seen:

- Skin warts are common on the fingers and soles in school-age children.
- Plantar warts (verrucae) are flat, hyperkeratotic lesions on the soles of the feet.

Most viral warts resolve within a year when immunity develops.

Treatment options include:

- salicylic and lactic acid paint
- cryotherapy with liquid nitrogen

Repeat treatments over many weeks are required.
Viral warts also occur in other locations:

- Laryngeal papillomas are found on the vocal cords.
- Genital warts (condylomata acuminata) are papular or frond-like growths in the perineal area.

These can be a sign of sexual abuse in young children.

Molluscum contagiosum

This common eruption in children is caused by the molluscipox-virus. These are smooth, pearly papules with an obvious central dimple that arise in crops (often on the trunk). They are not irritating and are of low infectivity. The papules resolve spontaneously without scarring usually within 6 months to 2 years and treatment is not required, although cryotherapy can be used if rapid removal is required.

Fungal skin infections

These include dermatophytosis (ringworm) and candidiasis (thrush).

Dermatophytoses (tinea capitis, corporis, pedis and unguium)

Dermatophytes are filamentous fungi that infect the outer layer of the skin and also the hair and nails. They also affect some animal species (e.g., cattle and cats). Clinical features vary with the site of infection.

- Tinea capitis (scalp ringworm) – on the scalp, tinea causes patchy alopecia and occasionally a boggy inflammatory mass called a 'kerion'.
- Tinea corporis (body ringworm) – on the trunk, tinea appears as annular lesions with central clearing and a palpable, erythematous border.
- Tinea pedis (athlete's foot) – this presents as itchy, scaling and cracking of the skin of the feet, especially between the toes.

Examination under ultraviolet light (Wood's) shows a green–yellow fluorescence of infected hairs with certain fungal species. Diagnosis can be made by microscopic examination of skin scrapings for fungal hyphae.

Treatment varies with the severity of infection:

- Mild infections are treated with topical antifungal preparations such as clotrimazole or miconazole.
- Severe infections and tinea capitis require systemic treatment with oral antifungals (griseofulvin or terbinafine) for several weeks.

Candidiasis (thrush)

Candida albicans, a yeast (budding, unicellular organism), is the most common pathogen. The organism colonizes the skin and mucous membranes. Transmission is via person-to-person contact, contaminated feeding bottles, etc. In infants, candidal infections frequently involve the oral cavity (thrush) or the nappy area. It is acquired from the mother's vaginal flora. It can also affect the nipples of breastfeeding mothers.

Diagnosis is clinical:

- Oral thrush presents as white plaques on the tongue and buccal mucosa.
- Monilial dermatitis: localized shiny redness typically affecting moist areas and *not* sparing flexural skin creases (this may occur in the absence of oral thrush).

Management involves topical nystatin as first-line therapy. Oral treatment should be given as well as direct treatment to lesions in perineal disease.

Prevention requires good hygiene and rigorous disinfection of feeding bottles and dummies.

Chronic or recurrent mucocutaneous candidiasis should raise the suspicion of immunodeficiency.

INFESTATIONS

Scabies

Scabies is a skin infestation caused by the mite *Sarcoptes scabiei.* It is transmitted by prolonged skin-to-skin contact. The fertilized adult female mite burrows deep in the stratum corneum laying two or three eggs a day until she dies after about 5 weeks. The eggs hatch after a few days and larvae move on to the skin surface, maturing into adults in 10 to 14 days.

Clinical features

The key symptom is severe itching, caused by hypersensitivity to the mite/its faeces, typically worse at night. The rash consists of vesicles, weals, papules and burrows which are pathognomonic.

Common sites for burrows are the interdigital webs and the anterior aspects of the wrists. In infants, the soles of the feet, head and neck are commonly affected (Fig. 12.7).

The rash may become excoriated and secondarily infected.

Management

Diagnosis is clinical and can be confirmed by identification of mites or ova in scrapings from burrows or vesicles. Treatment is permethrin cream 5%, applied to the entire body, with two treatments 1 week apart. It can take several weeks for the pruritus to subside after successful treatment as hypersensitivity persists. This can be managed with oral antihistamines and topical steroids.

HINTS AND TIPS

It is important to treat all contacts. Parents should also be advised to wash all clothes and bedding to prevent reinfection.

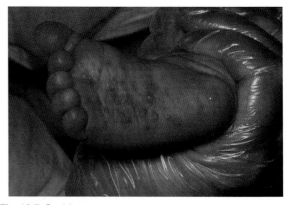

Fig. 12.7 Scabies.

Headlice (*Pediculosis capitis*)

Headlice (nits) is infestation with Pediculosis capitis, a blood-sucking arthropod that infests the scalp. Transmission is by head-to-head contact, explaining its prevalence in nurseries and schools.

Clinical features

The louse egg is attached to the base of the scalp hair and is visible as a small, white, grain-like particle (the 'nit'). Eggs hatch after a week and the louse lives for 2 to 3 months. Many infestations are asymptomatic but the most common manifestation is severe itching of the scalp, sometimes accompanied by enlarged cervical lymph nodes.

Management

Finding a louse is diagnostic. Lice can be removed by wet combing with a fine-tooth comb or by applying dimeticone to the hair. The whole family should be treated.

Chapter Summary

- Rashes are very common in paediatrics, and skill is needed to ascertain those signalling underlying illness.
- Dermatological conditions can have significant psychological impacts which should be assessed and appropriate support given.
- When treating infestations such as scabies and headlice, it is vital to treat the whole family or they will recur.

UKMLA Conditions
Atopic dermatitis and eczema
Urticaria

UKMLA Presentations
Acute rash
Chronic rash

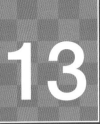
INTRODUCTION

This chapter covers a range of topics within paediatric neurology. It looks at distinguishing fits, faints and funny turns in addition to the diagnosis and management of epilepsy. It covers common and serious causes of headache. It also looks at central nervous system (CNS) infections, cerebral palsy, neurocutaneous syndromes and CNS malformations.

FITS, FAINTS AND FUNNY TURNS

Transient episodes of altered consciousness, abnormal movements or abnormal behaviour are common presenting problems. There are many causes, which range from benign (e.g., vasovagal episodes) to potentially serious (e.g., cardiac causes or epileptic seizures). A thorough history including events before, during and after is essential.

History

Provoking events

Exactly when and where the episode occurred and what the child was doing just before it happened could help identify the cause. For example:

- trauma (head injury)
- flashing lights
- unwell with fever
- during exercise
- symptoms of anxiety (e.g., hyperventilating, paraesthesia)

Description of the episodes

An accurate witness account is helpful when trying to identify the type of event that occurred. Ask specifically about:

- loss of consciousness/awareness
- abnormal movements (unilateral or bilateral, limb involvement, facial movements, e.g., twitching, lip smacking)
- duration of the episode
- altered tone (rigidity or sudden fall)
- associated features (e.g., incontinence, foaming at the mouth, breath holding, pallor or cyanosis, eye moment)

Other important features

Investigate about:

- birth history
- developmental history
- family history (specifically of epilepsy and febrile convulsions)

COMMUNICATION

A good description of the event is sometimes all you need, and parents can often demonstrate what happened. Some may have even recorded the event on video (e.g., on their mobile phone). It is helpful to advise them to do so if the event ever happens again. If the parent did not witness the event, try to speak to who did (e.g., call the school to ask a teacher).

Examination

The well child

Physical examination is often normal in idiopathic epilepsy (the majority). However, particular attention should be paid to:

- Skin: neurocutaneous syndromes are associated with epilepsy, especially tuberous sclerosis and neurofibromatosis.
- Optic fundi: fundal changes may occur in congenital infections and neurodegenerative diseases.
- Lying and standing blood pressure.

Acute presentations

Physical examination of an infant or child presenting acutely following generalized tonic-clonic seizures (particularly the first episode) has a different emphasis, reflecting the likely causes (Box 13.1). Important features on examination include:

- fever: febrile convulsions or intracranial infection
- altered level of consciousness
- anterior fontanelle: tense or bulging if the intracranial pressure (ICP) is raised
- optic fundi: papilloedema (Fig. 13.1) in raised ICP
- focal neurological signs
- meningism
- signs of systemic illness (e.g., rash, signs of tonsillitis, nasal congestion)

BOX 13.1 CAUSES OF SEIZURES

Common	Uncommon
Febrile seizures	Head injury
Epilepsy	Hyponatraemia
Meningitis/encephalitis	Space-occupying lesion
Hypoglycaemia	Metabolic disorders

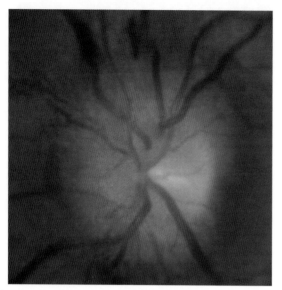

Fig. 13.1 Papilloedema is an important clinical sign in raised intracranial pressure. This photograph shows a raised optic disc with burred margins and peripapillary haemorrhages.

Seizures

Many other events can be mistaken for seizures. The key differentials to include are listed by age in Table 13.1.

Table 13.1 Differential diagnosis of seizures by age

Age	Differential diagnosis
Infants	Jitteriness Benign sleep myoclonus Apnoeas Gastro-oesophageal reflux (Sandifer syndrome)
Toddlers	Breath-holding attacks Reflex anoxic seizures Rigors Masturbation
Children	Vasovagal syncope (faints) Behavioural (e.g., day-dreaming, tantrums) Tics Panic attacks Migraine Night terrors

The classification system has changed over the years and the most recent approach by the International League Against Epilepsy classifies seizures according to the area of the brain in which the electrical activity started, if known.

See the 'Epilepsy' section for further detail.

Faints (vasovagal syncope)

This is a common, benign event which must be carefully distinguished from other more worrying causes of collapse. Syncope is common amongst teenagers, and other features include:

- provoked by emotion, hot environment
- preceded by nausea, dizziness, gradual loss of vision
- sudden loss of consciousness and posture
- rapid recovery

An ECG is mandatory to exclude evidence of a significant cardiac dysrhythmia.

Funny turns

Breath-holding attacks

These typically occur in toddlers and can be frightening for the observer, usually the parents:

- Provoked by temper, frustration or strong emotion.
- The screaming toddler holds his or her breath, leading to cyanosis and potentially loss of consciousness.
- Rapid recovery.

Reflex anoxic seizures

This is a condition that occurs due to increased vagal tone whereby there is a brief, paroxysmal episode of asystole triggered by pain or emotion. It is more common in infants up to 2 years and children will usually outgrow it. They have the following characteristics:

- The infant or toddler becomes pale and loses consciousness (syncope secondary to vagal-induced bradycardia).
- The subsequent hypoxia might induce a tonic-clonic seizure.

Rigors

Rigors are transient exaggerated shivering in association with high fever, often mistaken by parents and health professionals as a seizure.

Table 13.2 Causes of coma

Cause	Differential diagnosis
Infection	Meningitis Encephalitis
Trauma	Head injury
Metabolic	Hypoglycaemia
Primary central nervous system disorder	Seizures (e.g., epilepsy)
Drugs	Opiates Lead

Table 13.3 The Glasgow Coma Scale

		Glasgow Coma Scale	
Score	Eye opening	Best motor response	Best verbal response
1	No response	No response	No response
2	Open to pain	Extension	Nonverbal sounds
3	Open to verbal command	Inappropriate flexion	Inappropriate words
4	Open spontaneously	Flexion with pain	Disorientated and conversing
5		Localizes pain	Orientated and conversing
6		Obeys command	

THE UNCONSCIOUS CHILD

The acute development of a diminished level of consciousness is a medical emergency. In the majority of cases a systemic problem rather than a primary brain disorder is responsible (Table 13.2). The cause might be evident from the history but, if not, clinical evaluation is the key after emergency management. See Chapter 20 for investigation and management. It is important not to perform lumbar puncture (LP) in an acutely comatose child as raised ICP is likely. It can always be performed later if a diagnosis is required.

Examination

Systemic examination
The priorities are:

- airway, breathing and circulation
- temperature
- blood glucose
- hypertension, bradycardia, irregular respiration (signs of coning, Cushing's triad)
- signs of physical abuse or injury

Neurological examination
For a neurological examination, the AVPU is a quick and simple scoring system. There are four categories:

- A = *a*lert
- V = responds to *v*oice
- P = responds to *p*ain
- U = *u*nresponsive

A more formal assessment of the level of consciousness is the Glasgow Coma Scale (GCS) score (Table 13.3) A patient scoring a P on the AVPU scale is usually a GCS score of 8 or less. Other features in the neurological examination should include:

- The pupils: these might be small (suggests opiate or barbiturate poisoning), large (suggests a postictal state) or unequal (suggests severe head injury or intracranial haemorrhage).
- Signs of meningism.
- The fontanelle.

EPILEPSY

Epilepsy is common, affecting 5 per 1000 school-age children. It is a chronic disorder characterized by recurrent, unprovoked epileptic seizures.

A diagnosis of epilepsy is made in a patient in whom epileptic seizures recur spontaneously. However, it is important to recognize that an 'epileptic seizure' can be provoked in individuals who do *not* have epilepsy (e.g., with fever, hypoglycaemia or hypoxia).

Classification of seizures

The International League Against Epilepsy have recently revised their classification system for epileptic seizures. The goal in any patient should be to identify the types of seizure occurring and to diagnose the epilepsy or epilepsy syndrome present.

Seizures caused by an epilepsy syndrome are categorized as either an idiopathic generalized epilepsy syndrome, or by the age of onset (neonates and under 2, children under 12, variable – adults and children), then considering the nature of the seizure; these categories are used to direct treatment:

- generalized
- focal
- generalized and focal
- developmental impairment and epileptic encephalopathy

We consider these presentations below. Terms such as 'grand mal', 'petit mal', 'simple' and 'partial' are outdated and should be avoided.

Generalized seizures
These types of seizures originate from networks in both hemispheres. They can be motor (e.g., tonic-clonic and myoclonic) or nonmotor (e.g., absence seizures).

Tonic-clonic seizures

These are characterized by:

- tonic phase: loss of consciousness, rigidity with loss of posture
- clonic phase: jerking movements of all four limbs
- postictal drowsiness

These can be seen in epilepsy but also in febrile seizures and meningoencephalitis.

Absence seizures

These are characterized by:

- brief unawareness lasting a few seconds
- no loss of posture
- immediate recovery
- might be very frequent
- associated with automatisms (e.g., blinking and lip-smacking; in older children this can be mistaken for a focal seizure)

Focal seizures

These types of seizure originate from one hemisphere, either at a localized point or more widespread. They are characterized by:

- Involvement of only a particular part of the body.
- May be associated with an aura.
- Can have emotional, sensory or cognitive component.
- May spread to involve the entire body – focal onset to bilateral tonic-clonic.

Classification of epilepsies and epilepsy syndromes

Some forms of epilepsy may be classified into syndromes, which have a typical prognosis and respond to specific anticonvulsants. Some common and important types are listed in Box 13.2; however, this list is not exhaustive.

Childhood absence epilepsy

This relatively common variety of generalized seizure epilepsy has a peak onset at 6–7 years of age. The absence seizures comprise transient unawareness (blank spells), without loss of body tone. They typically last for 5 to 15 seconds but can be very frequent, with up to several hundred daily. Episodes can be induced by hyperventilation, occasionally used to help diagnosis. The electroencephalogram (EEG) is characteristic

---

BOX 13.2 TYPES OF EPILEPSY AND EPILEPSY SYNDROMES

Primary grouping/ age of onset	Generalized epilepsy	Focal epilepsy	Developmental and epileptic encephalopathies
Idiopathic Generalized epilepsy syndromes	– Childhood absence epilepsy – Juvenile myoclonic epilepsy – Epilepsy with generalized tonic-clonic seizures alone		
Syndromes that start in infants under 2 years of age	Self-limited neonatal epilepsy ('fifth day fits')		– West syndrome – Ohtahara syndrome – Dravet syndrome
Syndromes that start in childhood (2–12 years)	Childhood absence epilepsy	– Self-limited epilepsy with centrotemporal spikes (SeLECTS – previously benign rolandic epilepsy) – Self-limited epilepsy with autonomic seizures (SeLEAS previously Panayiotopoulos syndrome)	– Lennox-Gastaut syndrome – Epilepsy with myoclonic atonic seizures (Doose syndrome) – Laundau-Kleffner syndrome
Syndromes that can start at any age	Epilepsy syndromes in this category are numerous, but rare – Rasmussen syndrome		
Seizure not caused by epileptic syndrome	CNS infection Head trauma Arteriovenous malformations Tumours Cortical dysgenesis Hypoxic ischaemic encephalopathy		

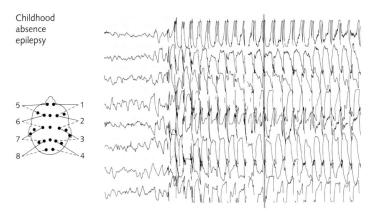

Childhood absence epilepsy

Fig. 13.2 Electroencephalogram in typical absence seizure. There is a three-per-second spike and wave discharge, which is bilaterally synchronous.

with generalized, bilaterally synchronous three-per-second spike–wave discharges (Fig. 13.2). The prognosis is good with spontaneous remission in adolescence in the majority of children. Sodium valproate and ethosuximide are the first-line drugs, although medication is not required for infrequent absences.

Infantile spasms (West syndrome)

This is an uncommon form of developmental and epileptic encephalopathy epilepsy with peak onset between 4 and 6 months of age. Myoclonic seizures occur, often as 'salaam spasms' – sudden flexor spasms of head, trunk and limbs followed by abduction and adduction of the arms. They are often multiple and can be misdiagnosed as colic. The EEG shows hypsarrhythmia, a chaotic pattern of large-amplitude slow waves with spikes and sharp waves. About 70% of the patients have the symptomatic form, and important causes include tuberous sclerosis and perinatal hypoxic-ischaemic encephalopathy. The prognosis is poor with often-intractable seizures and marked learning difficulties, but can be improved by early treatment. Treatment is with vigabatrin (alone initially in tuberous sclerosis) and prednisolone.

Aetiology

Epilepsy can result from a very diverse group of pathological processes (Box 13.3) but it is important to realize that in at least 50% of children no cause will be identified, even after extensive evaluation.

Diagnosis

A careful history is the mainstay of diagnosis. A detailed description is required of the events before, during and after a suspected seizure (a video recording is a useful adjunct). The first aim is to

> **BOX 13.3 CAUSES OF EPILEPSY**
>
> - Idiopathic (majority)
> - Cerebral malformations
> - Cortical dysgenesis
> - Tumours
> - Trauma
> - Central nervous system infection
> - Hypoxic-ischaemic encephalopathy
> - Chromosomal abnormalities (Down syndrome, Fragile X syndrome)
> - Neurodegenerative conditions
> - Neurocutaneous syndromes

distinguish true epileptic seizures from the many causes of faints, fits and funny turns.

Investigations

Epilepsy is primarily a clinical diagnosis (see epilepsy history and examination, discussed earlier in this chapter); however, there are some standard investigations, which can aid in diagnosis.

EEG

This may aid diagnosis by identifying a particular epilepsy syndrome, highlighting an anatomical focus point, or point towards a neurodegenerative disorder. A single EEG will be normal in up to 50% of children with epilepsy, especially since the child may not have a seizure during the test. In addition, nonspecific or even so-called epileptiform abnormalities can be found in 2% to 3% of normal asymptomatic children. A routine interictal EEG does not therefore prove or disprove a diagnosis of epilepsy. Additional information can be obtained from ambulatory EEG monitoring, video telemetry or recordings during sleep or after sleep deprivation.

Neuroimaging

Not all children with epilepsy require imaging. Indications for neuroimaging include:

- focal onset seizures
- seizures not responsive to first-line treatment
- a focal neurological deficit
- children less than 2 years old with afebrile convulsions

Magnetic resonance imaging (MRI) is the investigation of choice as it offers greater sensitivity in the detection of small lesions (e.g., in temporal lobe or subtle cortical dysgeneses).

Other investigations

Additional specific investigations might be appropriate if there is clinical suspicion of an underlying neurometabolic disorder. This is usually following discussion with a specialist centre, and may include:

- plasma and urine amino acids
- urine organic acids
- ammonia
- measurement of white blood cell enzymes
- DNA analysis
- biopsy of skin or muscle

Management of epilepsy

Effective management of a child with epilepsy involves far more than the prescription of antiepilepsy drugs (AEDs). Both the child and parents need to be educated about the condition and the prognosis of the particular epilepsy or epilepsy syndrome.

HINTS AND TIPS

Children with epilepsy should be encouraged to live a normal life including social activities. Certain activities, however, do require special precautions:

- Domestic bathing: children should be supervised in the bath; older children should be advised not to lock the door.
- Cycling: a helmet must be worn and traffic avoided.
- Swimming: never alone if seizures uncontrolled.

See www.epilepsy.org.uk for more practical and safety advice for patients and families.

It is important to consider the psychological and educational implications of anyone with a chronic illness. Behavioural and emotional difficulties can occur in the teenage years, with loss of self-esteem, anxiety or depression. This can have a knock-on effect on compliance with medication and seizure control. The diagnosis should be discussed with school staff and education provided about what to do in the event of a seizure. Learning difficulties are present in a proportion of children with epilepsy, but only a minority require special schooling.

Antiepilepsy drugs

Not all children with epilepsy require drug treatment. AEDs are not usually started after a first uncomplicated seizure and may not be needed for infrequent myoclonic or absence seizures. First-line treatment according to National Institute for Health and Care Excellence (NICE) is:

- sodium valproate, lamotrigine or levetiracetam for tonic-clonic seizures
- ethosuximide, sodium valproate, lamotrigine or levetiracetam for absence seizures

Monotherapy should be used wherever possible and achieves total seizure control in 70% of children. Many AEDs have side effects which should always be considered. Blood level monitoring is rarely needed, but may identify poor compliance.

HINTS AND TIPS

It is important to carefully consider the choice of antiepileptic drugs in sexually active girls. Sodium valproate should be avoided during pregnancy as it is teratogenic, therefore it may not be a good first-line approach in young women.

Carbamazepine is an enzyme inducer, hence increases the rate of metabolism of both progesterone and oestrogen. This means that a higher dose of the oral contraceptive pill and emergency contraception would be needed in girls taking carbamazepine.

Some children may be prescribed 'rescue medication' which their parents can administer at home in the event of a tonic-clonic seizure lasting over 5 minutes. This is usually rectal diazepam or buccal midazolam, which the parents are taught how to administer.

See Chapter 20 for management of status epilepticus.

FEBRILE CONVULSIONS

A febrile convulsion is a seizure associated with fever in a child between 6 months and 6 years of age in the absence of intracranial infection or an identifiable neurological disorder.

Febrile convulsions are the most common cause of seizures in childhood and occur in about 5% of children. There might be a familial predisposition. The seizures usually occur when body temperature rises rapidly.

Clinical features

They are typically brief (1–2 minutes), generalized, tonic-clonic seizures. The underlying infection causing the fever may be viral or bacterial (commonly otitis media, tonsillitis, pneumonia or urinary tract infection). It is important to identify the focus of the fever and to ensure there are no signs of meningitis.

Febrile convulsions are classified as:

- simple – less than 15 minutes, generalized, occurring once in 24 hours
- complex – longer than 15 minutes, focal or recurring within 24 hours

Management

Management includes:

- Identification and treatment of underlying infection: this might be apparent but investigations to consider include chest X-ray, blood culture, urine microscopy and culture and LP.
- Antipyretics do not prevent febrile convulsions, they should be used to manage distress in the context of fever.
- Prolonged convulsions are treated as per status epilepticus (see Chapter 20).
- Parental education.

Prognosis

In simple febrile convulsions the prognosis is very good, although parents should be warned that one-third of children will have further febrile convulsions in their lifetime. Children typically grow out of this by 6 years of age. In children presenting with a simple febrile convulsion, there is a slightly higher risk of developing epilepsy compared with that of the general public (1%–2%). In children presenting with a complex febrile convulsion, a family history of epilepsy or abnormal neurodevelopment, the risk is higher (5%–10%).

An EEG may be warranted in the event of a complex febrile convulsion or in the presence of risk factors.

HEADACHE

Headache commonly occurs as a nonspecific feature of many illnesses and is often self-limiting. By contrast, it can be a feature of meningitis which can be life-threatening. Recurrent headaches are very common in children and there are many differential diagnoses to consider (Fig. 13.3); serious causes are rare. Red flag symptoms for headaches in children vary with age; children displaying Red flag symptoms may need imaging.

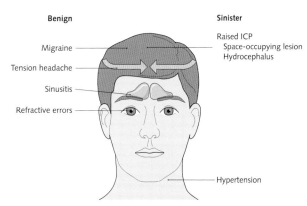

Fig. 13.3 Causes of recurrent headache. *ICP*, Intracranial pressure.

RED FLAG

Sinister causes include raised intracranial pressure, malignancy and intracerebral haemorrhage. Senior help and imaging should be considered in the presence of any of the following:

- sudden onset, severe headache
- morning headache and/or vomiting
- associated with straining (e.g., coughing or increased by lying down)
- weight loss
- progressing in severity
- associated seizures or focal neurology

History

The acronym SOCRATES can be useful for assessing pain and is easily applied to headache:

- *s*ite: frontal, temporal, bilateral or unilateral?
- *o*nset: gradual or sudden?
- *c*haracter: throbbing, tight, etc.
- *r*adiation: to the neck/face
- *a*ssociations: vomiting, photophobia, stiff neck, fever
- *t*ime course: duration of symptoms
- *e*xacerbating/relieving factors: analgesia, worse in the morning or with straining
- *s*everity: pain scoring (according to age)

Examination

Attention should be paid to the following signs in a child with headache:

- Blood pressure: hypertension (e.g., aortic coarctation is a rare cause of headache).

- Pulse: radial–femoral delay (coarctation).
- Visual acuity: refractive errors cause headache.
- Papilloedema: a late sign of raised ICP (Fig. 13.1).
- Focal neurological deficit: especially cerebellar signs (posterior fossa tumour).

Tension headaches

These are anxiety provoking but benign headaches affecting 10% of school children and can be difficult to treat. The aetiology is unknown but they are associated with stress. The classic history includes:

- felt across the forehead symmetrically
- band-like in nature
- gradual onset, duration less than 24 hours
- no associated nausea or vomiting
- often recur frequently

Management is mainly reassurance and to facilitate stress reduction. Simple analgesia can be used sparingly; however, overuse can exacerbate headache.

Migraine

The pathophysiology of migraine is poorly understood. It has a strong genetic predisposition and many sufferers are able to identify symptom triggers, which often include hormonal changes (menstruation), foods such as cheese and chocolate and stress.

Features of the headache typically include:

- unilateral and frontotemporal
- throbbing in nature
- with or without visual aura
- associated nausea, vomiting, abdominal pain, photophobia
- duration variable – hours to days

Migraine is classified by the International Headache Society into two main types: migraine with and without aura. Aura is defined as any reversible neurological features of gradual onset, which last less than 60 minutes.

Subtypes of migraine with aura include hemiplegic migraine and retinal migraine. Children are also susceptible to episodic syndromes associated with migraine which include cyclical vomiting, and abdominal migraine.

Management

Lifestyle advice including keeping well hydrated and ensuring good sleeping habits should be routine.

Medication options are limited in children with migraine. Start with simple analgesia such as paracetamol and ibuprofen. In acute management nasal triptans and antiemetics can be used. Preventative drugs such as propranolol should be guided by specialists.

Raised intracranial pressure

There are many causes of raised ICP including trauma, idiopathic intracranial hypertension, hydrocephalus, cerebral oedema and space-occupying lesions. Symptoms include:

- Headache worse in recumbent position (i.e., during the night or early morning).
- Pain is usually mild and diffuse.
- Nausea and vomiting.
- Visual disturbances.
- Personality changes may develop.

HINTS AND TIPS

Headache is rarely caused by a brain tumour but 70% of children with a brain tumour present with headache. The headache does not improve and gets progressively worse. It might wake the child at night, is worst in the morning and associated with vomiting. Most are in the posterior fossa and cause raised intracranial pressure.

Management

Acute management depends on the cause. General principles of emergency treatment are hypertonic saline and/or mannitol and steroids. More chronic conditions such as idiopathic intracranial hypertension and hydrocephalus are treated differently.

INFECTIONS OF THE CENTRAL NERVOUS SYSTEM

Meningitis

Acute meningitis is caused by a range of bacteria and viruses varying with age (Box 13.4), or more rarely by tuberculosis, fungal infections or malignant infiltration. The serious and potentially

BOX 13.4 PATHOGENS IN MENINGITIS

Bacterial	Viral	Other
Neonates:		
Group B streptococcus, *Escherichia coli*, *Listeria monocytogenes*		
	Children:	
Neisseria meningitidis, Streptococcal pneumonia, *Haemophilus influenzae* type B	Enteroviruses, Epstein-Barr virus, mumps	*Mycobacterium tuberculosis*, fungi (e.g., *Aspergillus* spp.), aseptic (no organism identified)

lethal nature of bacterial meningitis renders it most important. Viral meningitis is more common and, in the absence of encephalitis, is a less serious, self-limiting condition.

COMMON PITFALLS

The terms 'meningitis' and 'meningococcal disease' are often used incorrectly by health professionals and patients:

- Meningitis refers to inflammation of the meninges due to pathogens listed in Table 13.4.
- Meningococcal disease refers to a serious condition resulting from meningitis and *Neisseria meningitidis* bacteraemia.

Bacterial meningitis

The peak incidence is in under 5-year-olds with 80% of all cases in children under 16 years. Meningococcal meningitis accounts for over half of cases and in the UK subtype group B is the most common variety. Pneumococcal meningitis is uncommon but is associated with higher fatality and neurological sequelae.

The prevalence of different strains has changed over the years due to the availability of vaccines. The pathogens are carried in the nasal passages and invade the meninges via the bloodstream.

Clinical features

Early symptoms and signs are nonspecific, making diagnosis difficult, especially in infants.

Table 13.4 Differences between neurofibromatosis type 1 (NF1) and neurofibromatosis type 2 (NF2)

Feature	NF1	NF2
Incidence	About 1/5000	About 1/40,000
Inheritance	Autosomal dominant	Autosomal dominant
Family history	About 50% inherited	Mainly new mutations
Genetic cause	NF1 gene (chromosome 17q11.2)	NF2 gene (chromosome 22q11.2)
Café-au-lait spots	Characteristic	Uncommon
Skin neurofibromas	Common	Uncommon
Lisch nodules	Characteristic	Uncommon
Acoustic neuromas	Uncommon	Characteristic, often bilateral
Risk of central nervous system tumours	Common	Common

There might be irritability, poor feeding, vomiting, fever and drowsiness. More specific signs develop later, including:

- a bulging fontanelle
- neck stiffness and photophobia in the older child
- seizures
- nonblanching rash (see Fig. 20.10)
- septic shock (see Chapter 20)

Diagnosis

LP and cerebrospinal fluid (CSF) examination are the definitive tests. Blood cultures should be taken and LP performed as soon as possible if there are no contraindications; however, this must not delay treatment.

Contraindications to LP include signs of raised ICP (depressed conscious state, papilloedema or focal neurological signs), coagulopathy and septic shock. A computed tomography (CT) scan does not exclude raised ICP.

Other useful investigations include:

- full blood count
- C-reactive protein (may lag if caught early)
- coagulation screen
- blood cultures
- blood gas (to include lactate)
- blood glucose
- rapid diagnostic tests (e.g., meningococcal PCR; see Chapter 2)

Treatment

A high index of suspicion is necessary in young children in whom signs and symptoms are nonspecific.

Broad-spectrum intravenous antibiotic treatment is initiated using a third-generation cephalosporin (e.g., ceftriaxone or cefotaxime – in children under 3 months) or in infants under a month of age (not on NICU), amoxicillin and gentamicin. A febrile child with a purpuric rash in the community (i.e., suspected meningococcal disease) should be treated immediately with benzylpenicillin (intramuscularly or intravenously). This can be given by the general practitioner or by paramedics. They should then be transferred urgently to hospital.

Dexamethasone is used in children over 3 months to moderate the inflammatory response. This has been shown to reduce the incidence of some neurological sequelae (e.g., hearing loss).

HINTS AND TIPS

Meningococcal septicaemia can kill within hours and early antibiotic treatment significantly reduces mortality rates. Nothing should delay antibiotic treatment including lumbar puncture.

Children with signs of shock will need to be transferred to paediatric intensive care for ongoing management.

Prevention

Vaccines are available against the following causes of meningitis:

- *N. meningitidis* subtype C
- *N. meningitidis* subtype B
- *N. meningitidis* subtypes ACWY
- *Streptococcus pneumoniae*
- measles, mumps, rubella
- tuberculous (TB) meningitis

Many are now routinely within the vaccinations schedule; however, some are targeted to at-risk groups.

Complications

Acute complications include:

- cerebral oedema
- seizures
- syndrome of inappropriate antidiuretic hormone secretion (SIADH)

Late complications include:

- limb ischaemia
- neuropathic pain
- sensorineural deafness
- neurological sequalae (e.g., hemiplegia, epilepsy)

All children should have their hearing tested following confirmed meningitis.

All bacterial meningitis should be reported to the public health department (UK Health Security Agency) who will advise on prophylactic antibiotic cover for all household contacts to eradicate nasopharyngeal carriage.

Encephalitis

In encephalitis there is inflammation of the brain substance. Acute encephalitis is usually viral. The most common causes in the UK are:

- herpes simplex virus 1 and 2
- enteroviruses
- varicella

The common viral exanthems (measles, rubella, mumps and varicella) can all cause encephalitis by direct viral invasion of the brain or can be complicated by an immune-mediated postinfectious encephalomyelitis.

Clinical features

The clinical features include early nonspecific symptoms such as fever, headache and vomiting. This is then followed by the abrupt development of altered level of consciousness, personality change and/or seizures.

Diagnosis

Diagnosis is difficult acutely, and the workup is similar to that of suspected meningitis. EEG and MRI may show characteristic temporal lobe abnormalities. Isolation of the causative organism may be possible from CSF or blood, and it is especially important to send these for viral culture.

Management

Most children with encephalitis will be admitted to an intensive care unit. High-dose aciclovir should be given in all cases to cover herpes simplex until results of investigations are available.

Postinfectious syndromes

These can affect the brain or peripheral nervous system:

- Acute disseminated encephalomyelitis (postinfectious encephalomyelitis): demyelination of the brain and spinal caused by an immune-mediated inflammatory reaction to viral infection. It may follow any of the common viral exanthems.
- Acute cerebellitis: typically caused by varicella zoster.
- Acute postinfectious polyneuropathy: Guillain-Barré syndrome (see below).

Guillain-Barré syndrome

This demyelinating polyneuropathy follows 2 to 3 weeks after a viral infection with, for example, cytomegalovirus or Epstein-Barr virus, or infection with *Mycoplasma pneumoniae* or *Campylobacter jejuni*.

Clinical features

Guillain-Barré syndrome usually begins with fleeting sensory symptoms in the toes and fingers and progresses to a symmetrical, ascending paralysis with early loss of tendon reflexes. Autonomic involvement might occur, with dysrhythmias, and bulbar involvement can cause respiratory failure. The disease can progress over several weeks. The CSF protein is characteristically markedly raised without an increase in white cell count.

Management

Supportive care including assisted ventilation might be required. Respiratory function must be monitored closely by peak flow if the patient is not ventilated. Specific therapy includes immunoglobulin infusion and plasma exchange. Full recovery in children expected; however, there may sometimes be residual neurological impairment.

MALFORMATIONS OF THE CENTRAL NERVOUS SYSTEM

If severe, these cause foetal loss or early death. They encompass such important conditions as hydrocephalus and neural tube defects.

Hydrocephalus

Hydrocephalus is enlargement of the cerebral ventricles due to excessive accumulation of CSF.

The causes include congenital malformations as well as acquired conditions. Hydrocephalus may be caused by:

- overproduction of CSF
- impaired absorption of CSF
- obstruction (intraventricular or extraventricular; see Box 13.5)

Impaired CSF absorption is common and can be a result of a subarachnoid bleed or postmeningitis. Overproduction of CSF is rare and may be due to a choroid plexus tumour.

Clinical features

The presenting clinical features vary with age and can even be detected on antenatal ultrasound. In infants:

- Rapid and excessive growth of head circumference is noted.
- Anterior fontanelle is full or bulging.
- Sutures become separated.
- Scalp veins are prominent.
- Sun-setting sign (loss of upward gaze of the eyes, a late sign).

In older children, the clinical features are those of raised ICP (see Box 13.6).

BOX 13.5 CAUSES OF OBSTRUCTIVE HYDROCEPHALUS

Intraventricular obstruction	Extraventricular obstruction
Congenital malformations:	Congenital malformations:
• aqueduct stenosis, Dandy-Walker syndrome, intraventricular haemorrhage, ventriculitis, space-occupying lesions	• Arnold-Chiari malformation

BOX 13.6 SIGNS OF INCREASED INTRACRANIAL PRESSURE IN OLDER CHILDREN

- Altered sensorium.
- Headache.
- Vomiting (especially in the morning).
- Decerebrate/decorticate posturing.
- Abnormalities of pupillary size and reaction.
- Papilloedema (see Fig. 13.3).

Diagnosis

Diagnosis is confirmed by imaging. If the anterior fontanelle is still open, ultrasound is used to assess ventricular dilatation. A CT scan or MRI will establish the diagnosis and cause, and is useful for monitoring treatment and detecting complications.

Treatment

Treatment depends on the cause; however, insertion of shunt system is often required. These include ventriculoperitoneal or ventriculoatrial shunts. Complications of shunts include obstruction and infection.

Neural tube defects

These affect 2 in 1000 live births despite efforts to prevent the condition with folic acid and high-quality antenatal care. They are discussed in Chapter 15.

CEREBRAL PALSY

Cerebral palsy is a group of conditions affecting motor function and posture due to a nonprogressive lesion of the developing brain. It is useful to remember that although the lesion is nonprogressive, the clinical manifestations evolve as the child gets older. Children with cerebral palsy often have problems in addition to disorders of movement and posture, for example, with learning, reflecting more widespread damage to the brain.

The cause is unknown in many patients but identified risk factors can be categorized into antenatal, perinatal and postnatal insults (see Box 13.7). It is important to be aware that perinatal asphyxia is an uncommon cause (3%–21%) of cerebral palsy.

Clinical features

Cerebral palsy can present with:

- hypotonia in infancy
- feeding difficulties due to lack of oromotor coordination
- delayed motor milestones
- speech and language delay
- motor disorders (e.g., hypertonia, hemiplegia)

There is a vast spectrum of disease severity. Effects can range from having little to no physical disability and thriving in mainstream school to children who are nonverbal and have four-limb spastic quadriplegia.

Diagnosis

The diagnosis is clinical. Typically, there will be one or more of the following clinical signs:

- abnormal tone: hypertonia or hypotonia
- abnormal power (e.g., delay in motor milestones)

BOX 13.7 CAUSES OF CEREBRAL PALSY

Antenatal (80%)	Perinatal (10%)	Postnatal (10%)
Multiple gestations Congenital infection: • Rubella, cytomegalovirus, toxoplasmosis, cerebral dysgenesis • Shoulder dystocia, cord prolapse, antepartum haemorrhage (e.g., placenta praevia), hypoxic ischaemic encephalopathy	• Prematurity • Perinatal asphyxia • Intraventricular haemorrhage • Hyperbilirubinaemia (kernicterus) • Hypoglycaemia • Head injury • Central nervous system infection	• Meningitis, encephalitis • Late-onset IVH

BOX 13.8 PROBLEMS ASSOCIATED WITH CEREBRAL PALSY

Respiratory	Gastrointestinal	Musculoskeletal	Neurological/learning
Aspiration Recurrent pneumonia	Failure to thrive Feeding difficulties Gastro-oesophageal reflux Constipation	Delayed motor milestones Contractures Scoliosis	Learning difficulties Speech and language problems Hearing and visual impairment Seizures

---

• abnormal reflexes (e.g., brisk tendon reflexes or abnormal absence [or persistence] of primitive reflexes)
• abnormal movements (e.g., athetosis or chorea)
• abnormal posture or gait

Neuroimaging (e.g., MRI) may be indicated but is not diagnostic. Other investigations are often needed, for example, to exclude metabolic or genetic causes.

Classification

Cerebral palsy is classified according to the anatomical distribution of the lesion and the main functional abnormalities; 10% of cases are mixed.

Spastic cerebral palsy (70%)

Damage to the pyramidal pathways causes increased limb tone (spasticity), brisk deep-tendon reflexes and extensor plantar responses. Hypotonia might precede spasticity. The distribution of affected limbs allows further classification:

• Hemiplegia: paralysis affecting one side of the body.
• Diplegia: bilateral paralysis.
• Quadriplegia: all four limbs are affected. There is often truncal involvement, seizures and intellectual impairment. This is the most severe form.

Ataxic cerebral palsy (10%)

Caused by damage to the cerebellum or its pathways. Features include early hypotonia with poor balance, uncoordinated movements and delayed motor development.

Dyskinetic (athetoid) cerebral palsy (10%)

Caused by damage to the basal ganglia or extrapyramidal pathways (e.g., in kernicterus). The clinical presentation is often with hypotonia and delayed motor development. Abnormal involuntary movements, which include chorea (abrupt, jerky movements), athetosis (slow writhing continuous movements) or dystonia (sustained abnormal postures) might appear later.

Management

Management of cerebral palsy requires a multidisciplinary approach and a community paediatrician usually oversees the care. Prognosis in early infancy can be uncertain. Motor function may be worsened by hypertonia, which is treated by physiotherapy, muscle relaxants (e.g., baclofen), botulinum toxin injections to specific muscle groups or surgical intervention for severe contractures. Orthopaedic intervention is often beneficial (braces, surgery, special shoes). Attention must be paid to associated problems such as sensory deficits, learning difficulties and epilepsy (25%–50% of all children experience seizures), which are often difficult to control (see Box 13.8). An assessment of learning needs is important to optimize learning potential.

COMMUNICATION

A child with quadriplegic cerebral palsy requires round-the-clock care, which can put real strain on the whole family. Medical professionals should enquire about how

---

the family is coping, and signpost to services such as social and respite care. In addition, the history from a parent of a child with cerebral palsy is hugely important as they are the experts in their child and tend to know when something is not right.

NEUROCUTANEOUS SYNDROMES

Neurofibromatosis type 1 (von Recklinghausen disease)

Neurofibromatosis type 1 (NF1) is an autosomal dominant disorder affecting about 1 in 5000 live births. About 50% of cases result from new mutations of the NF1 gene (chromosome 17q11.2). Diagnostic clinical features include:

- an affected first-degree relative
- axillary or inguinal freckling
- café-au-lait patches on the skin (at least six must be present; 50% of normal individuals have at least one)
- Lisch nodules (pigmented hamartomas on the eye): usually seen after 5 years of age
- cutaneous neurofibromas (two or more)
- plexiform neurofibroma
- optic glioma
- characteristic bone/osseous lesion (typically include sphenoid dysplasia or pseudoarthrosis of a long bone)

Other features of NF1 include renal artery stenosis, macrocephaly, learning difficulties and seizures.

Neurofibromatosis type 2

Neurofibromatosis type 2 (NF2) is a distinct disease due to mutations in a different gene on chromosome 22. It is much rarer than type 1 (affecting 1 in 40,000 people) and is characterized by bilateral acoustic neuromata and other central nervous system (CNS) tumours.

The differences between type 1 and type 2 are outlined in Table 13.4. Management for both types includes annual surveillance including ophthalmology review, audiology, blood pressure and physical examination for signs of complications. An assessment of learning needs should also be undertaken.

Tuberous sclerosis

This is an autosomal dominant disorder affecting one in 7000 live births. Up to 75% of cases represent new mutations. It is genetically heterogeneous with one disease gene on chromosome 9 and a second gene on chromosome 16.

Classically it presents with seizures, learning difficulties and various cutaneous features including:

- facial angiofibromas (adenoma sebaceum)
- hypopigmented macules (ash leaf spots, seen with a Wood's light)
- shagreen patches
- periungual fibromas

It is a multisystem disease affecting not only the skin and brain but also the heart, lungs and kidneys (see Box 13.9).

Sturge-Weber syndrome

This sporadic disorder is characterized by:

- Unilateral facial naevus (port-wine stain) in the distribution of the trigeminal nerve.
- Angiomas involving the leptomeningeal vessels in the brain leading to seizures.
- Haemangiomas in the spinal cord.

There are abnormal blood vessels over the surface of the brain, which might be associated with seizures, hemiplegia and learning difficulties. Ocular involvement can result in glaucoma.

Brain imaging typically shows unilateral intracranial calcification with a double contour like a railway line and cortical atrophy.

ABNORMAL INVOLUNTARY MOVEMENTS

Abnormal involuntary movements in children may have many different aetiologies from metabolic movement disorders to simple tremors and can be part of syndromes. The different types of abnormal involuntary movements are detailed below:

- Tics (physical manifestation) and conversion disorders – will be covered in Chapter 18
- Tremors
- Dystonias
- Ataxia
- Myoclonus
- Choreas

Ataxia in childhood has many causes as in adulthood, however the incidence of these is different.

Creating a surgical/medical sieve to aid differential diagnoses can help when preparing for exams:

- Vascular disorders
- Brainstem encephalitis
- Trauma
- Autoimmune/postinfectious – acute cerebellar ataxia
- Inborn errors of metabolism
- Neoplastic – posterior fossa tumour
- Congenital – immunodeficiency (ataxia telangiectasia), Neurological (Friedrich's ataxia, spinocerebellar ataxia, Wilson disease)
- Degenerative – olivopontocerebellar degeneration, adrenoleucodystrophy
- Functional – conversion disorder

Chorea in paediatric populations can be caused by:

- Drugs: anticonvulsants, neuroleptics, benzodiazepine withdrawal, psychostimulants
- Vascular: stroke, cerebral palsy with dyskinesis
- Mitochondrial: mitochondrial encephalopathy with lactic acidosis and stroke (MELAS)
- Autoimmune: poststreptococcal, Sydenham chorea, systemic lupus erythematosus
- Endocrine: hyperthyroidism

INTRACRANIAL HAEMORRHAGE

This is fairly uncommon and as in adults is made up of four types of bleeds: extradural, subdural, subarachnoid and parenchymal haemorrhage. In this chapter, we will focus on subdural and subarachnoid bleeds due to their serious and slightly more frequent nature.

- Subdural haemorrhage (SDH) – these injuries usually occur through trauma. The overall incidence in infants is around 12 to 25 cases per 100 000. Sadly, most SDH are related to nonaccidental injury (NAI), however, it is important to have a good understanding of the other causes of this, such as those detailed below:
  - Meningitis
  - Coagulopathy
  - Vascular malformations
  - Rare metabolic disorders
- If the cause is thought to be due to NAI, then NICE guidance should be followed.
  - This would involve ensuring the child is clinically stable, maintaining the child in a place of safety and discussing with a senior paediatrician.
  - This should be covered further in the safeguarding section of this book (Chapter 19).

- Management of this would depend on the clinical status of the child and the degree of haemorrhage seen. If felt appropriate, neurosurgical opinion should be gathered.
- Subarachnoid haemorrhage (SAH) – these are fairly rare within paediatrics, affecting roughly 0.5% to 4.6% of children. The most common causes of these are usually vascular (aneurysm, arteriovenous malformation) or neoplastic in nature.
- There are certain genetic disorders and syndromes that can predispose children to SAH, such as Sturge-Weber syndrome, tuberous sclerosis, Marfan syndrome and Moya Moya disease, to name a few.
- The further investigation and management of the haemorrhage will depend on the clinical scenario and differentials.

The key investigations and management will be related to clinical findings.

NEURODEGENERATIVE DISORDERS OF CHILDHOOD

A large number of individually rare but important inherited diseases are associated with progressive neurodegeneration in childhood. Most are autosomal recessively inherited and genetic and biochemical defects have been established at a molecular level in many cases. Acquired forms do occur, such as prion disease and subacute sclerosing panencephalitis. Loss of acquired skills is the hallmark of a neurodegenerative disorder. Parental consanguinity increases the risk of such disorders.

Examples include:

- lysosomal storage diseases
  - sphingolipidoses (e.g., Tay-Sachs disease)
  - mucopolysaccharidosis (e.g., Hurler syndrome)
- peroxisomal disorders (e.g., adrenoleucodystrophy)
- trace metal metabolism disorders (e.g., Wilson disease, Menke syndrome)

Clinical features

It is important to distinguish between developmental delay and developmental regression – in delayed development, milestones are not achieved in time, but once attained, they are not lost. In regression, there is a gradual loss of milestones that have already been attained. The child may have a normal initial development, only to lose those skills later, indicating a progressive disorder of the brain.

Features of neurodegenerative diseases include:

- regression of milestones
- progressive dementia
- epilepsy
- visual loss
- ataxia

- alterations in tone and reflexes (depending on the precise pattern of nervous system involvement)

NEUROMUSCULAR DISORDERS

These are best considered according to their anatomical site (see Box 13.10) in the lower motor pathway. Genetic, infective, inflammatory and toxic factors can cause this group of disorders.

Clinical features

The hallmark of these disorders is weakness. They can present with:

- hypotonia
- delayed motor milestones
- weakness
- fatigability
- abnormal gait

Clinical features on examination include hypotonia, muscle weakness or wasting, abnormal gait and reduced tendon reflexes.

Diagnosis

Special investigations useful in the diagnosis of neuromuscular diseases include:

- muscle enzymes: serum creatine kinase is elevated in Duchenne and Becker dystrophies
- electrophysiology: nerve conduction studies and electromyography
- muscle or nerve biopsy
- DNA analysis, and genetic studies
- imaging: ultrasound, CT or MRI of muscle
- serum anti-acetylcholine receptor antibody testing for myasthenia gravis

Muscular dystrophies

This group of inherited disorders is characterized by progressive degeneration of muscle. The most common is Duchenne muscular dystrophy.

Duchenne muscular dystrophy

This X-linked recessive disease affects 1 in 4000 male infants. About one-third of cases are new mutations. The disease gene encodes dystrophin, and causes reduced production of the dystrophin protein, resulting in loss of myofiber membrane integrity – causing repeated cycles of necrosis and regeneration; fat and connective tissue progressively replace muscle – responsible for the clinical features.

Affected boys usually develop symptoms between 2 and 4 years of age. Independent walking tends to be delayed and affected children never run normally. Patients require a wheelchair by 12 years of age and die from congestive heart failure or respiratory failure in the third decade.

Clinical features

Associated clinical features include:

- pseudohypertrophy of calf muscles
- proximal muscle weakness
- positive Gower sign (evident at 3–5 years): the hands are used to push up on the legs to achieve an upright posture, indicating weakness of the pelvic girdle muscles
- scoliosis and contractures
- dilated cardiomyopathy
- recurrent respiratory infections and restrictive lung disease
- mild learning difficulties

Diagnosis

Most cases are confirmed by DNA analysis. Other investigations include raised serum creatine kinase (10–20 times normal), muscle biopsy and electromyography.

Management

Treatment is supportive. Walking can be supported by provision of orthoses and scoliosis can be helped by a truncal brace or moulded seat, a powered wheelchair is needed between 9 and 12 years of age. Early diagnosis is important to allow identification of female carriers and genetic counselling. Respiratory symptoms can be helped with noninvasive respiratory ventilation. Cardiomyopathy worsens with age and is often the cause of death.

Becker muscular dystrophy

This disease is milder than Duchenne muscular dystrophy but is caused by a mutation in the same gene. Dystrophin is present but much reduced and females can have mild symptoms. The average age of onset is much later (in the second decade of life) and the life expectancy is slightly longer.

BOX 13.10 NEUROMUSCULAR DISORDERS

Anterior horn cell	Peripheral nerve	Neuromuscular junction	Muscle
Spinal muscular atrophy	Hereditary neuropathy	Myasthaenia gravis	Muscular dystrophies
Poliomyelitis	Guillain-Barré syndrome		Myotonia
	Bell palsy		Congenital myopathies

Myotonic dystrophy

This is an autosomal dominant, trinucleotide repeat condition. It is a multiorgan disorder affecting muscle, endocrine system, cardiac function, immunity and the CNS.

Clinical features

- Hypotonia.
- Progressive muscle wasting.
- Typical facial features: inverted V-shaped upper lip, thin cheeks and high-arched palate.
- Myotonia: a characteristic feature, usually seen beyond 5 years. This is a slow relaxation of muscle after contraction, demonstrated by asking the patient to make tight fists and then to quickly open the hands.
- Arrhythmias, endocrine abnormalities, cataracts and immunologic deficiencies can also occur.

Diagnosis is by DNA analysis to show the CTG repeat. Serum creatine kinase is usually normal. Only supportive treatment is available.

Spinal muscular atrophies

Spinal muscular atrophies (SMA) are progressive degenerative diseases of motor neurons that may onset as early as foetal life. The more severe forms present in early infancy with severe hypotonia and weakness, whereas the late-onset forms present in later childhood. These disorders are characterized by hypotonia, generalized weakness and absent or weak tendon reflexes. Fasciculations – seen in the tongue, deltoids or biceps – are characteristic and indicate denervation of the muscle. Previously, children with the severe early-onset type rarely survived beyond 2 years, whereas intermediate forms lead to severe motor disability. However, recently treatments (nusinersen) have become available for specific types of SMA; this emphasizes the importance of rapid diagnostic tests (DNA results can be available within a matter of days) to guide appropriate management.

PERIPHERAL NERVE PALSIES IN CHILDREN

Bell palsy is an acute, idiopathic unilateral LMN palsy of cranial nerve 7 (facial nerve).

Not associated with other cranial neuropathies or brainstem dysfunction; 70% to 90% has a good prognosis of resolution in a few months.

Must consider other sinister and serious causes of facial nerve palsy before diagnosis. Importantly, Bell palsy can occur in severe hypertension – always check the blood pressure.

Aetiologies: infective (HSV1, VZV, mumps, rubella, EBV, Lyme disease), trauma (base of skull fracture, forceps delivery), neurological (Guillain-Barré syndrome, MS, mononeuropathy), neoplastic (posterior fossa tumour, parotid gland tumour, leukaemia), hypertension, or inflammatory (HSP, Kawasaki syndrome).

RED FLAGS

- Insidious onset >2 weeks
- Forehead sparing
- Fever
- Rash
- Ear pain
- Bilateral facial palsy

Investigations and management are based on clinical history, but can range from:

Checking BP (?hypertension), FBC with blood film (?leukaemia), infective screen (?HSV, HIV, Lyme disease).

Basic management of Bell palsy – care for eye (prevent dryness + abrasions), Corticosteroids (within 3–7 days of symptom onset).

Erb palsy has been described in Chapter 15, 'Neonates'.

Klumpke's palsy – a less common neuropathy compared to Erb palsy. This is a palsy associated with brachial plexus injury to nerves C8 and T1. It is associated to difficult vaginal injuries where the extraction has caused some stretching to the inferior brachial plexus. It can also occur in later life through injury or tumours developing close to the inferior brachial plexus. The child adopts a 'claw-like hand' where the elbow is bent and the hand is supinated and the wrist and fingers flexed.

Management ranges from physiotherapy (mild cases) to surgical intervention (severe cases).

VISUAL FIELD DEFICITS

These will be, to a large extent, covered by your adult medicine training. The neurology will remain constant however the aetiology will be slightly different.

This book will not delve into the visual field pathway and specific lesions causing specific signs, but rather will focus on the differences between adults and paediatric populations.

Some causes of paediatric visual field defects fall into these areas:

- Perinatal/postnatal insults – Cerebral palsy, periventricular leukomalacia
- Epilepsy (treatment of – medical and surgical)
- Tumours – craniopharyngiomas, pituitary adenomas, optic gliomas, meningiomas, neurofibromas
- Hydrocephalus (Arnold-Chiari malformations, tumours, neonatal brain haemorrhage, infection)

BOX 13.11 VISUAL ASSESSMENTS IN CHILDREN	
Age	**Visual assessment techniques**
Birth:	Observation of eye movements Ophthalmoscopy – examining for red/white reflex
0–1 years	– Optokinetic nystagmus (measuring ability of a child to follow an object while head remains stationary – optokinetic reflex) – Visual evoked potentials
1–3 years	Picture tests and identification, cover/uncover test
3–5 years	HOTV chart (Sheridan Gardiner), tumbling E chart, picture tests, Snellen charts, colour testing

– Stroke (infarct or haemorrhagic – usually secondary to other conditions – heart issues, sickle cell, tumours)

Visual screening (for types of assessments, see Box 13.11) is completed through childhood at birth (on newborn screening), 6 weeks at GP check-up, 7 to 8 weeks via health visitors and 4 to 5 years via orthoptists.

– Secondary screening (orthoptic visual screening) can be performed when concerns are raised by parents and healthcare professionals.

SQUINT AND AMBLYOPIA

A squint (strabismus) can be divided up into two causes:

a) Nonparalytic (concomitant)
b) Paralytic (incomitant/noncomitant)

Technical terms used to describe a squint are as follows:

a) Latent – squint eye misalign during cover test, but normal during uncovered period
b) Manifest – squinting eye corrects position when straight eye covered to focus on object
c) Convergent – also called esotropia – squint eye deviates towards nose
d) Divergent – also called exotropia – squint eye deviates away from nose
e) Constant
f) Intermittent
g) Accommodative – convergent squint that can occur in children with refractive errors or amblyopia
h) Nonaccommodative – convergent squint not associated with visual accommodation
i) Congenital
j) Acquired

The aetiology can be broadly categorized into the following:

1) Idiopathic
2) Due to a refractive error – hypermetropia
3) Visual loss (retinoblastoma, cataract, ocular malformations, optic neuropathy, amblyopia)
4) Ophthalmoplegia – central or peripheral (congenital, brain tumour, hydrocephalus, myasthenia gravis, head injury, postviral problems)

To investigate which type of squint is present a few tests need to be done. This is done via a combination of the following:

1) History (remember red flags, risk factors and family history)
2) Inspection of the eye
3) Hirschberg test (corneal light reflex test)
4) Cover test
5) Cover/uncover test
6) Eye movement assessment

HINTS AND TIPS

Risk factors for squint are:

1) Low birth weight and prematurity
2) Maternal smoking during pregnancy
3) Anisometropia or hypermetropia
4) FHx of squint
5) Others: assisted deliveries (forceps/lower segment caesarian section [LSCS]), pseudo squint, neurodevelopmental disorders

RED FLAG

If a squint is not seen and managed early, it can lead to the following:

• Amblyopia
• Loss of binocular vision/failure to develop binocular vision
• Social, developmental and psychological problems

When to refer to ophthalmology:

1) If there is any child with suspected or confirmed squint they should be assessed in an eye clinic
2) If a child has any of the following they should be assessed by an ophthalmologist
   a. Limited abduction
   b. Double vision
   c. Headaches
   d. Nystagmus
   e. Constant squint/worsening squint from 2 months of age

General management of a squint:

1) Correct refractive errors (glasses)
2) Eye patch + cycloplegics to train the 'bad eye'
3) Eye muscle exercises
4) Surgery to eye muscles

5) Botox (in certain circumstances)

General management of amblyopia:

1) Correct refractive errors (glasses)
2) Eye patch and cycloplegics
3) Surgery to eye muscles

● Chapter Summary

- An eyewitness description of a fit, faint or funny turn should always be sought, as this can be key to determining the cause.
- Epilepsy affects 5 in 1000 children. Seizure types are characterized according to where the electrical activity started in the brain (e.g., focal vs. generalized).
- Febrile convulsions are the commonest cause of seizures in childhood. A third of children will have recurrent febrile convulsions.
- Meningococcal meningitis is a life-threatening emergency.
- Cerebral palsy is a result of a nonprogressive lesion in the brain. It requires a multidisciplinary team approach to management.

UKMLA Conditions

Cerebral palsy and hypoxic-ischaemic encephalopathy
Epilepsy
Febrile convulsion
Migraine
Muscular dystrophies
Non-accidental injury
Peripheral nerve injuries/palsies
Raised intracranial pressure
Subarachnoid haemorrhage
Subdural haemorrhage
Tension headache
Visual field defects

UKMLA Presentations

Abnormal involuntary movements
Fits/seizures
Headache
Squint

Musculoskeletal system

INTRODUCTION

This chapter covers common paediatric abnormalities of the lower limbs, upper limbs, and spine. It also looks at rheumatological presentations in children, and skeletal dysplasias.

The immature skeleton has several key differences to be aware of when learning about childhood musculoskeletal disorders, particularly in trauma. These include:

- the presence of growth plates
- increased bone elasticity (protective against fractures)
- extremely active periosteum (promotes fracture healing)

Young children are often not able to communicate the site of pain, which can present a diagnostic challenge. There are also congenital musculoskeletal disorders that are important to detect to optimize growth and development.

LIMP

This is an extremely common presentation for lower limb pain in children and many centres will have a proforma to follow for history, examination and investigations.

Differential diagnosis

The list of conditions that can present with limp is substantial (Table 14.1). Many will self-resolve with supportive treatment; however, it is important to be able to identify serious causes.

Table 14.1 Causes of limp in children of different ages

Age	Common causes
Toddler (<4 years)	Developmental dysplasia of the hip Transient synovitis (irritable hip) Toddler's fracture
Child (4–10 years)	Transient synovitis (irritable hip) Perthes
Adolescents	Slipped upper femoral epiphysis
Any age	Traumatic fractures Nonaccidental injury Septic arthritis Osteomyelitis Reactive arthritis

History

Key points to ask in the history are:

- duration of symptoms
- precipitating factors (e.g., any history of trauma or prodromal illness)
- symptom progress (e.g., is it improving, the same or worse?)
- red flags symptoms (see Table 14.2)
- birth and developmental history
- family history

Examination

Examination is key to identify the site of pain and to target investigations (i.e., imaging).

The paediatric Gait, Arms, Legs and Spine assessment is used as a standardized screening tool to identify an abnormal joint or painful area (see Further reading). This should be carried out in all children with limp as it will not only help identify the site of pain but also ensures the child is examined top to toe (important when considering many differentials including nonaccidental injury).

Specific signs to look out for in the limping child include:

- gait pattern (e.g., antalgic, toe walking, circumductive, Trendelenburg)
- deformity or swelling
- erythema or warmth
- bruising
- limb length discrepancy
- signs of hypermobility
- systemic features (tachycardia, fever, pallor, lymphadenopathy, eye involvement, rash)

Table 14.2 Red flags in the limping child

Symptoms	Associated conditions
Night-time wakening, night sweats, fatigue, anorexia, weight loss	Malignancy
Redness or swelling or fever	Infection (e.g., osteomyelitis, septic arthritis)
Unexplained rash, early morning pain/stiffness	Inflammatory bone disease
Unexplained bruising	Haematological disease (e.g., haemophilia) Nonaccidental injury
Severe pain or agitation following traumatic injury	Compartment syndrome

Investigations

In many cases of limp there is no need for investigations. When performing investigations, many are aimed at excluding serious causes requiring urgent attention.

Investigations to consider are described here.

Blood tests
- Full blood count.
- C-reactive protein (CRP), erythrocyte sedimentation rate (ESR).
- Blood culture.

Imaging
- Plain X-rays.
- Ultrasound.
- Computed tomography (CT).
- Magnetic resonance imaging (MRI).

DISORDERS OF THE HIP AND KNEE

Developmental dysplasia of the hip

This term has replaced the previous name of 'congenital dislocation' of the hip. Perinatal hip instability results in progressive malformation of the hip joint; it occurs in 1.5 in 1000 births.

Developmental dysplasia of the hip (DDH) represents a spectrum of hip instability ranging from a dislocated hip to hips with various degrees of acetabular dysplasia (in which the femoral head is in position but the acetabulum is shallow). It was previously thought to be entirely congenital, but is now known to also occur after birth in previously normal hips.

All babies are screened clinically but 40% will be missed and the use of national ultrasound screening remains controversial; 90% will spontaneously resolve without treatment.

Cause
The cause is unknown but risk factors for DDH include:
- breech delivery
- family history (there is a genetic predisposition)
- first born
- female sex
- race (lowest amongst Africans)
- oligohydramnios
- neuromuscular disorders
- syndromes
- congenital muscular torticollis
- congenital foot abnormalities

Warning signs might be:
- delayed walking
- a painless limp
- a waddling gait

Asymmetrical skin creases are found in 30% of all infants and are an unreliable guide; 10% of all babies have hip clicks and this is normal.

Diagnosis
Babies are screened at birth and at the 6-week check using the Barlow and Ortolani manoeuvres:
- *Barlow test* – apply backward pressure to each femoral head in turn and a subluxable hip is suspected on the basis of palpable partial or complete displacement.
- *Ortolani test* – apply forward pressure to each femoral head in turn, in an attempt to move a posteriorly dislocated femoral head back into the acetabulum.

With increasing age, contractures form and these tests are then unhelpful. Typically, on examination there is limited abduction (a supine child should be able to abduct fully the flexed hip up until the age of 2 years). The femur might be shortened (Allis sign). Ultrasound scanning is diagnostic. Hip X-rays are not useful until after 4 to 5 months of age when the femoral head has ossified (Fig. 14.1).

Management
This involves:
- Pavlik harness (fixing the hip in abduction, effective in <6-month-olds)
- reduction (open or closed)

For children in whom the diagnosis has been delayed, open reduction and derotation femoral osteotomy should be performed.

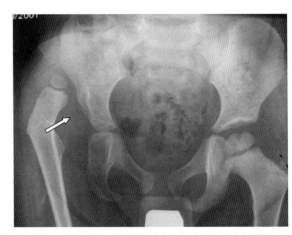

Fig. 14.1 X-ray of developmental dysplasia of the right hip in an older child.

In these cases, accelerated degenerative changes might necessitate total hip replacement in early adult life.

Transient synovitis (irritable hip)

This common self-limiting condition occurs in children between 2 and 10 years of age often following a viral infection. Typical features are:

- sudden onset of pain
- limp
- refusal to bear weight on the affected side

There is no pain at rest. Examination reveals limited passive abduction and rotation in an otherwise well and afebrile child. The critical differential diagnosis is septic arthritis, in which the child is febrile, unwell with pain at rest and refusal to move the affected joint.

Diagnosis

This is a diagnosis of exclusion and it is important to distinguish transient synovitis from septic arthritis and osteomyelitis:

- Acute-phase reactants: white blood cell count (WBC), CRP and ESR. These are raised in septic arthritis and osteomyelitis.
- Blood cultures: negative in transient synovitis.

Hip X-ray does not enable differentiation and therefore may not be useful; ultrasound is the preferred initial imaging modality. If there is doubt, the joint should be aspirated for culture followed by prompt administration of intravenous antibiotics.

HINTS AND TIPS

Irritable hip is a diagnosis of exclusion. Septic arthritis must always be considered, as the management is very different.

Management

Treatment is supportive (analgesia and avoiding strenuous activity) because the condition spontaneously resolves in 2 weeks.

National Institute for Health and Care Excellence (NICE) guidance on children with suspected transient synovitis states:

- Safety net (seek medical attention if the child becomes unwell or febrile).
- Regular analgesia (particularly nonsteroidal antiinflammatories).
- Review in 48 hours to check symptoms resolving.
- Review in 7 days from onset to check symptoms completely resolved.
- Undertake investigations (bloods, ultrasound, X-ray) if diagnostic uncertainty or any red flag symptoms.

Perthes disease

This idiopathic disorder is a result of a vascular injury causing osteonecrosis of the femoral head prior to skeletal maturity. This leads to flattening and fragmentation of the femoral head during a key period of growth in childhood. Revascularization and reossification occur with the restoration of blood supply, which may have resulted in deformity.

Risk factors include:

- a previous family history
- male sex: it is five times more common in boys

The incidence is 1 in 2000 and is most common amongst boys aged 4 to 8 years.

Clinical features

There is an insidious onset of limp between the ages of 3 and 12 years. Pain, which might be intermittent, can be felt in the hip, thigh or knee (known as referred pain). Between 10% and 20% of cases are bilateral. Abduction and rotation are limited on examination.

Diagnosis

Hip X-rays are diagnostic (Fig. 14.2). If there is doubt, then serial films or MRI might be necessary.

Management

The prognosis in most children is good, especially in those under 6 years of age or if less than half of the femoral head is involved. In younger children, only analgesia and mild activity restriction with bracing are needed.

In older children, and those in whom more than half of the epiphysis is involved, permanent deformity of the femoral head occurs in over 40%, resulting in earlier degenerative arthritis. In severe disease, the hip needs to be fixed in abduction, allowing the femoral head to be covered and moulded by the acetabulum

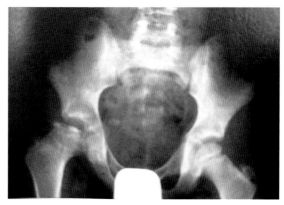

Fig. 14.2 Anteroposterior pelvic radiograph showing Perthes disease of the right hip: the process is in the fragmentation phase and the epiphysis appears to be in pieces.

as it grows. Plaster, calipers or femoral or pelvic osteotomy may achieve fixation.

Slipped upper femoral epiphysis

In this relatively uncommon condition of unknown aetiology, the femoral head slips off the metaphyseal head. Slipped upper femoral epiphysis occurs during the adolescent growth spurt and:

- Is most common in boys.
- Obesity is a risk factor.
- Is associated with endocrine disorders (hypothyroidism).
- Typically presents between 10 and 15 years of age.
- Presents with limp, hip pain or referred knee pain.

About 30% have a family history and 20% are bilateral, although not necessarily synchronous. Diagnosis is by plain radiographs (see Fig. 14.3) and unstable hips are an orthopaedic emergency. Complications are avascular necrosis and premature fusion of the epiphysis. Management is by pinning the femoral head or osteotomy. Nonsurgical treatment is ineffective and will result in deformity.

DISORDERS OF THE SPINE

Back pain

Back pain is uncommon before adolescence. In infants and young children it is usually associated with significant pathology such as connective tissue disorders or malignancy and referral is always warranted.

In adolescence back pain may be caused by:

- Muscle spasm or soft-tissue pain: this is usually a sports-related injury and should be treated with analgesia and physiotherapy.
- Scheuermann disease: osteochondrosis (idiopathic avascular necrosis of an ossification centre) of the lower thoracic vertebrae. This is the most common cause of hyperkyphosis in children. This is usually progressive and is treated with physiotherapy, bracing and surgery if severe.
- Scoliosis (see below).
- Spondylolisthesis: a defect in the pars interarticularis of (usually) L4 or L5 where there is anterior shift of the vertebral body on the one below.
- Vertebral osteomyelitis or discitis: these two conditions often present together, with severe pain on weight-bearing and walking, associated with local tenderness and grumbling fever.
- Tumours: these can be benign or malignant and might cause spinal cord compression.
- Idiopathic: this is a diagnosis of exclusion, but pain might be exacerbated by stress and poor posture.

HINTS AND TIPS

Think of malignancy in bone pain. Suggestive features include:

- nonarticular bone pain
- back pain
- pain out of proportion to swelling or at night
- weight loss

RED FLAG

Spinal cord compression is a surgical emergency and it may be the first presentation of a malignancy. Symptoms include:

- back pain
- lower limb weakness
- sphincter dysfunction (incontinence)
- sensory deficits
- abnormal gait

Any malignancy has potential to cause cord compression but neuroblastoma, sarcomas and non-Hodgkin lymphoma are commonly associated. The diagnosis is confirmed by urgent magnetic resonance imaging of the spine and treatment is with corticosteroids followed by either radiotherapy, chemotherapy and/or surgery.

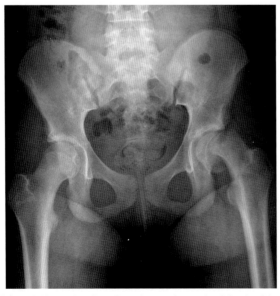

Fig. 14.3 X-ray showing slipped upper femoral epiphysis of the left hip.

Scoliosis

This is lateral curvature of the spine associated with a rotational deformity and affects 4% of children. It is classified according to cause:

- vertebral abnormalities (e.g., hemivertebra, osteogenesis imperfecta)
- neuromuscular (e.g., polio, cerebral palsy)
- miscellaneous (e.g., idiopathic (most common), dysmorphic syndromes)

Idiopathic scoliosis

As well as lateral curvature, there is rotation of the thoracic region, which can be demonstrated as the child bends forwards and a rib hump is noted (Fig. 14.4). More than 85% of cases occur in adolescence. It is more common in girls and often there is a family history. Pain is not a typical feature. The scoliosis is monitored clinically, radiologically and chronologically:

- Mild curves are not treated.
- Moderate curves are braced (23 hours a day until growing has stopped).

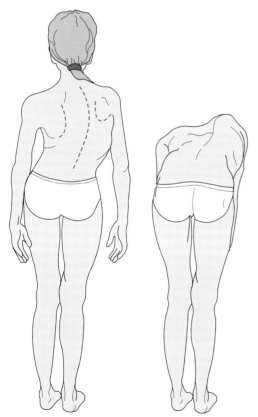

Fig. 14.4 Idiopathic adolescent scoliosis showing vertebral rotation (rib hump) when bending forward.

- Severe curves (>40°) require surgery that fuses the spine, and therefore terminates further growth. Untreated severe curves result in later degenerative changes, pain and unwanted cosmetic appearance.

Torticollis

Acute torticollis (wry neck) is a relatively common and self-limiting condition in young children, often associated with an upper respiratory tract infection.

The most common cause of torticollis in infants is a sternomastoid tumour. A mobile nontender nodule within the sternomastoid muscle is noticed in the first few weeks of life. The cause is unknown. It usually resolves by 1 year and is managed conservatively by passive stretching and physiotherapy. Surgery is reserved for persistent cases. There is an association with developmental dysplasia of the hip – and this is investigated for (usually by ultrasound) when recognized.

DISORDERS OF THE UPPER LIMBS

There are many abnormalities that affect the upper limbs, the majority of which are congenital and include:

- polydactyly (extra digits) – this can be isolated or as part of a syndrome
- syndactyly (fused digits)
- radial club hand – strong association with TAR syndrome (thrombocytopaenia and absent radius) and Holt-Oram syndrome (limb malformations and cardiac lesions)

It is important to fully consider function as well as aesthetic appearance before considering surgery. The management will likely be led by orthopaedic and/or plastic surgeons.

Pulled elbow

This is commonly seen in emergency departments and presents as a child suddenly unwilling to move their arm. This occurs when the radial head becomes subluxed, typically by swinging or picking up a child by their arms. Treatment is by reduction: the doctor holds and then supinates the arm whilst feeling for a clunk at the distal humerus.

DISORDERS OF THE SKULL

Craniosynostosis

This is premature fusion of the cranial sutures (Fig. 14.5). Most affected infants present soon after birth with an abnormal skull shape; the shape of the skull depends on which sutures have

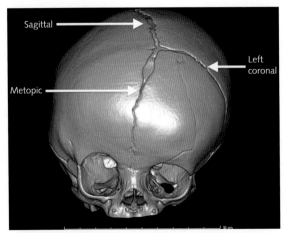

Fig. 14.5 Craniosynostosis on three-dimensional computed tomography reconstruction. This image shows fusion of the right coronal suture causing plagiocephaly.

fused. The sagittal suture is most commonly involved causing a long, narrow skull (scaphocephaly).

This can lead to raised intracranial pressure, affect neurodevelopment and have cosmetic implications and is therefore surgically corrected at around 10 months of age.

FRACTURES

Paediatric fractures have a unique classification system due to the presence of growth plates. This is known as the Salter-Harris classification (see Fig. 14.6). Type II is the commonest type and describes a fracture that goes through the physeal plate and involves part of the metaphysis.

Whilst fractures are common in children, it is important to identify those that are associated with child abuse. Some general rules are:

- fractures in nonmobile children
- spiral fractures of the femur/long bones (in children <15 months)
- rib fractures (and no history of major trauma)
- multiple fractures at different healing stages
- delay in presentation

BONE AND JOINT INFECTIONS

Osteomyelitis

This describes infection of the bone, usually by haematogenous spread. It may also be secondary to trauma or following surgery. Early recognition and aggressive treatment can be life- and limb-saving. Infection typically starts in the metaphysis where there is relative stasis of blood. Two-thirds of cases occur in the femur and tibia. The peak incidence is bimodal, occurring in the neonatal period and in older children (9–11 years).

In all age groups, the most common pathogen is *Staphylococcus aureus,* although group B *Streptococci* and *Escherichia coli* occur in neonates.

Children with sickle cell disease have increased susceptibility to *Salmonella* osteomyelitis. *Mycobacterium tuberculosis* should also be considered.

Clinical features

Infants present with fever and refusal to move the affected limb. Older children will localize the pain and are also systemically unwell with fever. Examination reveals exquisite tenderness over the affected bone usually with warmth and erythema. Pain limits movement.

Diagnosis

The acute-phase reactants (WBC, CRP and ESR) are usually significantly elevated (in comparison to in transient synovitis). Blood cultures are positive in more than half of the cases; however, aspiration of the bone may be necessary to identify the organism and its sensitivity. X-rays tend to be normal in the first 10 days, so MRI and ultrasound scans have become the chosen modalities of imaging. Periosteal elevation or radiolucent necrotic areas on plain X-rays can usually be demonstrated between 2 and 3 weeks.

Treatment

Early treatment with intravenous antibiotics is imperative until there is clinical improvement and normalizing of the acute-phase

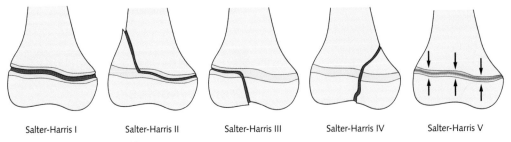

| Salter-Harris I | Salter-Harris II | Salter-Harris III | Salter-Harris IV | Salter-Harris V |

Fig. 14.6 Salter-Harris classification of fractures.

reactants. Several weeks of oral antibiotics follow. Failure to respond to medical treatment is an indication for surgical drainage.

Complications include:

- chronic osteomyelitis
- septic arthritis
- growth disturbance and limb deformity (occurs if the infection affects the epiphyseal plate)

Septic arthritis

Purulent infection of a joint space is more common than osteomyelitis and can result in bone destruction and considerable disability. The incidence is highest in children younger than 3 years of age and is usually haematogenous in origin. Other causes include:

- osteomyelitis
- infected skin lesions
- puncture wounds

In infants, the hip is the most common site (the knee is the most common site in older children). *S. aureus* is the most common pathogen in all age groups. The organisms are similar to those found in osteomyelitis and the conditions might occur together.

Clinical features

The typical presentation is a painful joint with:

- fever
- irritability
- refusal to bear weight

Infants often hold the limb rigid (pseudoparalysis) and cry if it is moved. There is tenderness and a variable degree of warmth and swelling on examination.

Investigation

The acute-phase reactants are usually elevated. Aspiration of the joint space might reveal organisms and the presence of white cells.

Ultrasound can identify effusions and X-rays are often initially normal or show a nonspecific, widened joint space.

Management

Early and prolonged intravenous antibiotics are necessary. Surgical drainage is indicated only if the infection is recurrent or if it affects the hip.

RHEUMATIC DISORDERS

There are many rheumatic disorders that can affect children. This book will consider the following conditions:

- juvenile idiopathic arthritis (JIA)
- juvenile dermatomyositis
- systemic lupus erythematosus (SLE)
- Postinfectious/reactive

Juvenile idiopathic arthritis

JIA has replaced the term 'juvenile chronic arthritis'. The incidence is 1:10,000 children and the term 'JIA' includes several clinically and genetically different disorders:

- systemic JIA
- polyarticular onset: rheumatoid factor (RF)-negative JIA
- polyarticular onset: RF-positive JIA
- oligoarticular arthritis
- enthesitis-related arthritis
- psoriatic arthritis

It is diagnosed after arthritis in one or more joints for 6 weeks after excluding other causes in a child and can then be subclassified according to mode of onset and disease pattern (see Table 14.3). Blood investigations for antinuclear antibodies (ANAs) and RF are helpful in classification but are not diagnostic.

Table 14.3 Classification of juvenile idiopathic arthritis

	Systemic	Polyarticular	Oligoarticular
Number of joints involved	Variable	More than four	Four or less
Joints involved	Knees Wrist Ankle and tarsal	Any joint	Knees Ankles Elbows Hips spared
Pattern	Symmetrical	Symmetrical	Asymmetrical
Rheumatoid factor	Negative	Positive or negative	Negative
Eye involvement	No	No	Yes in 30%
Clinical course	Poor in one-third	Good if rheumatoid factor negative	Good

Systemic JIA (previously Still disease)

This mainly affects children under 5 years. The arthritis primarily affects the knees, wrist, ankles and tarsal bones. Other features include:

- high daily spiking fever
- a salmon-pink rash
- lymphadenopathy and hepatosplenomegaly
- arthralgia, malaise and myalgia
- inflammation of pleura and serosal membranes (pleuritis, pericarditis)

There is often no arthritis at presentation. One-third will have a progressive course and the worst prognosis occurs in the younger age.

Polyarticular JIA

Polyarticular infers that five or more joints are involved, and it can be subdivided based on the presence or absence of RF.

Rheumatoid factor-negative polyarticular JIA

This affects all ages and all joints but spares metacarpophalangeal joints. Limitation of the motion of the neck and temporomandibular joints is seen. It has a good prognosis, but disease may be prolonged.

Rheumatoid factor-positive polyarticular JIA

This mainly affects females over 8 years and causes arthritis of the small joints of the hand and feet. Hip and knee joints are affected early and rheumatoid nodules are seen over pressure points. There might be a systemic vasculitis; functional prognosis is poor due to joint destruction.

Oligoarticular JIA

Early onset is the most common subtype and typically occurs in young girls under 6 years with asymmetric arthritis involving knees, ankle and elbows. ANAs are nearly always present and one-third will develop chronic iridocyclitis (inflammation of the iris and ciliary body, which comprise the anterior uveal tract: anterior uveitis). The definition 'oligoarticular' requires that the disease affects four or fewer joints and it has a good prognosis, but eye involvement is independent of the joints. There is a subclass called 'extended oligoarticular' in which more than four joints are affected after 6 months; this has a poorer prognosis.

HINTS AND TIPS

Ophthalmological screening with a slit lamp to detect anterior uveitis is especially important in children with oligoarticular juvenile idiopathic arthritis.

Diagnosis

Useful tests for the evaluation of JIA include:

- Full blood count: anaemia occurs in systemic disease.
- Acute-phase reactants: elevated.
- RF: negative in the majority.
- ANA.
- X-rays: soft-tissue swelling in early stages. Bony erosion and loss of joint space later.

Management

A multidisciplinary team approach is required. This will encompass:

- Physiotherapy: to optimise joint mobility, prevent deformity and increase muscle strength.
- Analgesia: pain control and suppression of inflammation are achieved by high-dose nonsteroidal antiinflammatory drugs (NSAIDs; e.g., ibuprofen and naproxen).
- Disease-modifying drugs (see Table 14.4).

COMMON PITFALLS

It is important not to forget that arthritis can be associated with other chronic diseases, for example, inflammatory bowel disease, cystic fibrosis and immunodeficiency syndromes. This highlights the need for a thorough systemic review within the history.

Table 14.4 Drugs used in treatment of juvenile idiopathic arthritis

Drug	Comments
Corticosteroids	First line, commonly required for symptom management. Can be given orally, intravenously or intraarticularly. Many side effects with prolonged use in high doses including stunted growth, Cushing syndrome and osteoporosis.
Methotrexate	Second line, for control of arthritis. Potentially serious side effects including myelosuppression, hepatotoxicity and Stevens-Johnson syndrome.
Biological agents	
For example, tocilizumab (anti-interleukin-6)	For prolonged systemic features in systemic juvenile idiopathic arthritis. Side effects include neutropaenia and abnormal liver function.
Antitumour necrosis factor-alpha agents (e.g., etanercept)	Alternative to methotrexate if not tolerated or for resistant arthritis.

Juvenile dermatomyositis

This is a rare disorder affecting 3 in 1 million children. The diagnosis is clinical and presents with:

- heliotrope facial rash (blue/purple rash over eyelids)
- periorbital oedema
- Gottron papules (thick, scaly and red rash over the small joints of the hand, elbows and knees)
- proximal muscle weakness

Raised muscle enzymes, myopathic changes on electromyography and a characteristic approach on muscle biopsy confirm the diagnosis. Management includes physiotherapy for strengthening and to prevent contractures, speech and language team involvement if palatal or oesophageal muscles are affected, long-term corticosteroids and immunosuppression. The disease can be difficult to control and can be associated with serious complications such as interstitial lung disease.

Systemic lupus erythematous

This often presents in childhood and is more common in girls and amongst the African race. It is a multisystemic, chronic autoimmune disease with a hugely variable clinical picture (see Table 14.5).

Diagnosis

This can depend on which systems are involved but commonly includes:

- Blood tests: 95% of patients are ANA positive and 65% are positive for antibodies to double-stranded DNA. Antiphospholipid antibodies infer thrombotic risk.
- Urine tests: proteinuria, albuminuria and casts confirm renal involvement.
- Renal biopsy.
- Imaging (brain MRI, ECHO as indicated).

Table 14.5 Clinical features of systemic lupus erythematosus by system

System involved	Description
Skin	Malar rash (erythematous rash over cheeks sparing nasolabial folds), photosensitivity
Constitutional	Fever, weight loss, fatigue
Musculoskeletal	Arthralgia, polyarthritis
Renal	Glomerulonephritis, renal failure
Cardiac	Pericarditis, myocarditis
Central nervous system	Depression, seizures, chorea
Haematological	Thrombotic risk (lupus anticoagulant), cytopaenias
Respiratory	Pneumonitis, interstitial lung disease, effusions

Management

Management is according to disease severity. Most will require NSAIDs, corticosteroids and hydroxychloroquine. A stepwise progression is then made to other immunosuppressants such as methotrexate and azathioprine and monoclonal antibody therapy. Antiplatelet treatment may be used prophylactically or warfarin for confirmed thrombosis.

Despite the advances in immunomodulating therapies, SLE is still associated with significant morbidity and mortality.

Postinfectious and reactive arthritis

These are a group of rheumatological processes that occur 3 days to 6 weeks after infection. Reactive arthritis typically occurs post-gastrointestinal (*Campylobacter* sp.) or urogenital infection (*Chlamydia trachomatis*). Postinfectious arthritis is usually caused postinfectious illness (not including gastrointestinal or urogenital). The joint inflammation is caused by immune complexes in the absence of any local pathogen.

Reactive arthritis may have a variable course which may remit or progress to chronic spondyloarthritis, whereas postinfectious are usually transient and short lived.

Classically reactive arthritis will affect males ages 20 to 40, is associated with being HLA-B27 positive and presents with a triad of symptoms:

- Arthritis – predisposition for lower limbs
- Urethritis
- Conjunctivitis/painful red eye

However, in children this triad is much more uncommon and may present with other features (dependent on age):

Dactylitis, enthesitis, keratoderma blennorrhagicum, and other systemic features such as fever, malaise and fatigue

Investigation

Bedside – urine and stool microscopy, culture and sensitivity, and urine for *Chlamydial* sp.
Bloods – FBC, CRP + ESR, U+E, LFTs, ASOT
Special – joint aspiration (if one swollen hot joint), HLA-B27 genetics

Management

NSAIDs.

Treatment of bacterial infection with appropriate antibiotics if still present.

GENETIC SKELETAL DYSPLASIAS

Achondroplasia

See Chapter 16.

Osteogenesis imperfecta (brittle bone disease)

Osteogenesis imperfecta (OI) is a heterogeneous group of disorders caused by mutations in type I collagen genes; the commonest (considered here) resulting from mutation in the COL1A1/2 genes. All are now recognized to have autosomal dominant inheritance (specifically, for types II–IV, a dominant negative effect, where mutations in the affected gene cause change in the protein structure and how it functions, a qualitative effect on collagen, rather than the quantitative effect with type I), characterized by fragile bones, frequent fractures and short stature.

- Classic nondeforming OI with blue sclerae (previously type I); fractures (varying from a few to 100) often start when starting to walk (and fall) are more easily managed, and heal without deformity; stature is normal – severity is considered mild.

- Perinatally lethal OI (previously type II) most dying from respiratory insufficiency (small thorax, flail chest) within the first week of life; the sclerae are dark blue.
- Progressively deforming OI (previously type III) fractures occur from birth with normal handling. Considered intermediate severity – death can occur from respiratory insufficiency (as type II), but otherwise individuals are typically of extremely short stature, most require mobility assistance. Fractures are very difficult to manage and heal with deformity.
- Common variable OI with normal sclerae (previously type IV); this is the most variable presentation from moderately severe to very mild short stature, multiple fractures that heal with mild to moderate deformity.

Management is by aggressive orthopaedic treatment of fractures to correct deformities and genetic counselling of the parents.

● Chapter Summary

- It is vital to ask about red flag symptoms when taking a history from a limping child to identify malignancy and bone infections.
- Children with osteomyelitis are typically unwell with fever and significantly raised inflammatory markers compared to those with transient synovitis.
- Screening in those high risk for developmental dysplasia of the hip is important as clinical examination may miss the diagnosis.
- Back pain is rare in young children and warrants referral. Idiopathic scoliosis is common in adolescent girls.
- There is a classification system for types of juvenile idiopathic arthritis which has implications for treatment and prognosis.

UKMLA Conditions
Idiopathic arthritis
Reactive arthritis
Septic arthritis

UKMLA Presentation
Acute joint pain/swelling
Musculoskeletal deformities

Foetal and neonatal life is best regarded as a continuum. Many factors from before conception to delivery influence the health of the newborn infant.

Definitions

'Neonate' refers to an infant less than 1 month old. Perinatal mortality rate is defined as the total number of stillbirths and neonatal deaths that occur per 1000 total births (see Fig. 15.1 for further definitions). In the UK although this rate has continued to fall, a national target has been set to half the rate by 2030. Social deprivation and babies of Black or Asian ethnicity continue to have the highest rates of perinatal and neonatal deaths in the UK.

MATERNAL AND FOETAL HEALTH

Many maternal conditions or lifestyle choices can affect the foetus. The chance of a good outcome can be enhanced by simple interventions, including prior to conception:

- Avoiding smoking and alcohol.
- Folic acid supplements: reduce risk of neural tube defects.
- Immunization: flu and whooping cough vaccines are routinely recommended for all pregnant women.
- Minimize infection risk: avoid exposure to toxoplasmosis (via cat's litter), listeriosis (unpasteurized dairy products) and chicken pox exposure if not varicella immune.
- Optimizing treatment of maternal conditions such as hypertension, diabetes mellitus and epilepsy.
- Genetic counselling for couples at risk of inherited diseases.

FOETAL ASSESSMENT AND ANTENATAL DIAGNOSIS

Several methods for assessing the growth, maturation and wellbeing of the foetus are available, including:

- ultrasound
- Doppler blood flow studies
- foetal echocardiography
- foetal magnetic resonance imaging (MRI)

Antenatal diagnosis is now available for many disorders using the methods shown in Fig. 15.2.

Screening for trisomy 21 (Down syndrome), 18 (Edwards syndrome) and 13 (Patau syndrome) is routinely offered. The combined test at 12 weeks includes:

- maternal age-related risk
- nuchal translucency (neck-skin fold thickness) on ultrasound
- pregnancy-associated plasma protein A levels
- free β-human chorionic gonadotrophin levels

Antenatal diagnosis can allow the option of termination to be offered, therapy to be given or neonatal management to be planned in advance.

MATERNAL CONDITIONS AFFECTING THE FOETUS

Organogenesis occurs during the embryonic period (weeks 2–9) with many organs structurally complete by the end of the second

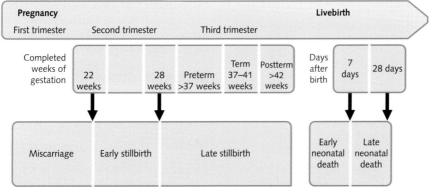

Fig. 15.1 Terminology used in antenatal and neonatal periods.

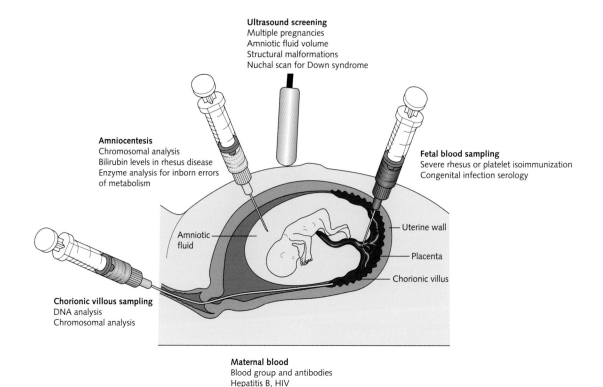

Ultrasound screening
Multiple pregnancies
Amniotic fluid volume
Structural malformations
Nuchal scan for Down syndrome

Amniocentesis
Chromosomal analysis
Bilirubin levels in rhesus disease
Enzyme analysis for inborn errors
of metabolism

Fetal blood sampling
Severe rhesus or platelet isoimmunization
Congenital infection serology

Amniotic
fluid

Uterine wall

Placenta

Chorionic villus

Chorionic villous sampling
DNA analysis
Chromosomal analysis

Maternal blood
Blood group and antibodies
Hepatitis B, HIV
Maternal serum α–fetoprotein for neural tube defects
Test for Down syndrome risk estimation

Fig. 15.2 Methods of antenatal diagnosis. *HIV,* Human immunodeficiency virus.

trimester. Therefore disease and medications affecting the first and second trimesters carry the highest risk of congenital anomalies.

Maternal diseases

Diabetes mellitus
Potential foetal problems include:

- Congenital malformations: there is a threefold increase (especially cardiac malformations).
- Macrosomia: the foetal insulin response to hyperglycaemia promotes excessive growth, which predisposes to difficulties during delivery.

Potential neonatal problems include:

- Hypoglycaemia: transient early hypoglycaemia occurs due to foetal hyperinsulinism; early feeding can usually prevent this.
- Respiratory distress syndrome (RDS).
- Polycythaemia (haematocrit >0.65).

Hypertension
High blood pressure can lead to preeclampsia and eclampsia, which carry significant maternal morbidity and mortality risks.

It also infers an increased risk of miscarriage, stillbirth, preterm delivery and intrauterine growth retardation.

Maternal thyroid disease
Transplacental thyroid-stimulating antibodies can be transmitted to the foetus from women with Graves disease causing neonatal thyrotoxicosis. Neonatal thyroid function tests should be checked at 7 to 10 days or earlier if symptomatic.

Other autoimmune disorders can affect the foetus such as systemic lupus erythematous, which is associated with increased risk of miscarriage and congenital heart block. Maternal thrombocytopaenia (most commonly idiopathic) can cause a transient thrombocytopaenia in the neonate, leading to intracranial haemorrhage.

Maternal drugs affecting the foetus

Several medications in addition to alcohol and narcotics have potential teratogenic effects (Table 15.1).

Maternal infections and the foetus

A number of infections acquired by the mother can affect the foetus. Transmission can occur in utero, during labour or postpartum (Box 15.1).

Table 15.1 Medications that can harm the foetus

Drug	Adverse effects
Cytotoxic agents (e.g., methotrexate)	Congenital malformations
Phenytoin	Foetal hydantoin syndrome (growth retardation, microcephaly, hypoplastic nails)
Sodium valproate	Neural tube defects
Carbamazepine	Growth retardation, craniofacial abnormalities
Lithium	Cardiac defects (Ebstein anomaly)
Isotretinoin	Congenital malformations, cardiac defects
Warfarin	Interferes with cartilage formation, risk of cerebral haemorrhage and microcephaly
Thalidomide	Limb shortening (phocomelia)
Drug abuse	
Alcohol	Foetal alcohol syndrome (characteristic facies, septal defects, learning difficulties)
Opiates (heroin/methadone)	Growth retardation, prematurity, drug withdrawal in neonate (tremors, hyperirritability, seizures)
Cocaine	Miscarriage, prematurity, cerebral infarction

BOX 15.1 INFECTIONS TRANSMITTED IN UTERO TO THE FOETUS: TORCH ACRONYM

T	Toxoplasmosis
O	
R	Rubella
C	Cytomegalovirus
H	Herpes simplex virus Human immunodeficiency virus
+ Others	Syphilis Listeria monocytogenes

Cytomegalovirus

Cytomegalovirus (CMV) is the most common congenital infection with an incidence of 3:1000 live births. About 1% of women acquire a primary CMV infection in pregnancy and it can be transferred in utero or via oral or genital routes. Many infants with congenital CMV are asymptomatic and develop normally; however, severe congenital infection causes:

- intrauterine growth restriction (IUGR)
- hepatosplenomegaly and jaundice
- thrombocytopaenia
- microcephaly, intracranial calcification and chorioretinitis

Long-term sequelae include cerebral palsy, epilepsy, learning difficulty and sensorineural hearing loss, which may develop later in childhood.

Diagnosis is made by virus isolation, especially from urine and saliva. To confirm congenital infection, specimens for viral isolation must be taken within 3 weeks of birth. Treatment is with ganciclovir; however, this is not curative and can cause bone marrow suppression.

Rubella

Congenital rubella is rare but causes severe defects especially during the first trimester. It should also always be thought of in the growth-restricted neonate with sensorineural deafness (see Box 15.2 for clinical features).

Rubella immunoglobulin G (IgG) is routinely screened for antenatally, and women who are seronegative should be immunized after delivery. Immigrants to the UK from countries where rubella vaccination is not routine are at particular risk.

Pregnant women exposed to rubella should be tested for rubella IgG and IgM regardless of previous serological testing. A high likelihood of congenital rubella infection early in pregnancy is an indication for offering termination.

Varicella zoster virus

Most women are immune from past infection with chickenpox and are therefore not at risk. The timing of infection corresponds to risk of severe disease or complications. Maternal risk of severe disease

BOX 15.2 CLINICAL FEATURES OF CONGENITAL RUBELLA

Growth retardation

Hepatosplenomegaly

Congenital heart disease:
- patent ductus arteriosus
- pulmonary stenosis

Eye:
- glaucoma
- cataract
- retinopathy

Ear:
- sensorineural deafness

is highest in the late second or third trimester. With maternal infection in the first 20 weeks of pregnancy 'congenital varicella syndrome' can occur, with an incidence of 1% to 2%; characterized by:

- cicatricial skin lesions (scars)
- malformed digits and limbs
- cataracts, chorioretinitis
- central nervous system damage

Infection one week before or after delivery results in the foetus receiving a high viral load but little in the way of maternal antibodies. Before varicella zoster immunoglobulin (VZIG) was introduced, 50% of deaths from varicella zoster virus (VZV) in children under one occurred in this group.

Exposed susceptible women can be treated with VZIG and aciclovir. Neonates exposed in the high-risk period should also be treated with VZIG. Intravenous (IV) aciclovir should be used if lesions develop in neonates and they should have ophthalmology follow-up.

Human immunodeficiency virus

Vertical transmission from mother to infant can occur in utero, during birth or postnatally by breastfeeding. The exact risk by each of these routes is uncertain but overall vertical transmission rate is now less than 1% and pregnant women are routinely screened for human immunodeficiency virus (HIV).

Prevention centres on reducing maternal viral load to undetectable and, if this is achieved, then vaginal delivery is possible. All newborns born to HIV-positive mothers receive zidovudine for the first weeks of life. Depending on the risk of vertical transmission and any drug resistance found in the mother, other agents such as lamivudine and nevirapine can be added. In the UK and other high-income countries, mothers are advised not to breastfeed, to reduce the risk of postpartum transmission. They should be provided with both free formula milk and lactation suppression. Babies are followed up until confirmed seronegative.

ETHICS

You should not assume that a mother has disclosed her human immunodeficiency virus status to her partner, family and friends. Paediatricians have a duty of care to the newborn, but this should not be at the expense of the mother's right to confidentiality and her autonomy. This must be handled sensitively.

Toxoplasmosis

Infection with the protozoan parasite *Toxoplasma gondii* occurs from the ingestion of raw or undercooked meat, or from oocytes excreted in the faeces of infected cats. Most infections are asymptomatic. Antenatal screening is not routine in the UK; surveillance data suggests congenital infection occurs in 3.4/100,000 live births. Transmission is unlikely where the mother has seroconverted prior to pregnancy. Transmission is more likely where seroconversion occurs later in pregnancy; however, more serious disease occurs when the transmission is in the first trimester. Clinical manifestations at birth can include:

- chorioretinitis
- hydrocephalus
- intracranial calcification
- neurological damage

Infants with asymptomatic infection may still develop chorioretinitis in later life.

NORMAL NEONATAL ANATOMY AND PHYSIOLOGY

There are characteristic features of newborn anatomy and physiology that are important and these are considered in turn.

Size and growth

The average infant born at full term in the UK, which includes any infant born between 37 and 42 weeks, weighs about 3500 g. Boys weigh approximately 250 g more than girls. Infants of 2500 g or less are classified as 'low birthweight'. During the first 5 days, up to 10% of birthweight is lost, especially in breastfed babies. This is usually regained by 7 to 10 days and the average weight gain is 200 g per week in the first month.

Skin

At birth the skin is covered with a greasy protective layer, the vernix caseosa. The underlying skin is immature, with a thin epithelial layer and incompletely developed sweat and sebaceous glands. Combined with the high surface area-to-body mass ratio, babies are prone to heat and water loss. Premature babies in particular can struggle to thermoregulate. There are numerous benign skin lesions that occur in the neonatal period (see Chapter 12).

Head

The average occipitofrontal head circumference (OFC) is 35 cm and this should be plotted on a growth chart. Moulding of the head might be present following vaginal birth; however, this resolves spontaneously and parents should be reassured. There are two soft spots (fontanelles) in the neonatal skull (see Fig. 15.3). The anterior fontanelle closes between 9 and 18 months of age and the posterior closes by 6 to 8 weeks.

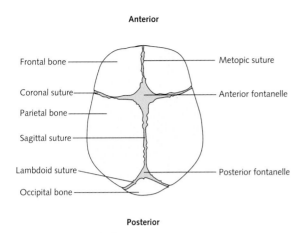

Fig. 15.3 Neonatal skull.

Respiratory system

Key changes must occur at birth to allow the newborn to convert from dependence on the placenta to breathing air:

- In utero, the airways and lungs are filled with amniotic fluid. Oligohydramnios can lead to small and underdeveloped lungs (pulmonary hypoplasia).
- The lung fluid is removed by squeezing of the thorax during vaginal delivery. There is also reduced production and increased resorption mediated by foetal catecholamines during labour and after birth.
- Surfactant lines the air–fluid interface of the alveoli and reduces the surface tension thereby facilitating lung expansion and the first breaths. This is associated with a fall in pulmonary vascular resistance.

Babies are obligate nose breathers and their respiratory rate is variable ranging between 30 and 50 breaths/min. Periodic breathing is normal and describes when a baby takes rapid shallow breaths followed by a pause of several seconds.

Cardiovascular system

Major changes in the lungs and circulation allow adaptation to extrauterine life.

In the foetal circulation, the right-sided (pulmonary) pressure exceeds the left-sided (systemic) pressure. Blood flows from right to left through the foramen ovale and ductus arteriosus (Fig. 15.4). At birth, these relationships reverse:

- Left-sided (systemic) pressure rises with clamping of umbilical vessels.
- Right-sided (pulmonary) pressure falls as the lungs expand and the rising partial pressure of oxygen (PO_2) triggers a prostaglandin-mediated vasodilatation.

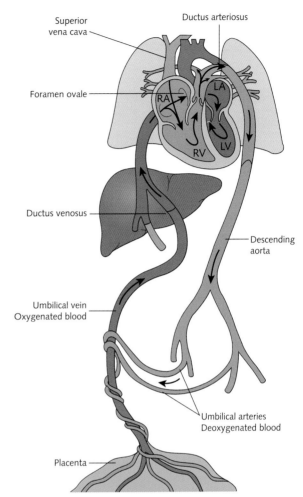

Fig. 15.4 Foetal circulation. *A,* Left atrium; *LV,* left ventricle; *RA,* right atrium; *RV,* right ventricle.

- The foramen ovale and ductus arteriosus close functionally shortly after birth. The ductus closes due to muscular contraction in response to rising oxygen tension.
- Certain forms of congenital heart disease are 'duct dependant', that is, flow through the duct is necessary for oxygen delivery and closure of the duct precipitates sudden deterioration (see Chapter 3).

Gastrointestinal system

Most infants over 35 weeks' gestation have developed the coordination necessary to 'latch on' and suck from breast or bottle. Meconium is usually passed on day 1 and delay beyond 24 hours is abnormal. With effective feeding meconium is replaced by yellow stool by day 3 or 4. Immaturity of the liver enzymes responsible for conjugation of bilirubin is responsible for 'physiological jaundice', which can occur from the second day of life.

RED FLAG

When there is delayed passage of meconium, you must exclude anorectal atresia. Once you have confirmed there is an anus, other differentials include meconium ileus, which is associated with cystic fibrosis, and Hirschsprung disease.

Genitourinary system

Urine production occurs during the second half of gestation and accounts for much of the amniotic fluid. The infant should void within the first 24 hours of life and this often occurs during delivery (thus can go unnoticed). Renal concentrating ability is diminished in neonates.

Haematopoietic and immune system

The newborn's red cells contain foetal haemoglobin, which has a higher affinity for oxygen than adult haemoglobin. The haemoglobin concentration of cord blood ranges from 150 to 200 g/L (mean 170 g/L). Delayed cord clamping is now recommended standard practice, reducing mortality (by 32% in preterm birth) and improving maternal and infant health, but it should not delay any required resuscitation.

The neonatal immune system is immature compared to older children and adults due to:

- impaired neutrophil reserves
- diminished phagocytosis and intracellular killing capacity
- decreased complement components
- low IgG_2, leading to infections with encapsulated organisms

Maternal antibodies (IgA) cross the placenta and are also found in breast milk, which provides some protection against infection.

Central nervous system

Myelination is incomplete at birth and continues during the first 2 years of life. A limited behavioural response repertoire is sufficient for survival and babies are born with primitive reflexes including rooting (searching for a nipple or teat), sucking and a startle (Moro) reflex. Newborn infants sleep for a total of 16 to 20 hours each day.

BIRTH

The short journey down the birth canal is potentially hazardous. Here we consider:

- normal care and resuscitation of the term newborn
- birth-related asphyxia
- birth injuries

Assessment and care at a normal birth

Even during normal birth there is a short period of oxygen deprivation; however, the baby then begins to breathe within a few seconds. The Apgar score is a commonly used assessment of the infant's condition (Table 15.2). The Apgar score is an indicator of intrapartum asphyxia but can also be influenced by maternal sedation or analgesia, gestational age and any cardiac, pulmonary or neurological disease of the infant. Most babies will establish respirations spontaneously after delivery, or if apnoeic, will respond to stimulation. However, a few will need more extensive resuscitation (Fig. 15.5).

Perinatal asphyxia

Perinatal asphyxia refers to a condition in which the foetus is acutely deprived of oxygen before, during or after birth. The majority of cases occur intrapartum, although 20% occur antepartum, and for a similar number it is not possible to determine the timing, a smaller number occur postnatally. Often the aetiology is unclear. Risk factors include preeclampsia, placental abnormalities, sepsis and IUGR. The incidence in developed countries has fallen to around 2 per 1000 live births.

The insult results in foetal hypoxia, hypercapnia and acidosis which manifest during labour as:

- foetal bradycardia (rate under 120 beats/min)
- foetal tachycardia (rate over 160 beats/min)

Table 15.2 Apgar score

Criteria	Score		
	0	1	2
Appearance (skin)	Blue or pale	Extremities blue	Pink
Pulse	Absent	<100 beats/min	>100 beats/min
Grimace (response to stimulation)	None	Weak	Cries
Activity (muscle tone)	Limp	Some flexion	Active movements
Respiratory effort	None	Weak	Cries

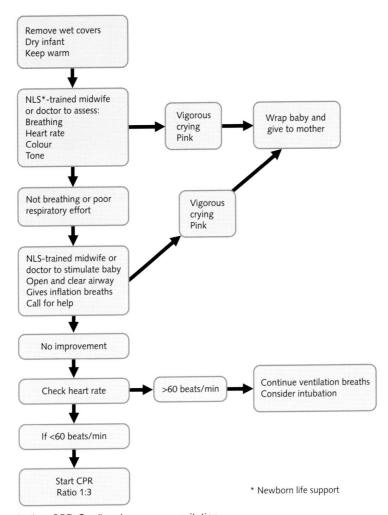

Fig. 15.5 Neonatal resuscitation. *CPR*, Cardiopulmonary resuscitation.

- abnormal pattern of deceleration during or after uterine contractions
- acidosis: pH <7.20 on foetal scalp blood sampling or cord blood gas
- meconium staining of the liquor

These signs are an indication for prompt delivery as hypoxic insults can affect all organ systems (Table 15.3). The brain is relatively protected due to autoregulatory mechanisms, however effects can be severe and irreversible.

Hypoxic-ischaemic encephalopathy

This describes the neurological manifestations of perinatal hypoxic injury. It may be classified using the Sarnat criteria as:

- Mild: lethargy followed by a period of hyperalertness with irritability but normal tone. There may be impaired feeding

Table 15.3 Complications of perinatal asphyxia

Organ	Complication
Brain	Hypoxic-ischaemic encephalopathy
Heart	Hypoxic cardiomyopathy, hypotension
Lungs	Persistent pulmonary hypertension
Guts	Ileus and necrotizing enterocolitis
Kidneys	Acute tubular necrosis
Blood	Disseminated intravascular coagulation

for 1 to 2 days. There are no focal signs or seizures. Prognosis is good.
- Moderate: hypotonia with reduced movements and conscious level. Seizures are often seen. Variable prognosis.

- Severe: coma with absence of spontaneous movement and reflexes. Seizures are usually seen and may be frequent. Multiorgan failure is often present. Morbidity and mortality are high.

Neuronal injury occurs in two phases: the acute injury caused by hypoxia at time of the event and the reperfusion injury which occurs between 6 and 72 hours post insult. Supportive care is therefore vital in minimizing damage and reducing morbidity. Total body cooling has been shown to reduce neurodisability in moderate to severe hypoxic-ischaemic encephalopathy (HIE; TOBY trial). This involves inducing hypothermia for 72 hours followed by gradual rewarming to protect the brain from reperfusion damage. It does not reduce mortality rates but improves outcomes in survivors. Neurological function and seizures can be monitored using an amplitude-integrated electroencephalogram (cerebral function monitor (CFM)) which provides some indication of prognosis.

In addition to cooling, close supportive management is needed including:

- respiratory support
- anticonvulsants for seizures
- fluid restriction
- circulatory support with inotropes if necessary

MRI and electroencephalogram can assist in predicting the outcome as cystic lesions or cerebral atrophy may appear in the ensuing weeks.

BIRTH INJURY

Physical injury during labour and delivery is relatively uncommon. Predisposing factors include:

- Breech presentation.
- Cephalopelvic disproportion.
- Macrosomia.
- Instrumental delivery (forceps or ventouse extraction). Injuries can occur to soft tissues, nerves or bones.

Common injuries include:

- Bruising.
- Cephalohaematoma: (haematoma of the scalp, limited by suture lines, usually benign) especially following ventouse delivery.
- Brachial plexus injury: for example, Erb palsy, especially following shoulder dystocia. The hand is held in the waiter's tip position (adduction and internal rotation of the arm, extension of forearm and flexion of the wrists and finger).
- Facial palsies: following forceps delivery (often resolves spontaneously, may cause feeding problems).

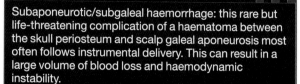

RED FLAG

Subaponeurotic/subgaleal haemorrhage: this rare but life-threatening complication of a haematoma between the skull periosteum and scalp galeal aponeurosis most often follows instrumental delivery. This can result in a large volume of blood loss and haemodynamic instability.

THE NEWBORN

Size and gestational age

Newborn infants might be small because they have been born preterm or because they are small in relation to their gestational age (small for dates). Some useful definitions are shown in Table 15.4.

Small for gestational age

This can be a normal occurrence as some babies are constitutionally small due to their genetics. Alternatively, it can represent IUGR, which can be caused by:

- Foetal problem: chromosomal disorders and congenital infections (more likely if the head circumference is also proportionally reduced, termed 'symmetrical IUGR').
- Placental/maternal problem: placental insufficiency caused by preeclampsia, advanced maternal age, smoking and multiple pregnancy (these cause asymmetrical IUGR, with brain growth relatively spared as an adaptive response).

The foetus with IUGR is at risk from hypoxia and death and is closely monitored using cardiotocography (CTG) and Doppler ultrasound to profile blood flow velocity in the uterine and umbilical arteries.

Postnatal problems encountered by the foetus with IUGR include:

- hypothermia
- hypoglycaemia from low fat and glycogen stores

Table 15.4 Definitions by weight

Term	Definition
Low birthweight	<2500 g
Very low birthweight	<1500 g
Extremely low birthweight	<1000 g
Small for gestational age	Birthweight <10th centile for gestational age
Large for gestational age	Birthweight >90th centile for gestational age

- polycythaemia (haematocrit >0.65)
- necrotizing enterocolitis (NEC)

Large for gestational-age infants

The most common cause of macrosomia is maternal diabetes mellitus. Potential associated problems include birth asphyxia from a difficult delivery and birth trauma, especially from shoulder dystocia, and neonatal hypoglycaemia if the mother had diabetes in pregnancy.

Feeding difficulties

Difficulty establishing feeding can occur with both breastfed and bottle-fed infants. This can be normal but can also be the first sign of an underlying problem.

Breastfeeding

There are many benefits to breastfeeding, which are listed in Chapter 21, and it should be encouraged by antenatal education. Potential problems include:

- Sleepy baby: newborns are often sleepy; however, jaundice, infection and hypoglycaemia can exacerbate this.
- Difficulty latching: this is common and midwives should support women by observing their technique. Look for inverted nipples, tongue-tie and cleft palate.
- Cracked nipples: this can cause severe discomfort for the mother.
- Poor milk supply: initially only drops of colostrum (early breast milk rich in protein, vitamins and immunoglobulins) are produced. This is replaced by full-fat breast milk usually by day 5.

Bottle feeding

Potential problems include:

- Incorrect reconstitution: electrolyte abnormalities which if severe could cause seizures.
- Overfeeding: this can cause reflux and vomiting.
- Inadequate sterilization: gastroenteritis (mainly in developing countries).

Weight gain in infants

Many babies lose weight in the first week. Full-term infants should regain their birthweight by day 7 to 10 and preterm babies by day 14.

> **HINTS AND TIPS**
>
> You should be familiar with how to plot a baby's growth on a centile chart and how to interpret it. There are different growth charts for boys and girls, preterm babies and Down syndrome.

Vomiting

Babies often regurgitate (posset) small amounts of milk during and between feeds. This is of no pathological significance and should not be confused with vomiting (the forceful expulsion of gastric contents).

Vomiting in the newborn could reflect systemic disease or intestinal pathology (Table 15.5). It is important to exclude serious causes, and some important radiological findings include:

- dilated bowel loops in obstruction (e.g., malrotation, volvulus)
- 'double bubble' in duodenal atresia
- pneumatosis (gas in bowel wall) in necrotizing enterocolitis
- free air in perforation (look under the diaphragm or request a lateral view)

> **RED FLAG**
>
> Bile-stained vomit indicates intestinal obstruction until proven otherwise: always ask if the vomit was green.

> **HINTS AND TIPS**
>
> Blood-stained vomit in the newborn might be due to swallowed maternal blood during delivery or from cracked nipples. It could also be due to haemorrhagic disease of the newborn caused by vitamin K deficiency, so check for other signs of bleeding.

Neonatal jaundice

Jaundice is common and occurs in most newborns, especially preterms. It can be classified as conjugated or unconjugated or by timing of symptom onset.

Recognition and treatment of severe neonatal hyperbilirubinaemia are important to avoid bilirubin encephalopathy or kernicterus (irreversible brain damage due to deposition of bilirubin in the basal ganglia). Early evaluation of conjugated hyperbilirubinaemia (>20 µmol/L) is important to allow early (<6 weeks) diagnosis and treatment of biliary atresia.

Jaundice in the first 24 hours

This is always pathological and must be investigated, the most common being excess haemolysis and sepsis. Neonatal haemolysis refers to the destruction of red blood cells by maternal IgG antibodies that cross the placenta during pregnancy resulting in disease.

Table 15.5 Vomiting in the newborn

Cause	Clinical signs	Examples
Intestinal obstruction	Bilious vomiting Abdominal distension High pitched or absent bowel sounds Tachycardia	Small bowel: – duodenal atresia (associated with Down syndrome) – malrotation ± volvulus – meconium ileus (associated with cystic fibrosis) Large bowel: – Hirschsprung disease – anorectal atresia
Necrotizing enterocolitis	Bilious vomiting Distended, shiny abdomen Haemodynamic instability	Associated with prematurity, perinatal hypoxia, congenital heart defects and infection
Tracheo-oesophageal fistula	Frothy mucoid vomiting Respiratory distress Failure to pass nasogastric tube	Many types
Infection	Vomiting and diarrhoea Temperature instability Rash Floppy	Gastroenteritis Urinary tract infection Meningitis Septicaemia
Raised intracranial pressure	Bulging fontanelle Sun-setting eye gaze	Brain tumour Hydrocephalus
Congenital adrenal hyperplasia	Vomiting Hyponatraemia Hyperkalaemia Ambiguous genitalia	21-Hydroxylase deficiency

Rhesus (Rh) haemolytic disease of the newborn

Rh status is determined by the presence or lack of major D Rh antigen on erythrocytes. Rh disease occurs when an Rh-negative mother is exposed to Rh antigen, either through pregnancy with an Rh-positive infant or through blood transfusion. The alloimmune response results in destruction of foetal red blood cells and the subsequent haemolysis, anaemia and jaundice can be severe. In some cases this can even result in foetal hydrops and death. The incidence has fallen since checking maternal Rh status has been made routine at antenatal booking. This allows for the administration of anti-D Ig, which is given to Rh-negative mothers shortly after giving birth to an Rh-positive infant. It is also given after potentially sensitizing events (e.g., antepartum haemorrhage). Disease typically affects the second pregnancy and severity increases with subsequent pregnancies.

ABO incompatibility

This occurs when there is a mismatch between the maternal and foetal blood group. ABO incompatibility is more common and less severe than Rh haemolytic disease, although they can present similarly with anaemia, jaundice and a positive direct antiglobulin test (DAT). The usual combination is a group O mother as they possess antibodies to both group A and group B antigens. No prior sensitization is needed in ABO incompatibility.

Jaundice at 2 days to 2 weeks

The most common cause is physiological jaundice. This is due to a combination of increased red cell breakdown and immaturity of the hepatic enzymes resulting in an unconjugated hyperbilirubinaemia. Prematurity, bruising, polycythaemia and dehydration can exacerbate it. Physiological jaundice usually peaks on the third day of life.

'Breast milk' jaundice affects 15% of healthy breastfed infants, although the cause remains unknown. Both physiological and breast milk jaundice usually resolve spontaneously but often require monitoring and occasionally treatment.

Prolonged jaundice (>2 weeks)

Prolonged jaundice (>2 weeks in term infants, >3 weeks in premature infants) is usually an unconjugated hyperbilirubinaemia, the causes of which are listed in Table 15.6. These infants must be examined for signs of dehydration, sepsis or obstructive jaundice.

Biliary atresia describes obliteration of all or part of the biliary tree and results in progressive liver disease. It is treated with surgery (the Kasai procedure; Fig. 15.6).

Investigations for babies presenting with prolonged jaundice include measurement of conjugated fraction, full blood count, blood group (mother and baby), DAT, urine culture and thyroid function. A glucose-6-phosphate dehydrogenase level may also be measured, particularly in infants of Mediterranean origin.

Table 15.6 Causes of neonatal jaundice

Onset	Cause
Less than 24 hours old	Excess haemolysis: • immune mediated – rhesus or ABO incompatibility • intrinsic red blood cell defects – glucose-6-phosphate dehydrogenase (G6PD), pyruvate kinase deficiency or hereditary spherocytosis Congenital infections
Between 24 hours and 2 weeks old	Physiological jaundice Breast milk jaundice Infection (e.g., urinary tract infection) Excess haemolysis, bruising or polycythaemia
Persistent jaundice after 2 weeks old	Unconjugated: • breast milk jaundice • infections (e.g., urinary tract infection) • excess haemolysis (e.g., ABO incompatibility) G6PD deficiency: • hypothyroidism (screened for in newborn) Galactosaemia Conjugated (>15% of total bilirubin): • biliary atresia • neonatal hepatitis • alpha-1-antitrypsin deficiency

Management of neonatal jaundice

Clinical estimation of the severity is unreliable and transcutaneous or plasma bilirubin must be measured. The bilirubin level must be measured and plotted on the treatment threshold graphs developed by National Institute for Health and Care Excellence (NICE). Treatment depends on the cause and may simply involve reassurance in physiological jaundice or feeding support in breast milk jaundice.

If the level is above the treatment threshold, the options are:

• phototherapy (sometimes with intravenous immunoglobulin in cases of rhesus or ABO haemolytic disease)
• exchange transfusion if above this threshold on the graph (whilst continuing phototherapy)

Babies may require several hours to several days of phototherapy. Phototherapy may be stopped when the serum bilirubin is more than 50 below the treatment line and a rebound bilirubin should always be checked after stopping.

Phototherapy

Blue light (not ultraviolet) of wavelength 450 nm converts the bilirubin in the skin and superficial capillaries into harmless water-soluble metabolites, which are excreted in urine and through the bowel. The eyes are covered to prevent damage and supplementary feeds are often given to counteract increased losses from skin.

Exchange transfusion

This is required if the bilirubin rises to levels considered dangerous despite phototherapy. It rapidly reduces the level of circulating bilirubin, and in isoimmune haemolytic disease also removes circulating antibodies and corrects anaemia. Techniques vary, but conventionally the exchange is done via umbilical artery and vein catheters. Aliquots of baby's blood (10–20 mL) are withdrawn, alternating with infusions of donor blood of the same volumes. It carries risks associated with transfusion, fluid overload, electrolyte imbalance and depletion of coagulation factors.

Complications

Bilirubin encephalopathy occurs when unconjugated bilirubin is deposited in the brain, especially in the basal ganglia and cerebellum. Early signs include lethargy and hypotonia and later they may develop seizures, irritability and hypertonia. The long-term sequelae include choreoathetoid cerebral palsy, sensorineural deafness and learning difficulties. Coexistent asphyxia, acidosis, hypoxia or sepsis increase the risk of developing kernicterus.

Biliary atresia

This is a rare disorder of unknown aetiology in which there is either destruction or absence of the extrahepatic biliary tree. It represents a rare but important cause of persistent neonatal jaundice (Fig. 15.6).

Clinical features

It presents with prolonged jaundice and is distinguished by being a predominant conjugated hyperbilirubinaemia accompanied by dark urine and pale stools. As the disease progresses there is failure to thrive due to:

• malabsorption
• enlargement of the liver and spleen

A bleeding tendency might develop due to vitamin K deficiency.

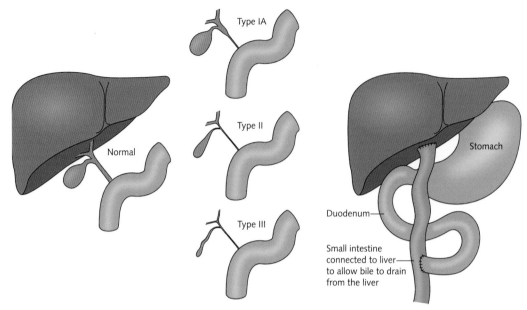

Fig. 15.6 Biliary atresia and the Kasai procedure.

Investigations
Abdominal ultrasound, liver biopsy and cholangiography might be required to clarify the diagnosis.

Management
Treatment consists of the Kasai procedure, which should ideally be carried out before the age of 6 weeks. Despite this the majority still require a liver transplant by age 20.

RED FLAG
Obstructive jaundice may present with pale stools and dark urine in addition to a conjugated hyperbilirubinaemia. Early diagnosis of biliary atresia is important because delay in surgical treatment beyond 6 weeks old compromises outcome.

DISORDERS OF THE TERM INFANT

Respiratory disorders

Respiratory distress in term infants is characterized by:

- tachypnoea: respiratory rate over 60 breaths/min
- recession: subcostal or intercostal
- cyanosis
- nasal flaring
- expiratory grunting

The most common causes are shown in Box 15.3.

BOX 15.3 CAUSES OF RESPIRATORY DISTRESS IN TERM INFANTS

Pulmonary	Nonpulmonary
Transient tachypnoea of newborn	Septicaemia
Pneumonia	Severe anaemia
Meconium aspiration	Congenital cardiac disease
Diaphragmatic hernia	
Choanal atresia	
Pneumothorax	

Transient tachypnoea of the newborn
Transient tachypnoea of the newborn (TTN) is a benign self-limiting condition believed to be caused by a delay in the normal reabsorption of the lung fluid at birth. It is more common after caesarean section and in infants of diabetic mothers. The chest X-ray (CXR) might show a streaky appearance with fluid in the horizontal fissure; it usually resolves within 48 hours.

Pneumonia
Risk factors for congenital pneumonia include prematurity, prolonged rupture of the membranes (over 24 hours) and maternal colonization of group B streptococcal infection (GBS). *Chlamydia* should be suspected if there is concurrent purulent conjunctivitis.

Neonates are also susceptible to community-acquired or nosocomial pneumonias in addition to viral causes (e.g., respiratory syncytial virus).

Management

This comprises:

- respiratory support with oxygen and ventilation if severe
- careful fluid balance
- IV antibiotics

Laryngomalacia

This manifests as stridor that is present from birth, which tends to resolve by 12 to 18 months of age. It usually does not require any specific treatment but symptoms can be more pronounced during an intercurrent illness when sleeping or when lying flat.

Pneumothorax

Spontaneous pneumothorax occurs in about 1% of term infants and does not always require intervention. In ventilated babies it is commonly iatrogenic and is diagnosed by CXR or transillumination of the chest.

Tension pneumothorax causes a sudden deterioration in the infant's condition with acute respiratory distress and necessitates urgent treatment by needle thoracocentesis followed by insertion of a chest drain.

Chylothorax

A rare cause of respiratory distress, due to accumulation of lymphatic fluid in the pleural cavity. Can be spontaneous (due to an anomaly of lymphatic drainage) or iatrogenic from birth trauma or thoracotomy. It needs drainage and occasionally dietary elimination of long-chain fatty acids may hasten resolution.

Meconium aspiration

Approximately 10% of term neonates pass meconium before birth. It is associated with foetal distress (e.g., hypoxic insult) and is more common in postdate babies. Inhalation of meconium results in bronchial obstruction and collapse, chemical pneumonitis and secondary infection – all leading to respiratory distress. There is also a high incidence of air leak (pneumothorax, pneumomediastinum) and pulmonary hypertension. Neonates may range from having mild symptoms to requiring ventilation.

Persistent pulmonary hypertension of the newborn

Pulmonary vascular resistance remains high after birth causing right to left shunting at both atrial and ductal levels with cyanosis. It can occur as a primary disorder but is more commonly a complication of perinatal asphyxia, meconium aspiration, severe sepsis or RDS. A CXR might show pulmonary oligaemia and the diagnosis is confirmed by echocardiography.

Management

Is mainly supportive but also includes:

- oxygenation
- assisted ventilation with good sedation
- inhaled nitric oxide and/or sildenafil for pulmonary vasodilatation
- extracorporeal membrane oxygenation (ECMO) for severe cases

Aspiration

Aspiration of milk or stomach contents into the lungs may occur especially in:

- infants with neurological problems (e.g., hypotonia)
- chronic lung disease (CLD) or RDS
- cleft palate
- tracheo-oesophageal fistula
- reflux

Gastrointestinal and hepatic disorders

Gastrointestinal disorders in the neonate can be congenital or acquired and can involve the length of the alimentary tract from the mouth to the anus.

Cleft lip and palate

This affects about 1:1000 babies. It manifests as:

- cleft lip alone: 35%
- cleft lip and palate: 25%
- cleft palate alone: 40%

Aetiology remains unclear but is thought to be polygenic. Some drugs are specifically teratogenic, including anticonvulsants and methotrexate. Cleft lip is usually diagnosed at the 18–20-week scan but isolated cleft palates are difficult to diagnose antenatally. Some infants can be breastfed; others require special teats, 'squeezy' bottles or temporary nasogastric feeding. Surgical repair is carried out at 6 to 12 months of age and it may need a staged approach.

Oesophageal atresia

The incidence is 1:3500 live births. A tracheo-oesophageal fistula is often also present (Fig. 15.7). As the foetus is unable to swallow during intrauterine life, there is polyhydramnios. Infants usually present with copious oral secretions and respiratory distress. The diagnosis is confirmed by attempting to pass a nasogastric tube, which would be coiled in the oesophagus on X-ray. About 50% of cases have other associated abnormalities (e.g., as part of the VACTERL association):

- **v**ertebral
- **a**norectal
- **c**ardiac

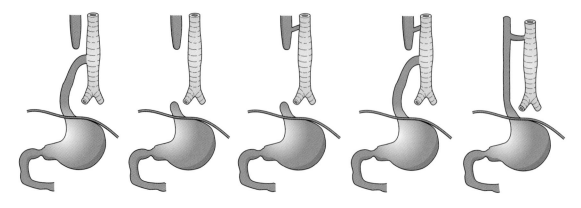

Oesophageal atresia with distal tracheo-oesophageal fistula (85%) Oesophageal atresia without tracheo-osophageal fistula (8%) Oesophageal atresia with proximal tracheo-oesophageal fistula (2%) Oesophageal atresia with proximal and distal tracheo-oesophageal fistula (1%) H-type tracheo-oesophageal fistula (4%)

Fig. 15.7 Oesophageal atresia and tracheo-oesophageal fistula.

- **t**racheo-oesophageal
- **r**enal
- **l**imb abnormalities

Initial treatment involves a Replogle tube, which is a suction catheter that clears the secretions that pool in the oesophageal pouch. Definitive treatment is surgical repair.

Bowel obstruction

Generally presents with:

- bile-stained vomiting
- absent or delayed passage of meconium
- abdominal distension

Diagnosis is made on clinical features and abdominal X-ray, and treatment depends on the cause. It can involve either the small or large bowel.

Small bowel obstruction
Duodenal atresia

Often associated with Down syndrome and diagnosed antenatally by a 'double bubble' or polyhydramnios appearance on ultrasound. Surgical repair is required.

Midgut volvulus and malrotation

Failure of midgut rotation in utero can result in duodenal obstruction. This may cause intermittent pain due to incomplete obstruction or present acutely with volvulus, which is a result of complete twisting of a bowel loop around its mesenteric attachment site.

Meconium ileus

This describes intestinal obstruction secondary to particularly thick meconium and is highly predictive of cystic fibrosis. Treatment with enemas can be attempted but surgery is often required as it can lead to perforation.

Large bowel obstruction
Hirschsprung disease

This occurs due to an absence of ganglion cells from the myenteric and submyenteric plexuses of a segment of the large bowel (usually the rectum and sigmoid colon). It can present acutely with bowel obstruction or insidiously with constipation.

Anorectal atresia

Can be isolated or part of VACTERL association. Surgical management may include a colostomy until a pull-through procedure can be performed. Some children remain faecally incontinent after repair, especially in high atresias.

Cardiovascular disorders

Congenital heart disease occurs in 8 of 1000 live births and is routinely screened for antenatally. They are discussed in detail in Chapter 3.

Haematological disorders

Vitamin K deficiency bleeding (previously known as haemorrhagic disease of the newborn)

This is caused by a relative deficiency of the vitamin-K-dependent coagulation factors II, VII, IX and X. It characteristically affects the fully breastfed infant between the third and sixth day of life, because breast milk does not contain adequate amounts of vitamin K. Mothers taking anticonvulsant drugs that interfere with vitamin K metabolism, such as phenytoin, are at increased risk.

Bleeding usually occurs from the gastrointestinal tract but infants can also present with intracranial haemorrhage.

A single intramuscular dose of vitamin K prevents this disease and is routinely offered. Alternatively, in well babies not at risk of bleeding disorders, oral vitamin K may be given – two doses within the first week, and a further dose (not if formula fed as formula feeds contain adequate vitamin K) at a month of age.

Neurological disorders

Neonatal seizures

Seizures are more common in the neonatal period than at any other time of life because the neonatal brain is mostly excitatory. The manifestations of neonatal seizures are rather different from those in older children, and it can be difficult to distinguish true seizures from normal baby movements.

COMMON PITFALLS

Neonatal episodes that are *not* seizures include:

- Jitteriness: the movement is a tremor – rhythmic movements of equal rate and amplitude (in seizures, clonic movements have a fast and slow component). There are no ocular phenomena. It is sensitive to external stimuli and is stopped by holding.
- Benign myoclonus: shock-like jerks when asleep.
- Startle reaction.

Neonatal seizures may be subtle in the form of eye deviation, apnoea, autonomic phenomena and oral movements. They may also be clonic (focal rhythmic and slow jerking), myoclonic (rapid isolated jerks) or tonic with abnormal posturing.

The antenatal and birth history together with clinical examination will often indicate the cause (Table 15.7) and help target your investigations.

Initial investigations

- Blood glucose, electrolytes, Ca^{2+}, Mg^{2+}.
- Cerebrospinal fluid (CSF) analysis for infection.
- Cranial ultrasonography for haemorrhages.

Table 15.7 Causes of neonatal seizures

Hypoxia	
Electrolyte and metabolic abnormalities	Hypoglycaemia Hyponatraemia Hypo/hypercalcaemia Inborn errors of metabolism
Central nervous system	Haemorrhage Infection Structural abnormality Epilepsy syndromes
Drug withdrawal	Opiates Benzodiazepines
Genetic disease	Neurocutaneous diseases
Hyperbilirubinaemia	Bilirubin encephalopathy

As indicated:

- Inborn error of metabolism: blood ammonia, lactate and amino acids, urine amino acids, organic acids, IV pyridoxine test:
- congenital infection screen (TORCH)
- cross-sectional cranial imaging: MRI or CT may be appropriate

Neonatal abstinence syndrome

Neonatal abstinence syndrome is a cluster of withdrawal symptoms that develop in babies of substance-abusing mothers. This may be due to heroin use or in those on a methadone programme.

Clinical features

This includes yawning, sweating, jitteriness, high pitched or inconsolable crying, diarrhoea and vomiting and pyrexia. More severe symptoms include seizures.

Diagnosis

This should be confirmed by urine toxicology in both mother and infant. Scoring charts are used to monitor infants at risk and dictate management. These babies are also at high risk of other diseases like hepatitis B, C and HIV, so the mother's serology should be checked.

Management

If withdrawal scores are high, treatment is initiated with oral morphine and gradually weaned over the next few days to weeks. It is also important to evaluate the social situation and liaise with drug and alcohol services, social services and the health visitor.

Infections

Congenital infections are discussed earlier in this chapter; however, there are other acquired infections that can carry significant morbidity and mortality, particularly bacterial infections.

Important bacterial pathogens in the neonate include:

- group B β-haemolytic streptococci (GBS)
- *Escherichia coli*

Minor infections
Skin pustules and paronychia

These are caused by staphylococcal infection and typically occur in moist areas such as the groin and axillae. Inflammation of the skin in the area of a nail fold can progress to become pustular. Treatment with flucloxacillin is sometimes necessary.

Conjunctivitis

A 'sticky eye' in the first day or two of life is often due to chemical irritation and clears spontaneously. Conjunctivitis with a purulent discharge might be due to:

- Staphylococci, streptococci, *E. coli*
- Gonococci: ophthalmia neonatorum
- *Chlamydia trachomatis*

Gonococcal and chlamydial infections are notifiable diseases and need systemic antibiotic treatment because the risk of scarring and blindness is high. IV antibiotics are used and ophthalmological review is mandatory. It is also important to treat the parents.

Thrush (moniliasis)

Infection with *Candida albicans* can affect the mouth or nappy area. Oral thrush appears as white plaques on the tongue and inside of the mouth. Nystatin drops for 7 to 10 days is usually effective and perineal thrush responds to topical antifungals.

Major infections

Sepsis

Neonatal sepsis carries a high mortality and morbidity and can be rapid and fulminant. As signs are nonspecific (Box 15.4), a low threshold for investigation and empirical treatment with antibiotics is needed. The overall incidence of serious acute infections in the newborn period is about 6 per 1000 live births in the UK. Risk factors for neonatal sepsis are discussed in Chapter 1in the neonatal history.

In addition to the signs mentioned in Box 15.4, signs relating to a site of infection may emerge. These include:

- tense fontanelle, seizures: meningitis
- respiratory distress: pneumonia

Diagnosis. If systemic infection is suspected, prompt investigation to identify a causative agent is essential:

- 'septic screen': blood, urine and CSF cultures
- consider CXR
- an FBC and CRP are helpful

Group B streptococcal infection

About 20% to 30% of pregnant women are colonized with GBS. Although women are usually asymptomatic, GBS sepsis in the neonate can be fatal. It may present early (within the first week) or later. Early disease is associated with a worse outcome but can be reduced with preventive measures including intrapartum antibiotic treatment of mothers, careful observation and early treatment of symptomatic neonates. Vaccines are under development.

Treatment. GBS infection is usually sensitive to penicillin. Aminoglycosides (e.g., gentamicin) are added for additional synergistic effects.

Meningitis

Neonatal meningitis is usually due to a different range of pathogens from that in the older child. In infants, the infective organisms include:

- GBS
- *E. coli*
- *Listeria monocytogenes*

Meningeal infection usually follows septicaemia. Clinical features include poor feeding, irritability and temperature instability. Fullness of the anterior fontanelle and seizures are late signs.

Diagnosis. CSF cultures are required to confirm the diagnosis.

Treatment and outcome. High-dose IV antibiotics for 14 days are required. Mortality has reduced from around 30%–60% to 10%–15% in developed countries, but morbidity remains unchanged with a high incidence of neurological impairment in survivors.

Urinary tract infection

The most common pathogen is *E. coli,* with other gram-negative organisms occasionally responsible. All neonates with a confirmed urinary tract infection should have an ultrasound of their renal tract to exclude structural abnormalities and hydronephrosis.

Symptoms and signs are usually nonspecific. Urine must be cultured in all infants with poor feeding, lethargy, vomiting, failure to thrive and jaundice.

Urine is obtained by clean catch for microscopy and culture; any bacteriuria or pyuria is considered diagnostic of urinary tract infection.

IV antibiotics are used for treatment (see Chapter 6 for up-to-date guidance).

THE PRETERM INFANT

About 8 in every 100 babies are born prematurely (before 37 weeks gestation) and are, therefore, 'low-birthweight' babies. Problems associated with prematurity are the leading cause of death in children under 5 years.

Table 15.8 Major problems in preterm infants

Temperature	Hypothermia
Respiratory	Respiratory distress syndrome Pneumothorax Chronic lung disease Pneumonia Pulmonary hypertension
Cardiac	Patent ductus arteriosus Hypotension
Gastrointestinal	Feed intolerance Vomiting and gastroesophageal reflux Jaundice Necrotizing enterocolitis
Infection	Group B streptococci *Staphylococcus epidermidis* Gram-negative cocci Fungi (e.g., *Candida* species)
Nervous	Intraventricular haemorrhage Retinopathy of prematurity Developmental delay Cerebral palsy
Bone	Osteopaenia of prematurity
Fluids and electrolytes	High transepidermal water loss Hypoglycaemia
Haematology	Anaemia

The major problems encountered by preterm infants are determined by the immaturity of their organ systems, particularly the lungs (Table 15.8).

ETHICS

The birth of a baby before 27 completed weeks gestation is termed extreme preterm birth. These babies have the greatest burden of mortality and morbidity with earlier gestations being associated with poorer outcomes, recognizing that other factors are important. Decision-making for these infants, particularly at the earliest gestations, is medically complex and ethically controversial. In the 1960s, birth before 28 weeks gestation was considered 'previable' but by the 1990s, 40% of babies born at 24+ weeks survived following neonatal intensive care. The threshold for active treatment is now between 22 and 23 weeks gestation following assessment of risk (stratified into extremely high, high or moderate risk) and multiprofessional discussion with the family.

General care of the preterm infant

Some basic principles apply to the care of all preterm infants.

Predelivery care

NICE guidance reflects increasing evidence for the effectiveness of prophylactic vaginal progesterone or prophylactic cervical cerclage in preventing preterm birth for those women with identified risk factors (history of spontaneous preterm birth up to 34 weeks gestation, or loss up to 16 weeks gestation, or cervical shortening). Antibiotics are used in women with preterm prolonged rupture of membranes. Once labour has started, it can be delayed for a short time (hours to days) by using tocolytic drugs (e.g., nifedipine) to allow time for corticosteroids and magnesium sulphate (respectively to reduce need for respiratory support, and for neuroprotection in preterm babies) to be administered.

COMMUNICATION

Parents should be given the opportunity to speak to a paediatrician prior to the delivery of a premature infant and, if possible, visit the neonatal unit. They should be sensitively counselled about the possible complications of preterm delivery and the chances of survival and disability. It is also important to tell them what happens soon after delivery and briefly about the resuscitation. They should also be prepared for a long stay in the neonatal intensive care.

Stabilization at birth

Delivery should ideally take place in a location with a neonatal intensive care unit. At birth the baby should be handled gently and kept warm. Babies of less than 32 weeks gestation are placed inside a plastic bag to minimize heat loss. Babies of later gestations should be dried and placed under a source of radiant heat.

Many preterm infants of 28 weeks gestation or less will not achieve adequate ventilation and will require intubation or nasal continuous positive airway pressure (CPAP). Surfactant administration is considered in infants <28 weeks at this stage.

COMMUNICATION

Some parents want to know the chances of survival of an extremely premature infant. MBRACE-UK data shows that babies alive at the onset of labour at 22 weeks have an overall survival of 5% but if well enough for active treatment this rises to 35%. At 24 weeks 60% of babies survive with 1 in 7 having a severe disability. By 28 weeks most babies survive and do not have major disability although learning difficulties can occur.

Body temperature

Preterm infants rapidly lose heat due to lack of brown fat, little muscle activity and high body surface area-to-volume ratio. Strategies for maintaining body temperature include:

- Radiant heat: used predominantly in resuscitation. Can cause excessive fluid loss over prolonged periods.
- Ambient temperature and humidity: incubators provide a controlled microenvironment.
- Insulation with clothing, including a hat to prevent excessive heat loss from the relatively large head.
- Plastic bags: when used the baby should not be covered by clothing and should be exposed to the heat source.

COMMON PITFALLS

Preterm babies are prone to hypothermia for many reasons; however, a low body temperature can also be a sign of sepsis. Temperature instability in a preterm baby should prompt a review and possibly a septic screen.

Avoiding infection

Meticulous attention to hand-washing before and after handling is the most important safeguard against transmitting infection. Good skin care will reduce the incidence of *Staphylococcus epidermidis* infection and regular review of any indwelling plastic such as cannulas, long lines, endotracheal tubes, as these are a source of infection.

Nutrition and fluids

Infants of 34 weeks' gestation or more are usually able to feed orally. Although preterm infants can digest and absorb enteral feeds, their sucking and swallowing reflexes are immature and some or all of the feeds might be delivered through a nasogastric tube. The approach to giving nutrition and fluids therefore depends on the size and maturity of the individual baby.

Extreme preterm and very-low-birthweight babies (<1500 g at birth) might require their fluid and calories to be given intravenously during the first few days or weeks. This is in the form of IV dextrose or total parenteral nutrition (TPN).

Which milk for preterm infants?

Breast milk has many benefits including protection against necrotizing enterocolitis and infection. Donor breast milk can be used in some cases, otherwise preterm formulas are available and breast milk fortifier can be used to provide extra calories.

Supplements

Preterm infants need supplements of phosphate and vitamin D to ensure adequate bone mineralization. A multivitamin preparation is usually given once full enteral feeding is established and continued until age 5, with an iron supplement from 4 weeks of age until weaned.

DISORDERS OF THE PRETERM INFANT

Respiratory disorders

Respiratory distress syndrome

This is caused by a deficiency of surfactant associated with immaturity of the type II pneumocytes. Surfactant is a lipoprotein that lowers surface tension in the alveoli and prevents collapse during expiration.

Clinical features

Signs might be present from birth or develop over the next 4 hours. The signs include:

- tachypnoea
- cyanosis
- subcostal and intercostal recession
- nasal flare
- expiratory grunting

The disease displays a spectrum of severity from mild to severe and life-threatening. A CXR will show a diffuse granular or 'ground glass' appearance of the lungs and an air bronchogram outlining the larger airways.

Management

Glucocorticoids given antenatally stimulate foetal surfactant production, but many preterm births progress too quickly. Effective stabilization at birth of infants at risk reduces the severity of the disease. The mainstays of management include:

- surfactant therapy
- oxygen
- assisted ventilation

Exogenous surfactant therapy given after birth via endotracheal tube reduces mortality and morbidity. Many babies can be rapidly weaned off ventilatory support after treatment; however, they may still require CPAP via the nasal airways or increased oxygen concentration – including high-flow oxygen.

Ventilation is guided by monitoring of the arterial blood gas tensions (partial pressure of oxygen in arterial blood [PaO_2] and partial pressure of carbon dioxide in arterial blood [$PaCO_2$]), high-frequency oscillatory ventilation can be used if conventional ventilation fails.

Surfactant deficiency itself resolves spontaneously in 3 to 7 days as endogenous surfactant is produced. Some extreme preterm infants require respiratory support for longer and go on to develop CLD.

HINTS AND TIPS

- Mechanical ventilation can cause acute lung injury.
- Overventilation (especially large volumes) is harmful and contributes to chronic lung disease.
- Oxygen should be used with care and a lower oxygen saturation limit is set to minimize retinopathy of prematurity and other adverse effects of hyperoxia.

Apnoeic attacks

Many small, preterm infants display 'periodic respiration' with some spells of very shallow breathing or complete cessation of breathing for up to 20 seconds. This reflects immaturity of the respiratory centre.

Apnoea is defined as cessation of respiration for at least 20 seconds. Predisposing factors include:

- RDS
- hypoxia
- sepsis – especially meningitis
- cranial pathology, especially haemorrhage

The differential diagnosis includes seizures, which can mimic apnoeic attacks.

Apnoea alarms are useful for alerting staff to the need for action. Breathing will usually start again with physical stimulation. Caffeine is used in premature infants to prevent apnoeic episodes (and seems to improve neurodevelopmental outcome). Ventilatory support might be needed if severe.

Cardiovascular problems

Patent ductus arteriosus

A patent ductus arteriosus is a common problem in preterm infants and is often associated with RDS. Failure of closure occurs because of gestational immaturity and hypoxia.

As the pulmonary vascular resistance falls, blood is shunted across the ductus from left to right. The clinical features are a widened pulse pressure with prominent peripheral pulses, tachycardia and a systolic murmur. This shunt often causes difficulty in weaning infants off the ventilator and it is diagnosed by echocardiography.

Management

Spontaneous closure may occur but treatment is used if the duct is causing significant problems (difficulty weaning ventilation, signs of heart failure, growth failure). Supportive management with fluid restriction and adequate oxygenation might be sufficient, but a prostaglandin inhibitor, such as ibuprofen, may be effective. Surgical ligation is occasionally required in ventilator-dependent infants.

Neurological problems

Intracranial haemorrhage

The germinal matrix is highly vascularized and damage to this area causes intracranial haemorrhage. Preterm babies often endure rapid changes to cerebral blood flow, which is a risk factor. Prognosis is poorer if the bleed is large enough to cause ventricular dilatation or if it extends into the parenchyma. Posthaemorrhagic hydrocephalus is a late complication of severe bleeds. Most events occur within the first 24 hours of life but infants continue to be at risk especially if unwell; for example, a preterm baby requiring high-pressure ventilation. Babies at risk are monitored by serial cranial ultrasound.

Periventricular leukomalacia

This describes necrosis of haemorrhagic areas that then undergo cystic change and ultimately cerebral atrophy. Hypoxia, ischaemia and infection are all risk factors. Prognosis is poor with most children having spastic diplegia or tetraplegia. Learning difficulties and cortical blindness also occur.

Gastrointestinal problems

Jaundice

Because of immaturity of hepatic enzyme there is a build of bilirubin causing clinical jaundice in the majority of preterm infants. This is discussed earlier in this chapter.

Necrotizing enterocolitis

Necrotizing enterocolitis involves inflammation and necrosis of the intestine, usually the distal ileum or proximal colon. The aetiology is uncertain but established predisposing factors include:

- preterm birth
- IUGR
- absent or reversed end diastolic flow on Doppler scans
- polycythaemia
- patent ductus arteriosus
- asphyxia
- early feeding with formula milk (early feeding with breast milk is protective)

Clinical features include apnoea, abdominal distension, vomiting and bloody stools. Abdominal X-ray might show dilated, thick-walled bowel loops, free air or intramural gas (a pathognomonic finding). Mortality ranges between 10% and 50% and is improving, but in severe cases with bowel wall destruction, perforation and peritonitis, mortality can approach 100%.

Management

Medical management includes:

- nil by mouth, nasogastric tube on free drainage
- parenteral nutrition or IV dextrose
- antibiotics: penicillin, gentamicin and metronidazole

Surgical resection of necrotic bowel might be required in severe cases or if perforation has occurred. If this is extensive, the infant could be left with short gut syndrome and long-term PN requirement.

Long-term prognosis

Although many preterm infants survive intact without sequelae, a number of significant problems can persist, especially in the very-low-birthweight group. These include:

- retinopathy of prematurity (ROP)
- CLD of prematurity
- neurodevelopmental problems

Retinopathy of prematurity

This occurs in premature infants whose retinas are incompletely vascularized at birth. There is abnormal vascular proliferation in response to insults including hyperoxia (but also hypotension and hypoxia). This may progress to fibrosis, retinal detachment and blindness.

All infants weighing less than 1500 g, <32 weeks' gestational age or requiring significant respiratory or cardiovascular support should have their eyes screened 6 to 8 weeks after birth. Most cases resolve spontaneously but laser therapy might be indicated for severe disease.

Chronic lung disease

CLD or bronchopulmonary dysplasia is often defined as requiring supplemental oxygen beyond 36 weeks' corrected gestation or 28 days of age, although this may change to account for better survival of extreme preterm infants. It occurs in newborns who, for any reason, require prolonged assisted ventilation with high pressures and high concentrations of oxygen. It is particularly common in very low-birthweight infants. Positive pressure ventilation causing volutrauma, barotrauma, oxygen toxicity and inflammation (possibly secondary to infection) are all believed to contribute. The CXR shows widespread opacities with patchy translucent areas.

Management

- Respiratory support: mechanical ventilation or CPAP and supplemental oxygen as needed, with efforts to minimize further damage.
- Steroids: effective in weaning from ventilatory support but controversial as they can increase the risk of neurodevelopmental impairment.
- Strict attention to nutrition.
- Prophylaxis against respiratory syncytial virus.

Bronchiolitis, particularly due to respiratory syncytial virus, is a major risk to infants with CLD; in recent years a monoclonal antibody (palivizumab) has been developed as prophylaxis and is recommended for vulnerable infants during the winter months.

Complete recovery of lung function may occur as the child grows; however, a proportion of children will continue to have reduced lung function and increased incidence of asthma and respiratory infections.

Neurodevelopmental problems

The prospects for normal survival in preterm infants are improving. However, very-low-birthweight infants and those with a gestation period of under 28 weeks are at risk of a range of neurodevelopmental problems including:

- cerebral palsy
- cognitive delay
- visual impairment
- hearing loss
- seizures
- behavioural problems
- educational difficulties

Infants born prematurely should be followed up by a paediatrician in a neurodevelopmental clinic usually up to 2 years of age.

CONGENITAL MALFORMATIONS

COMMUNICATION

Congenital refers to any condition present at birth. The cause might be genetic, environmental, infectious or idiopathic. Parents are often worried if a condition is the result of something they did during pregnancy and also about the chances of its recurrence in subsequent children. Eliciting these concerns and providing reassurance and offering genetic counselling are crucial.

Up to 70% of major congenital malformations can now be detected antenatally using ultrasound. There are too many to cover in this book but some of the most important are listed in the following sections:

Craniofacial

Craniosynostosis

Premature fusion of one or more of the cranial sutures results in an abnormal shaped head. Infants are at risk of raised intracranial pressure and impaired neurodevelopment in addition to cosmetic implications.

Cleft lip and palate

This is described earlier in this chapter and can be isolated or associated with other abnormalities such as Pierre Robin sequence. This is an association of micrognathia (small jaw), posterior displacement of the tongue and a cleft of the soft palate. Prone positioning maintains airway patency until growth of the mandible is established; however, some infants require a nasopharyngeal airway or even a temporary tracheostomy. The cleft is surgically repaired at 6–12 months.

Respiratory

Cystic adenomatoid malformation of the lung
Presence of a cystic, nonfunctioning area of lung (often a whole lobe).

Congenital diaphragmatic hernia
Occurs in 1 in 3000 live births. Fortunately, most are diagnosed on antenatal ultrasound scan, as this allows for appropriate early management: early intubation and nasogastric aspiration (to avoid inflation of the bowel). Around 80% are left sided and there is often pulmonary hypoplasia and therefore a high mortality rate. Treatment is surgical repair once stable enough.

Gastrointestinal

Gastroschisis (1:5000)
The bowel protrudes without any covering sac through a defect in the anterior abdominal wall adjacent to the umbilicus. This is usually an isolated anomaly.

Exomphalos (1:2500)
The abdominal contents herniate through the umbilical ring and are covered with a sac formed by the peritoneum and amniotic membrane. It is often associated with other major congenital abnormalities such as trisomy 13 and 18.

Central nervous system

Neural tube defects
These arise from failure of fusion of the neural plate in the first 28 days after conception. The incidence in the UK has fallen dramatically since the 1970s because of improved maternal nutrition, folic acid supplementation and better antenatal screening.

> **HINTS AND TIPS**
>
> Folic acid supplements should ideally be taken preconception and during the first trimester. Some women take a higher dose such as those with a personal or family history of neural tube defects, women with diabetes or women taking antiepileptic medicines as they are at increased risk.

The three main types are:

- spina bifida occulta
- meningocele
- myelomeningocele

They are usually in the lumbosacral region (Fig. 15.8).

Spina bifida occulta
The dorsal vertebral arch fails to fuse. There may be an overlying skin abnormality such as a tuft of hair or small dermal sinus. Tethering of the cord (diastomyelia) can cause neurological deficits with growth.

Meningocele
This describes a CSF-filled cystic protrusion with intact overlying skin (5% of neural tube defects). There is no neurological deficit or hydrocephalus, and it is surgically excised at around 3 months.

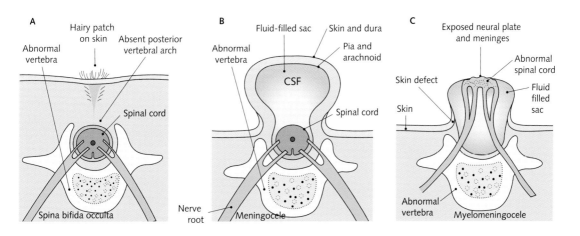

Fig. 15.8 Types of neural tube defects. *CSF,* Cerebrospinal fluid.

Myelomeningocele

This accounts for more than 90% of overt spina bifida. These are open with herniation of both the cord and meninges; there is commonly leaking of CSF. Neurological deficits are always present and can include:

- motor and sensory loss in the lower limbs
- neuropathic bladder and bowel

In addition, there is often scoliosis and associated hydrocephalus due to the Arnold-Chiari malformation (herniation of the cerebellar tonsils through the foramen magnum). Surgery prevents infection but does not restore neurological function.

Neural tube defects also include:

- Encephalocoele: extrusion of the brain and meninges through a midline skull defect.
- Anencephaly: the cranium and brain fail to develop (detected on antenatal ultrasound and termination of pregnancy is usually offered).

Urogenital

Visible abnormalities of the external genitalia range from the common (e.g., hypospadias; see Chapter 6) to complex genital anomaly where the sex of the individual is unclear. Around 1 in 4500 infants have complex genital anomaly at birth. It is a very difficult area raising strong emotions in families and great care should be taken when discussing investigation and management. The most common cause of ambiguous external genitalia is congenital adrenal hyperplasia leading to a virilized female (see Chapter 7).

Musculoskeletal

Congenital talipes equinovarus (club foot)

The entire foot is fixed in an inverted and supinated position. This should be distinguished from 'positional talipes', in which the deformity is mild and can be corrected with passive manipulation. Referral should be made to orthopaedic surgeons and physiotherapy, as early treatment (including serial casting where appropriate) is important to prevent disability.

HINTS AND TIPS

Features of talipes equinovarus:

- 1.5 per 1000 live births

- male-to-female ratio: 2:1
- 50% bilateral
- multifactorial inheritance
- associated with oligohydramnios, congenital hip dislocation and neuromuscular disorders (e.g., spina bifida)

Developmental dysplasia of the hip

Congenital instability or even dislocation of one or both of the femoral heads from an often-shallow acetabulum. The aetiology is unclear but it is associated with ligamentous laxity and a genetic predisposition. Bracing with a Pavlik harness is usually the first line of treatment but open reduction may be required. Without treatment significant leg length discrepancy and painful gait disturbances can occur.

THE CRYING BABY

Infant crying is normal but can cause familial distress and may be an indicator of ill health. At 6 to 8 weeks of age, a baby cries on average 2 to 3 hours per day; this usually improves by 3 to 4 months of age. Red flags for crying include sudden onset and persistence. Commonly, babies will cry because they are hungry or have a wet or dirty nappy.

If crying is related to feeding, gastrointestinal causes such as gastro-oesophageal reflux disease (GORD) and cow's milk protein allergy (CMPA) should be considered. Sometimes, crying is due to medical illness. Causes may include sepsis, meningitis, injury (e.g., NAI), arrhythmias and abdominal issues (e.g., incarcerated hernia and intussusception).

If the history is typical and examination normal, no investigations are required. As mentioned above, persistent crying can be a sign of nonaccidental injury; this is important to keep in mind for all professionals.

Once medical causes have been excluded, parental education and reassurance is all that is needed. Follow up with the health visitor may be useful to help support parents. Postnatal depression can contribute to parental anxiety around crying; this is important to identify for both mum and baby.

Chapter Summary

- Many aspects of maternal health have important influences on the foetus. Examples include medications such as antiepileptics, which can be teratogenic, and maternal conditions like diabetes mellitus and its association with multiple congenital anomalies particularly cardiac defects.
- There are many causes of respiratory distress in the term infant including transient tachypnoea of the newborn, which is usually self-limiting.
- Respiratory distress in the preterm is most commonly a result of respiratory distress syndrome, which arises from a lack of surfactant.
- Jaundice is a common problem seen in term and preterm infants and may require treatment such as feeding support, phototherapy or exchange transfusion if severe.
- The management of a preterm baby is different due to their small size and immature lungs and gut. They are also at increased risk of patent ductus arteriosus and intraventricular haemorrhages.
- The newborn and infant physical examination (NIPE) programme aims to identify all children with congenital abnormalities, where detectable, within 72 hours of birth. A further examination between 6 and 8 weeks of age is performed to identify abnormalities detectable by this time allowing referral for early clinical assessment.

UKMLA Conditions

Biliary atresia
Cerebral palsy and hypoxic-ischaemic
 encephalopathy
Intestinal obstruction and ileus
Meningitis
Peripheral nerve injuries/palsies
Pneumothorax
Rubella
Urinary tract infection
Volvulus
Down's syndrome

UKMLA Presentations

Congenital abnormalities
Crying baby
Difficulty with breast feeding
Fits/seizures
Jaundice
Prematurity
Vomiting

The human genome comprises 46 chromosomes, which include 22 pairs of autosomes and one pair of sex chromosomes. With the mapping of the human genome, our understanding of genetics has increased exponentially and continues to develop at a rapid rate. Many genetic disorders are encountered in paediatrics and it is important to remember that those that are associated with a poor prognosis and a short lifespan are not seen during adulthood. As our understanding of genetics has advanced, many new diagnostic technologies have become clinically relevant and therapies for genetic diseases are emerging.

Clinical manifestations are highly variable but it is worth remembering that many dysmorphic syndromes have a genetic basis.

COMMON PITFALLS

- Dysmorphism is an abnormality in form or structural development, often manifested in the facial appearance and often due to an underlying genetic disorder.
- A syndrome is a recognizable pattern of structural and functional abnormalities or malformations known or presumed to be the result of a single cause. Dysmorphism is often a feature.

BASIC GENETICS

Some useful definitions are shown in Table 16.1. A family tree is a tool often used when thinking about inheritance patterns. The key symbols used in drawing a family tree are shown in Fig. 16.1.

SINGLE-GENE (MONOGENIC) DISORDERS

Disorders of single nuclear genes are recognizable because of their Mendelian pattern of inheritance, which can be:

- autosomal dominant (AD)
- autosomal recessive (AR)
- X-linked

More than 13,000 single-gene disorders have been identified so far; with the molecular basis known in over 2000. Examples of important single-gene disorders are shown in Table 16.2.

Table 16.1 Basic genetics: some definitions

Term	Definition
Karyotype	A display of the set of chromosomes extracted from a eukaryotic somatic cell arrested at metaphase.
Genome	The totality of the DNA contained within the diploid chromosome set of a eukaryotic species.
Gene	A sequence of DNA occupying its own place (locus) on a chromosome and containing the information necessary for biosynthesis of a gene product such as a protein.
Allele	Any one of the variations of a gene or polymorphic DNA marker found in the members of a species. Numerous alleles may exist, but any individual usually possesses at most two alleles of the gene or polymorphic marker.
Genotype	The pair of alleles of a variable gene possessed by an individual, or the pairs of alleles of any number of variable genes possessed by an individual.
Phenotype	The entire physical, biochemical and physiological make-up of an individual as determined by genotype and environment.

Individually these are very rare, but collectively a single gene disorder affects around 1% of the population.

AUTOSOMAL DOMINANT DISORDERS

Alleles are variants in a particular gene at a particular locus – some alleles are dominant, others are recessive. In autosomal dominant disorders conditions, only one dominant allele is necessary to cause the disorder/phenotype; an affected person has just one copy of the abnormal gene (is heterozygous). Each offspring has a 50% chance of inheriting the abnormal gene, and thus, being affected. A typical pedigree of an AD disorder is shown in Fig. 16.2. The features of an AD pedigree are:

- Several generations with affected individuals.
- Equal numbers of males and females are affected.
- Male-to-male transmission occurs.

Several complicating factors can occur:

- Sporadic or 'de novo' mutations: a new mutation can occur in the parental gonads or the developing foetus – this isn't inherited (it is sporadic) meaning the risk to siblings of the disorder is low.

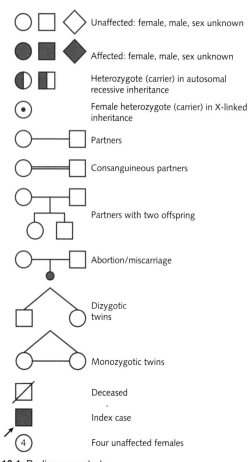

Fig. 16.1 Pedigree symbols.

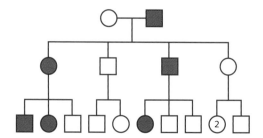

Fig. 16.2 Typical pedigree of an autosomal dominant condition.

- Variable expression: the pattern and severity of disease can be very variable for individuals in the same family/'pedigree' inheriting the affected allele.
- Reduced/incomplete penetrance: Penetrance is measured as the number of individuals who inherit a disordered allele AND manifest the disorder/phenotype; not all individuals inheriting the disordered allele to manifest/express the clinical disorder – but can still transmit the disordered allele to offspring.

Achondroplasia

This AD disorder is a skeletal dysplasia affecting 1 in 15,000 to 40,000 births. It is the commonest cause of short-limbed dwarfism; intelligence is normal. Most cases (80%) of Achondroplasia arise from sporadic/ 'de novo' mutations. The gene is found on the short arm of chromosome 4 and is a fibroblast growth factor receptor gene (FGFR3 gene). The typical clinical features are shown in Table 16.3.

Table 16.2 Examples of single-gene disorders

Mode of inheritance	Disorder	Frequency (carrier frequency in highest risk ethnic/geographic group); Gene involved
Autosomal dominant	Neurofibromatosis type 1	1/3000–5000; NF1
	Myotonic dystrophy	1/9000; DMPK
	Marfan syndrome	1/10,000; FBN1
	Tuberous sclerosis	1/15,000; TSC1 or TSC2
	Achondroplasia	1/15,000–40,000 FGFR3
Autosomal recessive	Sickle cell disease	1/600 (1/12 Africa, Mediterranean, India, Middle East, Central and South America); β-globin
	Cystic fibrosis	1/2500 (1/25 Caucasians); CFTR
	Alpha-thalassaemia	1/2500 (1/25 South East Asia); α-globin
	Beta-thalassaemia	1/3600 (1/30 Mediterranean, SE Asia); β-globin
	Congenital adrenal hyperplasia	1/10,000 (1/50); 21-hydroxylase
	Inborn errors of metabolism (majority), for example, phenylketonuria	1/10,000 (1/50); PAH
X-linked recessive	Glucose-6-phosphate dehydrogenase deficiency	1/2000 (Africa, Mediterranean, Asia); Gd
	Fragile X syndrome	1/4000; FMR1
	Haemophilia A	1/4000–10,000 mild-severe; F8 (factor VIII)
	Duchenne muscular dystrophy	1/5000; dystrophin
	Haemophilia B	1/30,000; F9 (factor IX)
	Colour blindness (red–green)	1/30,000; numerous, commonly CNGA3 or CNGB3

Table 16.3 Clinical features of achondroplasia

Body system	Clinical features
Musculoskeletal	Shortened limbs: proximal > distal Bow legs
	Short stature
	Thoracolumbar kyphosis
	Lumbar lordosis
Neurological	Hydrocephalus
	Motor developmental delay
Other	Macrocephaly Maxillary hypoplasia Recurrent otitis media

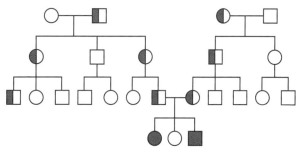

Fig. 16.3 Typical pedigree of an autosomal recessive condition.

Marfan syndrome

This is an AD connective tissue disorder caused by a defect of the FBN1 gene. Marfan disease is a good example of variable expressivity. Some individuals have mild symptoms (being tall, with long fingers), while others experience more serious/life-threatening complications; cardiac complications such as coarctation of the aorta, aortic regurgitation and mitral valve prolapse. Spinal deformities (e.g., scoliosis and pectus excavatum), restrictive airway disease and superior retinal detachment are also associated and affected individuals may have mild learning difficulties. Patients are typically tall with long limbs (arm span > height), arachnodactyly, joint laxity and a high arched palate.

AUTOSOMAL RECESSIVE DISORDERS

An affected individual has two copies of the abnormal gene inherited from each parent and is said to be homozygous for the disease alleles. Heterozygotes are carriers (i.e., carry only one abnormal copy) and are often unaffected, but may display a mild phenotype in some conditions. Many AR disorders are caused by mutations in the genes coding for enzymes. As half of the normal enzyme activity is usually sufficient, a person with only one mutant allele will not normally be affected.

A typical pedigree of an AR disorder is shown in Fig. 16.3. The features of an AR pedigree are:

- The risk of each child being affected when both parents are carriers is 25%.
- Males and females are equally likely to be affected.
- Parental consanguinity increases the risk of recessive conditions.

HINTS AND TIPS

- Autosomal dominant disorders are often caused by mutations in a gene encoding a structural protein.
- Autosomal recessive disorders are often caused by mutations in a gene encoding a functional protein, such as an enzyme.

Everyone probably carries at least one recessive disease gene allele. A couple who are first cousins are more likely to have inherited the same abnormal recessive disease gene allele from their common ancestor.

Certain recessive disorders show a founder effect. Affected individuals have inherited a founder mutation that occurred on an ancestral chromosome many generations ago. Carrier rates may be high within certain populations (e.g., Tay-Sachs disease in Ashkenazi Jews).

Important AR diseases are described elsewhere, including cystic fibrosis (Chapter 4), thalassaemia, sickle cell disease (Chapter 8), congenital adrenal hyperplasia and inborn errors of metabolism (Chapter 7).

X-LINKED DISORDERS

Several hundred disease genes are found on the X chromosome and give rise to the characteristic pattern of X-linked inheritance. Males transmit their X chromosome to daughters, and Y chromosome to sons; both sons and daughters receive an X chromosome from the mother. Females inactivate (randomly) one of their X chromosomes during embryonic development (Lyon's hypothesis).

Most X-linked disorders are recessive. Female carriers have an abnormal allele on one X chromosome but are protected by their second, normal allele. The male is hemizygous for the gene because he has only a single X chromosome. The abnormal allele is not balanced by a normal allele and he manifests the disease.

A typical pedigree for X-linked recessive inheritance is shown in Fig. 16.4.

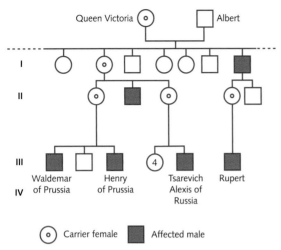

Fig. 16.4 The Royal Family pedigree demonstrating X-linked recessive inheritance of haemophilia A.

Waldemar of Prussia, Henry of Prussia, Tsarevich Alexis of Russia, Rupert

⊙ Carrier female   ■ Affected male

The features of an X-linked recessive pedigree are:

- Males only are affected.
- Carrier females might show mild signs of the disease depending on the pattern of X-chromosome inactivation – 'mosaicism'.
- Male infants of female carriers have a 50% chance of being affected; female infants have a 50% chance of being a carrier.
- All daughters of affected males are carriers.
- Sons of affected males are never affected because a father passes his Y chromosome to his son (i.e., there is no male-to-male transmission).

New mutations are common, so there might be no family history. Several important X-linked recessive diseases are discussed elsewhere, including haemophilia (Chapter 8) and Duchenne muscular dystrophy (Chapter 13). An additional example is fragile X syndrome.

Fragile X syndrome

This is an example of a trinucleotide repeat disorder. After Down syndrome, this is the most common cause of severe learning impairment with an incidence of 1 in 4000 males and approximately half this in females due to reduced penetrance. The disorder is due to expansion of a trinucleotide (CGG) repeat in gene FMR1.

The clinical features of fragile X syndrome are:

- learning difficulty (mean IQ 45; range 10 – normal range)
- autistic spectrum disorder (50%–70%)
- behavioural issues; ADHD, anxiety, temper tantrums and self-harm (hand biting)
- dysmorphic facial features (large forehead, long face, large prominent ears, macrocephaly) developing with age and often not readily recognizable in preschool children
- macro-orchidism

Table 16.4 Conditions with multifactorial inheritance

Type	Clinical condition
Congenital malformations	Neural tube defects
	Cleft lip and palate
	Pyloric stenosis
	Talipes
Medical conditions	Asthma
	Diabetes mellitus type 1 and 2
	Epilepsy
	Hypertension
	Atherosclerosis

The number of repeats determines status: unaffected individuals have fewer than 50 triplet repeats, carriers with a 'premutation' have 50 to 200 triplet repeats and affected men or women have over 200 triplet repeats.

MULTIFACTORIAL DISORDERS

Although some conditions result from a single gene mutation others have more complex causes. These diseases are influenced by the interaction of a number of genes (polygenic), one's environment and lifestyle. Multifactorial disorders include several common birth defects as well as a number of other important diseases with onset in childhood or adult life (Table 16.4).

A feature of the familial clustering of multifactorial diseases is that the recurrence risk is low, often in the range 3% to 5% (most significant for first-degree relatives and decreases rapidly with more distant relatedness). Factors that increase the risk to relatives include:

- Severely affected proband (e.g., greater in bilateral cleft lip and palate than unilateral cleft lip).
- Multiple affected family members.
- The affected proband is of the less often affected sex (if there is a difference in the M:F ratio of affected individuals).

In many multifactorial disorders, the environmental factors remain obscure.

CHROMOSOMAL DISORDERS

An alteration in the amount or nature of the chromosomal material is seen in 5 in 1000 live births and is usually associated with multiple congenital anomalies and learning difficulties. A high proportion (40%) of all spontaneous abortions are caused by chromosome abnormalities.

Most chromosome defects arise de novo. They are classified as abnormalities of number or structure, and might involve either

Table 16.5 Classification of chromosomal disorders

Type	Class	Name (live birth frequency)	Chromosomal abnormality
Numerical	Autosomal	Down syndrome (1/700) Edwards syndrome (1/5000) Patau syndrome (1/5000)	Trisomy 21 Trisomy 18 Trisomy 13
	Sex chromosomes	Klinefelter syndrome (1/500–1000) Turner syndrome (1/2000)	47,XXY 45,XO
Structural	Deletions	DiGeorge syndrome (1/6000) Prader-Willi syndrome (1/20,000) Cri-du-chat syndrome (1/15,000–50,000)	22q11.2 deletion 15q11–13 deletion 5p deletion

the autosomes or the sex chromosomes. Examples of important chromosomal disorders are shown in Table 16.5.

The indications for chromosome analysis include:

- phenotype consistent with known chromosomal disorder
- multiple congenital anomalies
- spontaneous abortion or stillbirth
- leukaemia and some solid tumours
- ambiguous genitalia

Chromosome studies are carried out on dividing cells. Most commonly, T cells from peripheral blood are used after stimulation of mitosis with phytohaemagglutinin.

Chromosomal abnormalities

Three autosomal trisomies are found in live-born infants; others are not compatible with life and are found only in spontaneously aborted foetuses. These are:

- Down syndrome: trisomy 21 (1:700 live births)
- Edwards syndrome: trisomy 18 (1:5,000 live births)
- Patau syndrome: trisomy 13 (1:5,000 live births)

Trisomy refers to the fact that three, rather than the normal two, copies of a specific chromosome are present in the cells of an individual. Trisomies commonly occur because of a meiotic error called 'nondisjunction' in the gamete of mother or father.

Down syndrome (trisomy 21)

Trisomy 21 is the most common autosomal trisomy compatible with life. The extra chromosomal material can result from nondisjunction, translocation or mosaicism.

Nondisjunction

About 95% of children with Down syndrome have trisomy 21 due to nondisjunction. The pair of chromosome 21 fails to separate at meiosis, so one gamete has two copies of chromosome 21. Fertilization of this gamete gives rise to a zygote with trisomy 21.

About 90% of nondisjunctions are maternally derived and the risk rises with maternal age, increasing steeply in mothers over 35 years (Table 16.6).

However, because a higher proportion of pregnancies occur in younger women, most children with trisomy 21 are born to

Table 16.6 Risk of Down syndrome (for live births) by maternal age at delivery

Maternal age (years)	Risk
All ages	1:700
20	1:1500
30	1:900
35	1:380
40	1:85
44	1:35

women under 35 years of age. The recurrence risk for parents of children with trisomy 21 increases to 1% to 2% (unless the age-related risk is higher).

Translocation

About 2% of Down syndrome children have 46 chromosomes with a Robertsonian translocation of the third chromosome 21 to another chromosome (most commonly 14). Three-quarters of cases are de novo and, in one-quarter, one of the parents has a balanced translocation involving one chromosome 21. If the mother is the translocation carrier, the recurrence risk might be as high as 15%; if the father is the carrier, the risk is 2.5%.

Mosaicism

In 2% of cases the nondisjunction occurs during mitosis after formation of the zygote so that some cells are normal and some show trisomy 21. The phenotype might be milder in mosaicism.

Clinical features

Down syndrome is often suspected at birth because of the characteristic facial appearance, but the diagnosis can be difficult on clinical features alone. A senior paediatrician should confirm clinical suspicion. Rapid chromosomal analysis is performed via fluorescence in-situ hybridization, but a complete karyotype is required if a translocation is suspected and should be used to confirm the initial result. The phenotypic

Table 16.7 Clinical features and associations with Down syndrome

Category	Clinical feature
Dysmorphic facial features	Brachycephaly Up slanting palpebral fissures Epicanthic folds Fat nasal bridge Protruding tongue Small ears Brushfield spots on the iris
Other dysmorphic features	Single palmar creases Incurved little fingers (clinodactyly) Gap between first and second toes (sandal toe gap) Short stature
Structural defects	Cardiac defects in 50% Duodenal atresia
Neurological features	Hypotonia in infancy Developmental delay Learning difficulties
Late medical complications	Increased risk of leukaemia Respiratory infections Hypothyroidism Coeliac disease Alzheimer disease Atlantoaxial instability

features are listed in Table 16.7. The risk of significant congenital anomalies is doubled in trisomy 21. See Chapter 15 for antenatal screening. Fig. 16.5 shows an image of a child with trisomy 21.

HINTS AND TIPS

- The mnemonic A TRISOMY CHILD can be used to help recall some of the clinical features associated with Down syndrome:
  - Atlanto-axial instability
  - Tongue protrusion
  - Respiratory infections
  - Incurved fifth finger
  - Single palmar crease/short stature
  - Obstructive sleep apnoea
  - Mental health conditions – anxiety and depression
  - Y – male infertility
  - Congenital heart disease/cataract
  - Hypotonia/hypothyroidism
  - Increased risk of leukaemia
  - Learning difficulty
  - Duodenal atresia

Management and prognosis

Parents need information about the implications of the diagnosis and access to support from professionals and support groups (e.g., Down syndrome association). Feelings of disappointment, anger and guilt are common. Genetic counselling for recurrence risks will be required. A cardiology review and echocardiogram should be arranged shortly after birth because of the association with cardiac defects. Screening for diseases associated with Down syndrome should be performed throughout life (e.g., hypothyroidism, coeliac disease). Patients may require support in later life with issues relating to education, employment and living arrangements. The average life expectancy has improved to around 60 years.

Edwards syndrome (trisomy 18)

The characteristic phenotype for Edwards syndrome includes microcephaly and micrognathia with associated cleft lip/palate, and ocular abnormalities (including short palpebral fissures, epicanthic folds, hypertelorism, microphthalmia and ptosis). The hands are often clenched with overlapping fingers and talipes, rocker bottom feet and absent radii may also feature. Systemic abnormalities include congenital cardiac malformations in 90% (ventricular septal defects most common), renal disease, exomphalos, atresia and developmental delay. The majority die in infancy.

Patau syndrome (trisomy 13)

Patau syndrome is associated with multiple major congenital anomalies including holoprosencephaly, exomphalos, cardiac and renal malformations. The phenotype may include microcephaly, microphthalmia, cleft palate, low set ears, polydactyly and talipes. A small proportion survive to adulthood – those with mosaicism have better prognosis but most die in early childhood.

Sex chromosome disorders

Turner syndrome

In this condition, there are 44 autosomes and only one normal X chromosome. It affects 1 in 2500 live-born females. Various underlying chromosomal defects are seen:

- In 55% of girls, the karyotype is 45,XO (true monosomy).
- In 25%, there is a deletion of the short arm of one X chromosome.
- In 15%, there is mosaicism.

The incidence does not increase with maternal age and the recurrence risk is the same as the general population risk.

Clinical features and diagnosis

The clinical features are listed in Table 16.8. Diagnosis may be made:

- prenatally by ultrasound scan
- at birth by presence of puffy hands and feet (lymphoedema) or a cardiac abnormality
- during childhood because of short stature

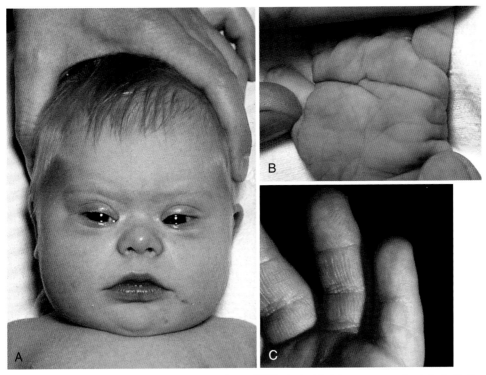

Fig. 16.5 Image of an infant with classical features of Down syndrome. (A) The typical facial appearance of an infant with Down syndrome shows the upward slant of the canthal folds of the eyes; protruding tongue; and short, thick neck. (B) The straight simian crease in the palm of the hand is a typical finding in children with Down syndrome. (C) A short little finger is a typical finding in children with Down syndrome. The tip of the little finger does not extend to the distal joint of the adjoining (ring) finger. (From Zitelli, B. L., & Davis, H. W. *Atlas of pediatric physical diagnosis.* 6th ed. St. Louis: Mosby; 2012.)

Table 16.8 Clinical features and associations with Turner syndrome

Category	Clinical feature
Dysmorphic facial features	Ptosis Neck webbing Low hairline
Other dysmorphic features	Neonatal lymphoedema Short stature Wide carrying angle (cubitus valgus) Widely spaced nipples Hypoplastic/hyperconvex nails Short 4th/5th metacarpals Multiple naevi
Structural defects	Cardiac defects (coarctation of the aorta) Horseshoe kidneys
Neurological features	Developmental delay Normal intelligence or mild learning difficulties
Late medical complications	Amenorrhoea Primary ovarian failure and infertility Hypothyroidism

- in adolescence because of primary amenorrhoea and lack of pubertal development

Diagnosis is confirmed by a blood karyotype. Fig. 16.6 shows an image of a child with Turner Syndrome.

Management

Therapy with growth hormone improves final height. Ovarian hormones are not produced due to the gonadal dysgenesis (streak ovaries). Oestrogen therapy is given at the appropriate age (11 years) to induce maturation of secondary sexual characteristics including breast development. Towards the end of puberty, progestogen is added to maintain uterine health and allow monthly withdrawal bleeds (periods). Although pregnancy can occur naturally, most patients are infertile. Pregnancy can be achieved with in vitro fertilization. Treatment may also be necessary for other abnormalities (e.g., surgical correction of coarctation of the aorta).

Klinefelter syndrome

Klinefelter syndrome is characterized by one or more extra X chromosomes, most commonly 47 XXY karyotype. The phenotype is of:

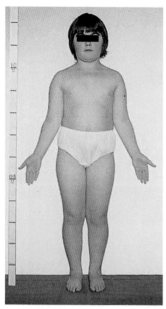

Fig. 16.6 Image of a child with Turner syndrome. (From Patton KT, Thibodeau GA. *Anatomy & physiology*, 8th edition. St. Louis: Mosby; 2013.)

- tall stature with long legs
- small testes
- gynaecomastia
- learning difficulties

Treatment with testosterone may be needed to stimulate development of secondary sexual characteristics.

Structural chromosomal abnormalities

These arise from chromosome breakage and include deletions, duplications, inversions and unbalanced translocations. Deletions are the most common. Most arise de novo, but they can also arise from inheritance of an unbalanced translocation. Examples of conditions associated with chromosomal deletions include:

- DiGeorge syndrome: caused by microdeletions of chromosome 22q11. The condition is associated with cardiac defects, cleft palate, hypocalcaemia, immunodeficiency and learning difficulties.
- Prader-Willi syndrome: caused by deletions of the paternal copy of 15q11–13. In childhood this causes insatiable appetite and obesity, with associated hypogonadotropic hypogonadism and learning difficulties.
- Angelman syndrome: caused by deletions of the maternal copy of 15q11–13. These children have significant developmental delay and learning difficulties, and

characteristically appear happy with frequent laughter. They often have seizures and ataxic gait.
- Cri-du-chat syndrome: caused by deletion of the short arm of chromosome 5 (5p–). Affected children have significant learning difficulties and a characteristic 'cat-like' cry.

MITOCHONDRIAL INHERITANCE

Mitochondrial disorders are inherited maternally. Examples include:

- mitochondrial encephalopathy, lactic acidosis, stroke-like episodes
- mitochondrially inherited diabetes mellitus

A mixture of normal and abnormal mitochondria (heteroplasmy) can exist within tissues. Most conditions that are mitochondrially inherited present in late childhood and so diagnosis may be delayed. Genetic counselling is of particular importance in these conditions.

GENETIC COUNSELLING

This is usually carried out as a specialist service by trained medical staff. The main aim is to provide information about hereditary disorders so that parents will have greater autonomy and choice in reproductive decisions.

The basic elements of counselling include:

- Establishing a diagnosis: this might involve physical examination of the affected child (proband) and family members and undertaking special investigations including DNA, cytogenetic and biochemical analysis.
- Estimation of risk: the risk for future offspring is determined by the mode of inheritance of the disease.

Table 16.9 A summary of common genetic tests in clinical practice

Test	Summary	Use in paediatrics
Karyotype	Identifies loss or gain of entire chromosomes and translocations from one chromosome to another.	Aneuploidy assessment (e.g., trisomies 21, 18) or a sex chromosome aneuploidy (e.g., 45,XO).
Fluorescence in situ hybridization (FISH)	Karyotyping is limited to the detection of large chromosomal rearrangements. FISH is able to detect much smaller changes. It involves the hybridization of fluorescently labelled DNA sequence probes with patient DNA. It identifies abnormal copy number or pathological location of a given fluorescence signal.	It is quicker than karyotyping for detecting aneuploidy. It can also confirm a suspected diagnosis of a well-described, specific syndrome, such as Di George syndrome or Williams syndrome.
Comparative genomic hybridization (CGH) array	Array CGH compares the patient's genetic code against a control and identifies differences between the two. It identifies copy number variations (CNVs).	Array CGH/SNP is indicated as first-line testing for unexplained learning difficulties, developmental delay, suspected autistic spectrum disorder, dysmorphism and multiple congenital abnormalities.
Single nucleotide polymorphism (SNP) array	SNP, a variation at a single site in DNA, is the most frequent type of variation in the genome. Advantage of SNP array over CGH array is that it can determine both CNVs and LOH (loss of heterozygosity i.e., loss of genetic material).	
Whole-genome sequencing (WGS)	WGS is the sequencing of all DNA present including chromosomal and mitochondrial DNA. This test has recently been introduced on the NHS and is seeing increased utility in paediatrics.	WGS is frequently used where the above tests have not yielded results despite strong clinical suspicions of an underlying genetic diagnosis.

- Communication: information must be conveyed in an unbiased and nondirective way. This should include magnitude of risk, severity of disorder and availability of treatment. Parental cultural, religious and ethical values should be explored, and all the possible options should be discussed.

Genetic tests

Table 16.9 summarizes common forms of genetic testing used in paediatric clinical practice.

HINTS AND TIPS

Options arising from prenatal genetic counselling:
- Decision not to have offspring.
- To accept the risk.
- Antenatal diagnosis and possible termination of pregnancy.
- Preimplantation diagnosis.
- Artificial insemination by donor or ovum donation.

Chapter Summary

- There are many types of genetic disorders, which include single-gene, chromosomal, mitochondrial and multifactorial disorders.
- There are different modes of inheritance amongst single-gene disorders, specifically autosomal dominant, autosomal recessive and sex linked.
- Trisomies 13, 18 and 21 are examples of chromosomal disorders; the only trisomies compatible with life. They are all associated with varying degrees of learning difficulties and major congenital anomalies.
- Genetic counselling involves identifying the diagnosis and then providing parents with information regarding future risk, severity of the disorder and treatment options.

UKMLA Condition
Down's syndrome

UKMLA Presentations
Congenital abnormalities
Dysmorphic child

Development

Normal development depends on genetic potential (nature) and on the environment (nurture). Studies over many years have established the average rate and pattern of development and there is a wide variation in normal rates of development in all domains. A child might be far from average but still normal. A major challenge in paediatrics is to distinguish such normal variation from a significant problem requiring investigation.

Developmental screening is offered routinely to all children in the UK. The aim of developmental surveillance is to identify developmental problems at an early stage to allow appropriate intervention. Any delay might be global or specific, but it is important to bear in mind interrelationships (e.g., hearing impairment can cause a delay in speech and language, with consequent disruption of social interaction and behaviour; visual impairment can affect fine motor skills and communication).

Clinical assessment of a child's developmental status is based on a thorough history, physical examination and observation of the child's performance and play.

HISTORY

This should encompass:

- antenatal history, including birth history
- family history (i.e., of learning disability or significant medical conditions)
- social history: risk factors (e.g., psychosocial deprivation)
- developmental milestones
- specific parental concerns

In particular, it is important to document any 'risk factors' that contribute to vulnerability and poor outcome, for example, prematurity, birth asphyxia, any chromosomal abnormalities or psychosocial deprivation, such as neglect.

HINTS AND TIPS

Milestones reflect the average age that a child acquires a particular ability:

- Motor problems often manifest in the first year.
- Talking and coordination problems often manifest in the second year.
- Behavioural and social problems often manifest in the third year.

EXAMINATION

This should include the following:

- appearance (i.e., are there dysmorphic features, visual or hearing aids)
- height and weight (plotted on a centile chart)
- head circumference
- systemic examination
- developmental assessment (observation and play)

Four aspects of development are routinely assessed:

1. gross motor
2. fine motor and vision
3. hearing and speech
4. social behaviour and play

Routine surveillance is carried out at recognized stages of development up until age 5 years or sooner if concerns are raised.

The general milestones expected according to age are described in the following section.

Key gross motor milestones

These include:

- primitive reflexes (e.g., Moro, asymmetrical tonic neck reflex, Babinski (newborn))
- head control when pulled to sitting (2 months; see Fig. 17.1)
- transient head control when held supine (2 months; see Fig. 17.2)
- rolls front to back (4 months)
- rolls back to front (6 months)
- loss of primitive reflexes (6 months)
- sits unsupported (6–9 months)
- crawls (9 months)
- cruises (10–12 months)
- walks (12–15 months)
- runs (18 months)
- jumps (2 years)
- climbs stairs, alternating feet (3 years)
- hops (4 years)
- rides a tricycle (5 years)

HINTS AND TIPS

The Moro response consists of extension of the arms, then brisk adduction towards the chest when the infant

---

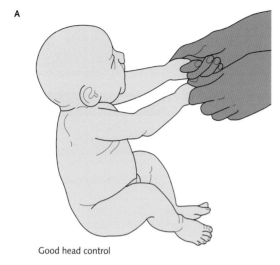

Good head control

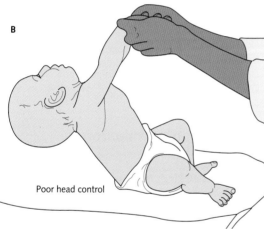

Poor head control

Fig. 17.1 (A) Good head control compared with (B) poor head control when pulled to sit.

is startled or the baby's head allowed to drop back slightly. It should be symmetrical and should have disappeared by 6 months. Persistence of this or any of the primitive reflexes beyond 6 months might indicate a cerebral disorder.

Key fine motor and visual milestones

These include:

- grasp reflex (newborn)
- palmar grasp (4 months)
- reaches for objects (4 months)
- fine pincer grip (12 months; see Fig. 17.3)
- uses spoon (15 months)
- builds tower of four blocks (18 months; see Fig. 17.4)
- tower of six blocks (2 years)
- tripod pencil grip (5 years)

HINTS AND TIPS

Hand preference develops at 18 to 24 months of age and is fixed at 5 years of age. Handedness before 12 months indicates a problem with the nondominant side.

Key speech and hearing milestones

These include:

- startles to loud noise (newborn)
- coos (2 months)
- laughs (4 months)
- babble (6 months)
- first word (12 months)
- 50 + words (2 years)
- knows name and age (3 years)
- tells a story (4 years)

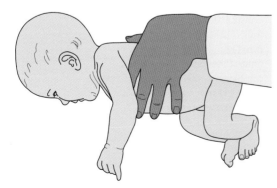

Fig. 17.2 Transient head control is seen when held in ventral suspension at 2 months.

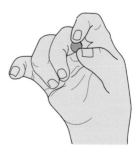

Fig. 17.3 Pincer grip.

FINE MOTOR TASKS

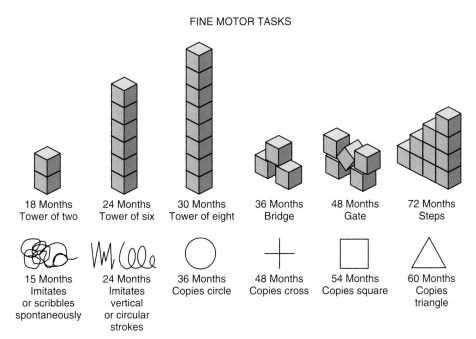

Fig. 17.4 Expected fine motor skills by age. (From *Zitelli and Davis' Atlas of Pediatric Physical Diagnosis*, 8th ed. Elsevier, 2021.)

All newborn babies are tested as part of the Newborn Hearing Screening Programme. The automated otoacoustic emission (AOAE) screening test is used, which is a simple, painless test that produces immediate results and can be carried out while the baby is asleep. If two AOAE test results are unsatisfactory, then brainstem auditory evoked potentials are performed.

Key social and cognitive milestones

These include:

- prefers colour, light and faces (newborn)
- follows beyond midline (2 months)
- social smile (2 months)
- stranger anxiety (6 months)
- symbolic play (i.e., tea party; 18 months)
- tantrums (2 years)
- shares toys (3 years)
- play games with rules (5 years)

SIGNS OF ABNORMAL DEVELOPMENT

Any parental or carer concerns about an infant or child's development (either slow progress or regression of skills) should be taken seriously and warrant prompt assessment and referral to the local community paediatric team. Concerns may also be raised by health visitors or teachers, or picked up by routine surveillance.

RED FLAG

The red flags listed below are well recognized as indicators of abnormal development and should prompt referral to paediatrics:

- Excessive head lag beyond 8 weeks.
- Not smiling by 10 weeks.
- Persistence of primitive reflexes beyond 6 months.
- Hand preference before 12 months.
- Not walking at age 18 months.
- Not knowing a few words by 18 months.
- Not interacting with other children at 3 years.

Poor tone, that is, head lag, may indicate a chromosomal problem or neuromuscular disorder. Persistence of primitive reflexes, early hand preference or delayed walking can be early signs of neurological conditions such as cerebral palsy. Poor social or communication skills may suggest either autism or possible audio-visual problems.

HINTS AND TIPS

Babies who were preterm need their development monitored. This is initially corrected according to their gestational age, but becomes less important after 2 years.

Table 17.1 Causes of global developmental delay

Type	Causes
Perinatal	Hypoxic-ischaemic encephalopathy Intracranial haemorrhage Teratogens
Infection	Toxoplasmosis, other (syphilis, varicella-zoster, parvovirus B19), rubella, cytomegalovirus and herpes (TORCH) infections Post central nervous system infection (meningitis, encephalitis)]
Metabolic	Hypothyroidism Inborn errors of metabolism (e.g., phenylketonuria)
Chromosomal disorders	Trisomy 13, 18 and 21 Fragile X syndrome
Neurodegenerative disease	Sphingolipidoses (e.g., Tay–Sachs disease) Mucopolysaccharidosis (e.g., Hurler syndrome) Peroxisomal disease (e.g., adrenoleucodystrophy)

Global developmental delay

This umbrella term describes when a child is not achieving their expected developmental milestones across several or all of the domains. Not all children with global delay are intellectually impaired. There is often a specific underlying aetiology (Table 17.1) with 40% due to a chromosomal abnormality (e.g., trisomy 21).

Investigation and management

This will depend on the setting and what tools are available for assessment (e.g., outpatient clinic is preferable to emergency department).

Community paediatricians are best equipped and more experienced in carrying out the detailed assessment that is required to identify if there is either specific or global developmental delay.

In addition to a thorough history and examination, they may request investigations, which might include:

- audiology assessment
- ophthalmology assessment
- brain imaging
- blood tests

Blood tests are directed towards identifying a specific aetiology and could include:

- Genetic testing (see Chapter 16)
- thyroid function tests

- congenital infection (toxoplasmosis, other (syphilis, varicella-zoster, parvovirus B19), rubella, cytomegalovirus and herpes (TORCH)) screen
- Lead and biotinidase
- plasma and urine amino and organic acids
- creatinine kinase

They will also arrange appropriate follow-up for monitoring progress and relaying results back to the parents. A crucial job is to help families to access the support they need (e.g., social care for children with disabilities, or to arrange an assessment of the child's educational needs).

HINTS AND TIPS

It is important to distinguish developmental delay from actual regression. Loss of previously acquired skills suggests a serious disorder and warrants urgent referral. Regression can be associated with rare diseases such as Rett syndrome, Landau-Kleffner syndrome and other neurodegenerative syndromes.

Specific developmental delay

Two common and important examples of delayed development in specific areas are discussed below.

Delayed walking

About 50% of children walk unsupported by 12 months and 90% by 15 months; further assessment is indicated if a child is not walking unsupported by age 18 months. Many will be normal late walkers, especially if a 'bottom shuffler', but a small percentage will have an underlying problem. Such problems include cerebral palsy, congenital developmental dysplasia of the hip or Duchenne muscular dystrophy.

Examination

- Locomotion: 'commando crawler' or 'bottom shuffler'?
- Musculoskeletal: check the hips for signs of dislocation (waddling gait, leg length discrepancy, limited abduction). Check the spine and overlying skin. Observe for foot deformities or signs of calf pseudohypertrophy.
- Neurology: check tone, power and tendon reflexes in all limbs.

Investigations

If indicated:

- imaging of hips or spine
- creatine kinase (raised in Duchenne muscular dystrophy)
- vitamin D level and bone profile

Management depends on the specific cause identified.

Speech and language delay

The development of normal speech and language requires:

- adequate hearing
- cognitive development
- coordinated sound production

Speech refers to the meaningful sounds that are made, whereas language encompasses the complex rules governing the use of these sounds for communication. Language can be further divided into comprehension and expression, and independent delays can occur in either aspect. As might be expected, the development of language is highly dependent on general intellectual development.

The causes of delay in speech and language development include:

- global delay: the most common cause
- hearing impairment
- environmental factors: lack of stimulus
- social and communication disorders: autism
- familial
- bilingual household

It is worth distinguishing between delay and actual disorders of speech and language such as stammering, dysarthria due to mechanical problems (e.g., cleft palate) or neuromuscular problems (e.g., cerebral palsy). In any case, speech and language therapists are invaluable in maximizing a child's potential.

● Chapter Summary

- The four developmental domains are gross motor, fine motor and vision, speech and hearing, social and cognitive.
- Developmental progress is assessed as part of routine surveillance.
- Children with suspected developmental delay and/or developmental red flags should be referred to community paediatricians for assessment.
- Global developmental delay may be secondary to a chromosomal abnormality and describes a child who is delayed in several developmental domains. It is important to request investigations and imaging to help identify the underlying cause.
- Loss of skills (regression) warrants an urgent referral and is often associated with neurodegenerative disease.
- Delayed walking may be normal but can indicate underlying cerebral palsy, developmental dysplasia of the hip or Duchenne muscular dystrophy. Initial investigations should include hip imaging, creatine kinase and vitamin D levels.

UKMLA Conditions
Muscular dystrophies
Down's syndrome

UKMLA Presentations
Abnormal development/developmental delay
Developmental delay
Dysmorphic child
Speech and language problems

A joint position statement from the Royal Colleges (Paediatrics & Child health – RCPCH, Emergency Medicine RCEM and Psychiatrists RCPsych) in 2021 recognized 'unprecedented demand' in children and young people presenting distressed with mental ill-health – since the pandemic onset. Behavioural and emotional problems are increasingly prevalent, with a spotlight on self-harm and suicide. Adolescence is a period where important disorders present, including major psychoses although these are rare. Complex psychosocial crises require multi-agency collaboration to support patients.

A child's personality, behaviour patterns and emotional responses are determined by an interplay between nature (genetic predisposition) and nurture (predominantly parenting).

ATTACHMENT

Secure early attachment is very important for emotional development. Separation anxiety when separated from the primary caregiver typically becomes evident at about 6 months to 1 year of age. By the second year, emotional attachments are extended to other family members, and by the age of 4 to 5 years, separation from parents can be tolerated for several hours as occurs with school attendance. With entry into school, the importance of others – such as teachers and fellow school children – in shaping the child's psychosocial development increases.

RED FLAG

Risk factors for disturbed emotional and behavioural development:
- parental mental health problems
- parental substance use
- domestic violence
- abuse or neglect
- divorce or bereavement
- intrusive overprotection or emotional rejection
- lack of or inconsistent boundary setting
- socioeconomic deprivation

PROBLEMS OF EARLY CHILDHOOD

Behavioural problems in early childhood can relate to sleeping or eating, and tantrums are common.

Babies

An average baby sleeps for 15 hours a day in the first 2 to 3 months of life, sleeping for about 4 hours and waking for 3 hours at a time. After about 4 months, night-time feeds may no longer be needed and the baby may start to sleep through the night. The main problems encountered are infants who seem to sleep all day and awake all night. The other major problem encountered is inconsolable crying which can be due to a myriad of reasons.

Toddlers

Sleep-related problems

Problems include:
- difficulty in settling to sleep at night
- waking at night
- nightmares and night terrors

Difficulty in getting to sleep at night

A child might not settle at night for many reasons including:
- separation anxiety
- fear of darkness and silence
- erratic bedtime routine

Helpful strategies include creating a predictable structure around bedtime and leaving the child alone to settle for lengthening periods.

Nightmares and night terrors

Nightmares are bad dreams that can be recalled by the child. They are common and normal unless very frequent or stereotyped in content. Reassurance is usually sufficient.

Night terrors are a form of parasomnia in which there is rapid emergence from the initial period of deep, slow-wave sleep, into a state of high arousal and confusion. The child usually cries out and is found sitting up with open eyes but disorientated and unresponsive. The child settles, with no subsequent recall of the episode. They often occur at the same time each night and waking the child briefly before the night terror is expected to occur might break the pattern.

Food refusal

Meal times can easily become a battleground. Parents often find that their toddler refuses to eat the meals provided or is a fussy eater. The child is usually well nourished with a normal rate of weight gain. Advice can be given to:

- Avoid snacking between main meals.
- Keep regular family meal times.
- Do not prolong mealtimes – if the child does not finish the meal within 20 minutes, take it away but do not give any other food as a replacement.
- Try to avoid turning meals into a battleground.

Small amounts of food with gradual introduction of new foods in a relaxed, nonbargaining atmosphere is the best approach. No preschool child will voluntarily starve himself or herself, although some mothers find this difficult to believe.

Tantrums

Toddlers normally go through a period in which they are disinclined to comply with their parents' demands; this phase is sometimes referred to as 'the terrible twos'. Temper tantrums can occur in response to frustration. Parents might become demoralized in their attempts to assert control.

Management strategies include:

- Praising compliance and rewarding good behaviour.
- Avoiding threats that cannot be carried out.
- Setting reasonable limits.
- Giving clear commands.

A tantrum itself can be dealt with by ignoring it (this can be difficult, especially in a public place) or by giving the child 'time out' (removing him or her from social interaction for a short period, e.g., in a separate room).

Breath-holding spells

These occur in children between 6 months and 2 years of age and are triggered by high emotion (tantrums, etc.). The child holds their breath, becomes pale or cyanotic, loses consciousness and falls to the floor. There may be tonic-clonic movements. History is vital in distinguishing this from other forms of syncope.

Intellectual disabilities

From mild to profound intellectual disabilities affect the way in which children through to adults learn new things. Individuals may experience problems ranging from being unable to understand complex information to unable to look after themselves. Some intellectual disabilities are tied with an organic medical condition or genetic diagnosis and in others they are not. Due to the diversity of how these disabilities affect individuals, careful assessments and care plans may be required to assist these individuals to give them the best chance throughout their development and future life.

Speech and language problems

During our early years we develop our receptive and expressive language. Alongside this, we develop the ability to phonate and articulate different sounds. When considering speech and language delay, you must think about what enables appropriate development of language and speech. This is made up of hearing (receptive), appropriate neural networks and phonation skills. If these are disrupted, then speech delay can occur.

Causes of speech and language delay and impairment can be sub-divided into:

- Global developmental delay
  - Down syndrome
  - Fragile X
  - Neglect
- Isolated speech and language delay
  - Hearing loss/impairment
  - Autistic spectrum disorder
  - Cleft palate

AUTISM SPECTRUM DISORDERS

Autism (also referred to as autism spectrum disorder) refers to a pervasive developmental disorder (or difference), which presents in early childhood and is lifelong. Autism describes qualitative differences in reciprocal social interaction and communication combined with restricted interests and repetitive behaviours. Autism is thought to affect about 1% of the population, is more common in boys than girls, and usually presents by the age of 3 years; however, girls are often diagnosed later or go undiagnosed.

Autism is found more commonly if there is:

- first-degree relative with autism
- parent with schizophrenia or affective disorder
- maternal sodium valproate administration in pregnancy
- gestational age less than 35 weeks
- children with:
  - learning difficulty
  - congenital central nervous system malformation, cerebral palsy or neonatal encephalopathy
  - Down syndrome, fragile X and other chromosomal/genetic conditions
  - tuberous sclerosis or neurofibromatosis
  - muscular dystrophy

HINTS AND TIPS

There is no evidence to link the measles, mumps and rubella (MMR) vaccine with autism – the original work which found this has been discredited. Autistic features often become noticeable at around the time the MMR vaccination is routinely given. Parents should be reassured and the risks associated with MMR discussed.

Clinical presentation

The core features of autism are:

- Impaired reciprocal social interaction – this may include difficulty in forming social relationships, avoiding eye contact and reduced response to other's emotions (e.g., difficulty in sharing enjoyment).
- Impaired communication – this can include delayed speech and language development, stereotyped or repetitive use of language and difficulty with initiating or sustaining reciprocal communication with others.
- Restricted interests and repetitive behaviours – this can include specific interests, attachments to unusual objects, reliance on routines or rituals with distress if these are altered and motor mannerisms (e.g., hand flapping).

Note that autism is described as a spectrum as many children will not have significant impairment in all these categories. Those with Asperger syndrome or 'high-functioning autism' may have a normal intelligence quotient (IQ) and speech development, having specific difficulties with social and communication skills, or obsessional interests.

It is very common for children with autism to also have significant learning difficulties: approximately 50% have an IQ of less than 70, and there is a 70% coincidence of psychiatric conditions including attention deficit hyperactivity disorder (ADHD), conduct disorders, depression and obsessive-compulsive disorder.

Around 25% will develop a seizure disorder.

Assessment and diagnosis

Assessment is comprehensive, focusing on the core features of autism, the child's home and school life, birth and developmental history, and clinical observation and examination. A collateral history from the school and from other agencies such as social care if involved can be very helpful. The first assessment may be by a paediatrician alone, but children should be referred to a multidisciplinary autism team consisting of a child and adolescent psychiatrist, clinical or educational psychologist and speech and language therapist, with input from other professionals as appropriate, such as a paediatric neurologist or occupational therapist.

> **COMMON PITFALLS**
>
> Autism cannot be ruled out in a child who smiles, makes eye contact or is affectionate with their families – it is a myth that children with autism do not display these behaviours.

Management

A multidisciplinary approach to management is key to offer holistic support to children and young people with autism, as well as their caregivers. Play therapists, speech and language therapists and clinical and educational psychologists play a key role in supporting development of communication, social and life skills. National Institute for Health and Care Excellence (NICE) is clear that there is no role for medication in managing the core features of autism, nor for intensive approaches such as neurofeedback.

Behaviour that is challenging should first be addressed with a psychosocial approach which identifies and addresses underlying stressors. Where this is unsuccessful, antipsychotic medication can be considered. This should be prescribed by an expert and closely monitored. Coexistent medical and psychiatric conditions should be assessed and treated as appropriate.

Families should be supported both psychologically and with practical help such as with respite for carers. Charities such as the National Autistic Society in the UK (www.autism.org.uk) can provide additional support. Significant input is needed around the time of transition to adult services which can be very disruptive and difficult if not managed effectively.

> **COMMUNICATION**
>
> While a diagnosis of autism can be difficult for families to accept, some families will feel a sense of relief at identifying an explanation. While it is important to be clear that there is no 'cure' for autism, it is important to be positive and explain that there is a lot which can be done to support people with autism, to give a good quality of life and increased independence.

ATTENTION DEFICIT HYPERACTIVITY DISORDER

The three hallmarks of ADHD are:

- inattention
- hyperactivity
- impulsiveness

Incidence and aetiology

ADHD is thought to affect 2% to 9% of schoolchildren in the UK. There is some variation in diagnostic criteria between the two systems (DSM-5 & ICD-11) commonly used. Current NICE guidelines direct that to diagnose ADHD requires fulfilling either ICD-11 or DSM-5 criteria for symptoms of hyperactivity/impulsivity and/or inattention that:

- persist in two or more settings (i.e., home and school)
- impair function, at least moderately, in multiple settings

Severe ADHD (hyperkinetic disorder) is a more severe subtype of ADHD with a prevalence of 1 in 200 – it is four times more common in boys than girls. Twin studies suggest a genetic contribution to aetiology. Perinatal problems and delays in early development appear to be more common in hyperkinetic disorder. Disturbed relationships, such as might occur with an emotionally rejecting parent or institutional upbringing, seem to exacerbate it.

Clinical features

Features of ADHD:

- Inattention: manifests as an easily distracted child who changes activity frequently and does not persist with tasks.
- Hyperactivity: an excess of movement with persistent fidgeting and restlessness.
- Impulsiveness: acting without reflection or prior thought.

These features are present in multiple settings and persist over time. They can be distinguished from normal high-spirited, energetic behaviour by the interference with normal social functioning.

Physical examination should include a search for:

- developmental delay, clumsiness
- deficits in hearing or vision and specific learning difficulties
- dysmorphic features

Investigations

Most children do not have a sudden onset or an identifiable brain disorder and do not need special investigations such as electro-encephalography or brain imaging. Up to 50% of children will have a comorbid psychiatric disorder.

HINTS AND TIPS

Parents may self-diagnose children with attention deficit hyperactivity disorder: it is important to have a definitive diagnosis made by a specialist to enable the child to access appropriate services, particularly in the school setting.

Management

A behaviour-modifying and educational approach is the mainstay of treatment but drug treatment should be considered if these strategies fail. It is important to explain the nature of the disorder to the parents and school staff. Parent support groups might provide reassurance and help.

Behavioural therapy

The first-line treatment for preschool children is group-based parent training and education programmes. In older children, individual psychological treatment may be more appropriate.

Key features are:

- a structured environment
- positive reinforcement
- cognitive approaches emphasizing relaxation and self-control

Extra help in the classroom and modification of the curriculum might be required.

Drug therapy

Where behavioural therapy is ineffective in children over 5 years old, central stimulant medication can be used in conjunction. First-line treatment is with methylphenidate which requires regular monitoring for side effects which include slowing of growth and hypertension. A medication break should be given at least once per year during the school holidays to assess whether it is still required. Lisdexamfetamine is used as a second-line treatment. Medication is not recommended in preschool children.

Alternative therapies

Numerous alternative therapies have been advocated; however, these have not been found to be evidence based. Many parents believe in a restricted diet or removing additives or colourings from the diet, but this is not recommended by NICE.

Prognosis

Symptoms diminish over time but approximately half will continue to have symptoms in adolescence and adulthood. Hyperactivity itself does not usually persist as a predominant feature into adulthood. However, ADHD can affect school performance and result in low self-esteem which can persist into adulthood.

BEHAVIOURAL PROBLEMS

Conduct disorder

Conduct disorders are the number one reason for referral to Child and Adolescent Mental Health Services (CAMHS). Conduct disorder describes persistent defiant or antisocial behaviour which violates age-appropriate social norms, for example, theft, truancy, destruction of property or violence to people or animals. They are more common in boys and more common in those with ADHD, autism or a mental health problem. Conduct disorders are strongly associated with poor educational outcomes, crime, substance use and mental health problems in adulthood. They should be managed with parent training and education programmes, and cognitive problem-solving approaches for the child or young person.

Oppositional defiant disorder

Oppositional defiant disorder is similar to conduct disorder, but it is not associated with severe antisocial or violent behaviour, and is more common in younger children (aged <8 years). It is highly predictive of developing conduct disorder.

CONTINENCE PROBLEMS

Enuresis (see Chapter 6)

Encopresis (faecal soiling)

Encopresis is voluntary or involuntary faecal soiling into a place other than a toilet for more than one time per month for at least 3 months at an age beyond which continence should have been achieved (normally about 4 years).

Children with encopresis fall into two main groups:

- retentive: rectum loaded with faeces, leading to overflow incontinence (the majority)
- nonretentive: without constipation (i.e., neurogenic sphincter disturbance or psychiatric illness)

A number of factors predispose to chronic stool retention. These include:

- environmental problems: lack of toilet facilities, harsh toilet training
- idiopathic: some children's rectums only empty occasionally, perhaps due to poor coordination with anal sphincter relaxation
- idiopathic constipation: for example, due to dehydration or an anal fissure leading to chronic retention
- organic constipation: associated with Hirschsprung disease, spinal cord abnormalities, anorectal malformations drugs or hypothyroidism

Once established, a large bolus of stool in the rectum might be impossible for the child to expel. The loaded rectum becomes dilated and might habituate to distension, so the child is unaware of the need to empty it. Psychological factors can be both a cause and a result of encopresis. Soiling disturbs the child and can have a profound impact in school, social life and in the family.

Onset of soiling in middle childhood, without coexistent constipation, suggests a primary psychiatric cause. It might occur in the setting of a chaotic family with high levels of emotional deprivation, neglect and disturbed behaviour.

History

Assessment must include a full bowel history and assessment of the family's psychological functioning.

Examination

It is important to perform systematic examination of the neurological system and abdomen. Abdominal palpation may reveal a faecal mass. Rectal examination is rarely indicated in children and, if needed, should only be done by an expert.

Management

The key objective in management of encopresis due to faecal retention is to empty the rectum as soon as possible. This is done via an escalating faecal impaction regimen of oral laxatives (e.g., macrogol). Regular defecation should then be encouraged by:

- regular laxatives
- star charts
- sitting on the toilet after meals
- dietary changes: increased fibre intake and adequate hydration

The distended rectum will take several weeks to shrink to normal size. It is unusual for the problem to persist into adolescence.

AFFECTIVE DISORDERS

Depression

Depression as a clinical syndrome is more than just a transitory low mood or feeling sad in response to adverse life circumstances. It is increasingly recognized in prepubertal children but is predominantly a problem in adolescence. Aetiology is multifactorial but there is a clear genetic contribution, and there may be a family history of depression or bipolar affective disorder. Contributory or causative factors include adverse social factors: explore any bullying at school or problems at home including parental relationship difficulty, abuse or neglect, parental mental health problems or substance use.

Clinical features

Depression can be categorized as mild, moderate and severe depression (with or without psychotic symptoms). For a diagnosis of depression, symptoms should be present for at least 2 weeks with symptoms present for most of the day.

It is characterized by:

- persistent feelings of sadness or unhappiness
- ideas of guilt, despair and lack of self-worth
- social withdrawal
- lack of motivation and energy
- biological symptoms with disturbances of sleep, appetite and weight

Management

General interventions should be offered for mild depression including advice on self-help information, exercise, sleep hygiene and anxiety management. If this persists or for moderate to severe depression, first-line treatment is psychological therapy – this can be in the form of cognitive behavioural therapy, family therapy or psychodynamic psychotherapy. Medication should be offered in conjunction with therapy where symptoms are severe or not improving, with fluoxetine recommended as first line.

Self-harm and suicide

The prevalence of self-harm and suicide in young people is increasing. Self-harm is an under-reported important clinical findings as nonfatal self-harm is the biggest risk factors for ensuing suicide in paediatric populations. The rough incidences in the UK from 2013 to 2021 are ~ 680 hospitalizations per 100,000 females and ~200 hospitalization per 100,000 males aged 10 to 24. Worryingly, this trend is on the rise according to recent studies.

Some common forms of presenting to hospital with deliberate self-harm are in the form of:

– Cutting or burning skin
– Poisonings (paracetamol overdose)
– Injured from purposeful risky behaviour

Young people who present with self-harm should be referred to CAMHS for comprehensive risk assessment and offered appropriate psychological support.

ANXIETY

Anxiety disorders are increasingly recognized as a problem in childhood and are more common in children with underlying depression. Although anxiety can occur as part of normal development, it is important to recognize where it becomes pathological, impacting on the child or young person's ability to take part in their normal activities. The mainstay of management is addressing underlying stressors and cognitive behavioural therapy.

School refusal

School refusal describes severe anxiety which presents as an unwillingness to attend school.

School refusal might be associated with:

• separation anxiety (under 11 years of age)
• adverse life events (bereavement, moving)
• stressors (bullying)

School refusers tend to be good academically. This should be distinguished from school absence due to truancy. Management requires an early, graded return to school with support for the parents and treatment of any underlying emotional disorder. Two-thirds of school refusers will return to school regularly.

Selective mutism

Selective mutism is an anxiety disorder where there is an inability to speak in specific social situations despite the ability to speak normally. It is rare, affecting around 0.5% children typically aged 3 to 6 years. The majority of cases resolve spontaneously; however, individual or family therapy may be required. It can be exhibited in response to abuse, especially sexual abuse.

PSYCHOSIS

Psychosis is uncommon in childhood and if it occurs, is more likely to be organic in origin, for example, the phenomenon of hyperactive delirium in some patients requiring paediatric intensive care. Chronic disorders such as schizophrenia and bipolar affective disorder can present in adolescence. In addition, drug-induced psychosis should be considered in the adolescent age group. Symptoms include delusions and abnormalities of perception (visual or auditory hallucinations).

EATING DISORDERS

Eating disorders are defined by negative beliefs related to eating and body image. Behaviours adopted include restriction of calorie intake (or binge eating), purging through vomiting or laxative use and excessive exercise. They most commonly present in girls aged 13 to 17 years but are increasingly recognized in boys (25% of all eating disorders according to recent studies) and in prepubertal children.

Aetiology

The aetiology is multifactorial. Risk factors include feeding difficulties in infancy, premorbid obesity and adverse life events or family history of eating disorders. There are several forms including anorexia nervosa, bulimia nervosa and binge eating. Eating disorders have many emotional, psychological and social consequences, and a high mortality rate due to physical complications or by suicide.

Substance misuse

Substance abuse is the misuse of substances other than the way intended to use them or using illegal substances in a harmful/detrimental way towards their body. This can cause disruption to the child or young person's mental and physical health alongside their social circumstances.

Misuse can take many forms from a child struggling with anorexia nervosa utilizing laxatives to a young teenager smoking cannabis and drinking alcohol excessively. An appropriate package needs to be sought for these individuals balancing effective, safe and least restrictive care.

> **COMMUNICATION**
>
> An important risk factor for eating disorders in adolescents is exposure to damaging content online – there are 'ana' (anorexia) and 'mia' (bulimia) sites where people are encouraged to persist with damaging behaviours. Make sure to discuss these with any young person presenting with low weight.

Anorexia nervosa

Anorexia nervosa is the maintenance of low bodyweight due to a preoccupation with weight and body image. It is characterized by:

- Weight less than 85% of expected bodyweight.
- Intense fear of gaining weight or being fat.
- Disturbed body image: believing they are fat when actually underweight.
- Denial of the danger of serious weight loss or low bodyweight.
- Amenorrhoea for at least three cycles (in postmenarchal girls).

It may present as failure to gain weight appropriately rather than loss of weight. The patient often displays obsessive, overachieving, perfectionist and controlling personality traits.

Clinical features

Physical examination may reveal:

- emaciation and muscle wasting
- fine lanugo hair over trunk and limbs
- bradycardia and poor peripheral perfusion
- slowly relaxing tendon reflexes

Investigations

Laboratory investigations may reveal:

- reduced plasma proteins, vitamin B12 and ferritin
- endocrine abnormalities: elevated cortisol, reduced T_4, luteinizing hormone and follicle-stimulating hormone

Management

The immediate aim is to make a therapeutic alliance with the patient to restore normal bodyweight. Most patients are managed on an outpatient basis, with goal setting and psychological interventions – NICE recommends family therapy first line, with alternatives including cognitive behavioural therapy or individual psychotherapy. Therapy must incorporate psychoeducation for the patient and their family. In severe cases, failing to respond to outpatient intervention, inpatient treatment is necessary. This can be difficult because affected young people might hide food and lie about their weight. Nasogastric feeding might be required if there is continued weight loss in hospital. Where there is severe malnutrition the patient should be monitored carefully for refeeding syndrome. Treatment will also encompass management of physical aspects of anorexia (e.g., gradual weaning off laxative and dental hygiene).

Prognosis

Prognosis is variable with a 5% mortality rate from malnutrition, infection or suicide. About 50% make a good recovery, 30% show partial improvement and 20% have a chronic relapsing course. Good prognostic factors are:

- young age at onset
- supportive family
- insight and improved self-esteem

Bulimia nervosa

Bulimia is a disorder characterized by abnormal body image, low self-esteem and regular binge eating with associated inappropriate behaviours to avoid weight gain (e.g., vomiting or laxative abuse). Weight may be low, but individuals are often in the normal range or overweight. Clinical features include hypotension, tachycardia, dry skin and menstrual abnormalities. In addition, where there is vomiting after binges there may be parotid enlargement or calluses on the fingers. Management is similar to anorexia nervosa with family therapy or cognitive-behavioural therapy playing a key role.

> **HINTS AND TIPS**
>
> There are high rates of eating disorders in young people with diabetes who may misuse insulin which can be very dangerous. This needs specialist management with increased monitoring of blood glucose and ketone levels.

Tics

These are habitual, paroxysmal, sudden and repetitive movements, gestures or noises. They can vary in presentation and disruption to one's life. Tourette syndrome is a tic-based disorder which involves both muscle and vocal components. The incidence of mild tics is roughly 1 in 10 children, whereas Tourette's is around 1 in 2000 children.

For tics which are believed to be transient in nature, these will disappear over time. However, for the more severe tic disorders, behavioural therapies and possibly neuroleptics (antipsychotics) can be utilized to improve the quality of life.

MEDICALLY UNEXPLAINED SYMPTOMS

Somatization and conversion disorders

Somatization is the development of physical symptoms secondary to psychological distress. This can be seen in children and young people with comorbid psychological conditions alongside stressful family situations and with family history of somatic issues. Some frequently seen somatic symptoms are abdominal pain, nausea, headaches, fatigue and limb pain. It is more commonly seen in girls.

This psychological distress can present in the way of a conversion disorder, which may appear as a child complaining of limb weakness or paralysis, seizure-like activity and an abnormal gait. The sensory distributions of these will not follow anatomical patterns of nervous distribution, but will tend to follow the child's understanding of the nervous system. Key clues about these diagnoses are related to inconsistent examinations and histories.

In any of these cases, it is vitally important to rule out any organic causes for these complaints before confirming it is secondary to psychological distress.

Management of these conditions is multifocussed and behavioural in nature. Parental therapy/counselling allows recovery to be facilitated in a supportive manner. Alongside this other behavioural therapies, such as cognitive behavioural therapy can play an important role together with physical rehabilitation.

Myalgic encephalitis/chronic fatigue syndrome (ME/CFS)

This refers to generalized debilitating fatigue persisting after routine tests and investigations have failed to identify an obvious underlying cause. It is classically exacerbated by mental and physical exertion and usually associated with nonspecific pain in muscles and joints. Headaches, sleep difficulties, depressed mood, sore throat, tender lymph nodes and abdominal pain can also occur.

Management

A full history and examination is important to characterize symptoms and basic screening tests are important to exclude other diagnoses (e.g., anaemia and hypothyroidism). Diagnosis requires persistent fatigue in combination with at least four associated symptoms for 3 months or more.

A multidisciplinary approach is valuable. Management includes:

- Energy Management (patient self-management, making the most of the energy a patient has, reducing the risk of worsening their symptoms – exceeding their limits; recognizing all types of activity – cognitive, physical, emotional and social).
- Caution incorporating physical activity and exercise into a management programme – individualizing this – explaining that this can help some patients, have no effect on others or can make symptoms worse.
- Medicines for symptom management.
- Advice and support around sleep hygiene, adequate hydration and a well-balanced diet.

Recurrent pain syndromes

Recurrent pain without an organic cause is not uncommon in children. The usual sites are the abdomen, head or limbs. A strict dichotomy between organic and psychological causation for recurrent pain is unhelpful and explains only a minority of cases.

Management

The history should establish:

- onset, frequency and duration of the pain and associated symptoms
- family functioning
- stressors (e.g., bullying at school)
- physical examination is directed towards excluding an organic cause (Table 18.1)

Measure the blood pressure and examine the fundi in a child with recurrent headaches. Investigations have a low yield if physical examination is normal and should be kept to a minimum. Full blood count, erythrocyte sedimentation rate and urinalysis might be indicated.

Table 18.1 Organic causes of recurrent pain

Site	Differentials
Abdominal pain	Genitourinary problems: urinary tract infection, obstructive uropathy Gastrointestinal disorders: constipation, inflammatory bowel disease, peptic ulcer
Headache	Refractive disorders Migraine Hypertension Raised intracranial pressure
Limb pain	Neoplastic disease: bone tumour, leukaemia Orthopaedic conditions (e.g., Osgood-Schlatter disease)

HINTS AND TIPS

Apley law: the further the pain is from the umbilicus, the more likely it is to be organic.

The more localized limb pain is, the less likely it is to be 'growing pains'.

It is key to acknowledge that the pain is real. Graded return to normal activity should be encouraged. Symptomatic relief should be offered (e.g., mild analgesics) and the patient should be encouraged to keep a symptom diary. It is important to provide psychological support.

Chapter Summary

- Emotional and behavioural problems are common in childhood – always consider the social context and possible underlying abuse or neglect.
- Support for children with neurodevelopmental or mental health problems should be holistic, with a multidisciplinary team approach and support for caregivers.
- Adolescence is a time when more serious mental health problems emerge – take self-harm or a change in eating pattern seriously and take a thorough social history.

UKMLA Conditions
Attention deficit hyperactivity disorder
Autism spectrum disorder
Eating disorders
Substance use disorder

UKMLA Presentations
Behavioural difficulties in childhood
Chronic abdominal pain
Learning disability
Self-harm
Speech and language problems
Substance misuse
Suicidal thoughts
Vomiting

Community paediatrics, public health and child protection

19

Social and preventative paediatrics encompasses the promotion of health and the prevention of illness through health surveillance, immunization, health education and injury prevention. In addition, community paediatric services are closely involved with working with children with disabilities and providing support in terms of child protection, foster care and adoption.

PREVENTION IN CHILD HEALTH

Many advances have been made in child health over decades; however, worldwide, including in the UK, there remains a high level of morbidity and mortality from preventable conditions including:

- infectious diseases
- congenital disorders
- unintentional injury ('accidents')
- malnutrition
- obesity

There is strong evidence that widening inequality underpins poor childhood health outcomes. For example, the highest socioeconomic groups have less than half the infant mortality rate than the lowest socioeconomic groups.

Strategies for prevention in child health include:

- immunization
- screening
- child health surveillance
- health promotion and education

Screening

An effective and worthwhile screening programme should satisfy certain criteria for the condition, test and intervention/treatment available.

- The **condition** screened for should be an important (frequent or severe) health problem.
- Primary prevention should be implemented as far as possible.
- The **test** should be simple, safe, sensitive and specific.
- There should be an agreed policy on further diagnostic tests and management choices for individuals testing positive on screening.
- **Early intervention** should improve the condition.
- The test and intervention/treatment should be cost-effective.

- The screening method should be acceptable to the child and parents.

Screening can be targeted at a 'high-risk' population (targeted screening) or carried out opportunistically when a patient presents for some other reason at the relevant age (population screening).

Child health promotion

A programme of health surveillance is undertaken to identify important conditions that have a better outcome if diagnosed and treated early (e.g., developmental dysplasia of the hip and deafness).

This programme includes:

- Newborn Infant Physical Examination (NIPE)
  - within 72 hours of birth (NIPE newborn)
  - at 6 to 8 weeks (NIPE infant)
- Newborn hearing screening
- Newborn blood spot screening
- One-year health review
- Two-year health review
- School entry health check
- National Child Measurement Programme (reception and year 6 only)

NIPE newborn examination

Full physical examination with particular emphasis on:

- eyes (presence of red reflex) – screening for congenital cataract(s)
- heart (presence of murmurs/absent femoral pulses)
- hips (presence of dislocated or dislocatable hip)
- testicles (undescended testes)

Newborn hearing screening

Newborn hearing is tested by otoacoustic emission and brainstem auditory evoked potentials in all babies in the first few days/weeks of life.

Newborn blood spot screening

Newborn blood spot screening ('Guthrie') ideally when 5 days old, screening for:

- sickle cell disease
- cystic fibrosis
- congenital hypothyroidism

- inherited metabolic disease:
  - phenylketonuria
  - medium-chain acyl-CoA dehydrogenase deficiency
  - maple syrup urine disease
  - isovaleric acidaemia
  - glutaric aciduria type 1
  - homocystinuria (pyridoxine unresponsive)
  - severe Combined Immunodeficiency (SCID; in some areas of England as a pilot study)

1–2-Week check

Performed by the midwife or health visitor: advice on safe sleeping, feeding, caring for the baby and immunizations.

NIPE infant (6–8-week check)

Usually performed by the general practitioner. Physical examination as per the neonatal examination. In addition:

- growth: weight, length and head circumference, which should be plotted on the growth charts
- development: alertness, eye contact, smiles, head control
- vision and hearing (explore parental concerns)

Assessment should also be made of the family's adjustment to the new infant, quality of parent–child interactions and signs of maternal mental health problems.

9–12-Month review

- general health
- assess growth and development
- health promotion to include accident prevention, dietary and dental advice
- parenting advice (boundary setting, encourage reading to child)

2–2.5-Year review

This is done by the health visitor but can also be done by nursery nurses, and includes:

- assessment of general health and growth
- assessment of development: with emphasis on social and communication skills
- parenting advice on toilet training, temperament and behaviour, early years education, tooth brushing and dental care, safety and accident prevention

School entry

- growth: height and weight
- hearing and vision tests
- review immunization status
- assess if any additional help will be required at school

Immunization

Immunization has conferred more benefits than any other medical advance or intervention. It has allowed the prevention of many major diseases such as diphtheria and polio, which previously caused death or long-term disability for millions, and the complete eradication of smallpox. Immunization is effective against a range of major bacterial diseases including *Haemophilus influenzae* type B (HiB; previously a major cause of meningitis and epiglottitis), diphtheria and tuberculosis (TB), as well as viral diseases such as measles, mumps, rubella (MMR) and hepatitis (A and B). In 2021 the World Health Organization recommended widespread use of the RTS,S (mosquirix) malaria vaccine in sub-Saharan Africa and other regions with moderate-high plasmodium falciparum malaria transmission, with funding of almost $160 million to facilitate this between 2022 and 2025.

Active immunization

Active immunization aims to provide long-term immunity through the generation of memory B cells. It can be induced by:

- a live, attenuated form of the pathogen (e.g., MMR or Bacille Calmette-Guérin (BCG) vaccine for TB)
- an inactivated organism (e.g., inactivated poliomyelitis vaccine, pertussis)
- a component of the organism (e.g., HiB, pneumococcal vaccine, hepatitis B and meningitis C)
- an inactivated toxin (toxoid), such as tetanus vaccine, diphtheria vaccine
- mRNA (Zika, COVID-19) translated by the host's cells to make a target protein (=intracellular antigen)

In many individuals, live, attenuated viral vaccines promote a full, long-lasting antibody response after one or two doses. Several doses of an inactivated version or toxoid are usually required.

Passive immunization

Passive immunization provides short-term immunity via the injection of human immunoglobulin. There are two main types:

- Human normal immunoglobulin which contains antibodies against hepatitis A, rubella, measles and many other viruses. It can be used to provide short-term immunity after infectious contacts in at-risk groups (e.g., infants, those with reduced immunity and pregnant women). An important paediatric use is in Kawasaki disease.
- Specific immunoglobulins for tetanus, hepatitis B, rabies and varicella zoster.

Routes of administration

Routes of administration are:

- by mouth: rotavirus
- intradermal: BCG
- intranasal: influenza
- subcutaneous or intramuscular injection: all other vaccines

In infants, the upper outer quadrant of the buttock or the anterolateral aspect of the thigh are the recommended sites for the injection of vaccines.

Immunization schedule

The updated UK vaccination schedule is shown in Table 19.1. Immunizations are carefully timed to ensure it is not so early that an inadequate immune response is generated but not so late that the child has a high risk of acquiring the disease before being protected. Equally live vaccinations should <u>not</u> be administered to those who are immunosuppressed/immunodeficient – this is why BCG (for those either living in areas with high TB incidence, or whose parents or grandparents were born in a country with

high TB incidence) administration is now delayed until 28 days of age allowing for the outcome of screening results (where available) into congenital immunodeficiency.

Additional hepatitis B vaccine is given at birth, 1 month and 1 year to babies born to mothers infected with hepatitis B.

> **HINTS AND TIPS**
>
> Premature infants should start the immunization schedule according to chronological age (i.e., 2 months from birth)

Indications and contraindications to immunization

Every child should have the opportunity to be protected against infectious diseases however, it is not a legal obligation. Providing information permitting a guardian with parental

Table 19.1 UK Immunization schedule

Age	Vaccine
Neonates at risk only	BCG (around 4 weeks, after Severe Combined Immunodeficiency (SCID) screening outcome, where tested)
2 months	Diphtheria, tetanus, acellular pertussis, inactivated polio, *Haemophilus influenzae* type B, hepatitis B (DTaP/IPV/HiB/HepB) Meningococcal group B (MenB) Rotavirus[1] (oral)
3 months	DtaP/IPV/HiB/HepB Pneumococcal conjugate vaccine (PCV) Rotavirus[1]
4 months	DTaP/IPV/HiB/HepB MenB
1 year	*H. influenzae* type B/meningitis C (HiB/MenC) PCV booster MenB booster Measles, mumps, rubella (MMR)
Preschool (approximately 3 years and 4 months)	Diphtheria, tetanus, acellular pertussis, inactivated polio (DTaP/IPV) MMR
For 2–3 years from Autumn 2022 All primary and secondary school children (reception to year 11) – subject to vaccine availability	Influenza vaccine – live attenuated nasal spray is recommended
Boys and girls aged 12–13 years	Human papillomavirus (types 16 and 18, which cause cervical cancer; types 6 and 11, which cause genital warts) – two doses 6–24 months apart
13–15 years	Meningococcal groups A, C, W and Y
13–18 years	Tetanus, diphtheria, inactivated polio (Td/IPV)

HepB, Hepatitis B; HiB, Haemophilus influenzae type B; IPV, inactivated poliomyelitis vaccine.
[1]*Check SCID screening outcome (where available)*

responsibility to make an informed decision regarding immunization, granting consent or declining consent is legally and ethically essential.

Widespread uptake of immunizations provides 'herd immunity', protecting those individuals who cannot be safely immunized (such as those with immunosuppression – see below). Special risk groups can be identified for whom the risk of complications from infectious disease is high and who should be immunized as a priority. These include children with:

- Chronic lung disease and congenital heart disease
- Down syndrome
- Absent or dysfunctional spleen
- Immunosuppression (including HIV) infection – **inactivated** vaccines only (see contraindications to live vaccine below)

General contraindications to immunization include:

- Acute illness with fever >38°C: postpone until recovery has occurred.
- A definite history of a severe general reaction, including anaphylaxis to a vaccine (previous dose) or vaccine component.

Anaphylactic reactions to MMR are not related to egg antigens; children with egg allergy should still receive MMR vaccination.

Contraindications to live vaccination – primary or acquired immunodeficiency:

- With impaired cell-mediated immunity (e.g., severe combined immunodeficiency – SCID).
- Being treated with immunosuppressive therapy (chemotherapy – including high-dose steroids, radiotherapy, biological therapies) for malignant or nonmalignant disease, including solid organ transplant – for between 3 and 12 months.
- Following stem cell ('bone marrow') transplant for at least 24 months
- Severe immunosuppression with HIV (BCG contraindicated in all HIV-positive individuals; infants born to mothers with HIV should have two negative HIV PCR tests before BCG)

'False' contraindications

The following are *not* contraindications to immunization:

- family history of adverse reactions to immunization
- prematurity (infants <28 weeks should have first immunization in hospital)
- stable neurological conditions (e.g., cerebral palsy)
- asthma, eczema, hay fever
- over the age recommended in the standard schedule
- minor afebrile illness
- child's mother being pregnant

COMMUNICATION

As discussed in Chapter 10, the measles, mumps and rubella vaccine is not linked to autism – this suggestion has been robustly debunked but careful communication is required to elicit parent concerns, reassure of the vaccine safety as well as educate on the danger associated with measles, mumps and rubella. Do not forget to provide practical advice on arranging catch-up vaccines at the general practitioner if these have been delayed due to parental fears.

Sudden unexpected death in childhood, sudden infant death syndrome

The death of a child during infancy or childhood is a tragedy; a thorough, compassionate investigation to understand why is an overwhelming need of bereaved families.

The term sudden unexpected death in childhood (SUDIC) includes all cases of a child's death, which was not expected in the 24 hours before. SUDIC can result from an unrecognized medical condition or unintentional incident. A rare minority result from child abuse or neglect. A sensitive, joint agency response is needed to understand and implement any lessons for other children and families; this includes counselling and bereavement support for the family.

SUDIC includes sudden infant death syndrome (SIDS) which is defined as the sudden death of an infant under 1 year of age, during sleep, which remains unexplained despite a complete postmortem examination, clinical history and review of circumstances surrounding the death. In the UK, around 200 infants die from SIDS each year. Although unexplained, we know factors to reduce the risk of SIDS:

- not smoking during pregnancy or breastfeeding; not allowing others to smoke in the same room as a baby
- always place a baby on their back ('back to sleep')
- not allowing a baby to overheat, or get too cold
- not sleeping with a baby on a sofa or armchair
- keeping a baby's head uncovered – tuck blankets no higher than shoulders

Brief resolved unexplained events

Previously known as 'apparent life-threatening events', a brief resolved unexplained event (BRUE) is a sudden event occurring in an infant (aged <1 year) which lasts less than 1 minute and involves one or more of:

- colour change: cyanosis or pallor
- alteration in breathing: absent, decreased or irregular

- change in tone: decreased or increased
- altered responsiveness

These are relatively common and require a careful history, thorough clinical examination, and a period of observation before discharge with advice if there are no concerning factors. Investigations should include a 12-lead electrocardiogram to rule out conduction problems and it is advisable to provide basic life support training to the carers. These events can be terrifying for caregivers who may require considerable reassurance.

CHILDREN WITH DISABILITIES

Many children have complex and long-lasting neurodevelopmental disabilities that require early identification and support in the community. With the increasing survival of extremely premature babies, there is an increased requirement for appropriate support for children with complex disabilities.

Disability is an overarching term which encompasses the following:

- impairment: a difference in body structure or function
- activity limitation: a difficulty in doing a particular task or action
- participation restriction: a barrier to being fully involved in life situations

Activity limitation and participation restriction are often caused by a lack of appropriate adaptation or inclusion methods, rather than because of the underlying impairment.

Causes of childhood disability

The causes of disability in childhood include:

- genetic conditions (e.g., Down syndrome, Prader-Willi syndrome)
- cerebral palsy
- global developmental delay (often idiopathic)
- hearing or visual impairment
- learning difficulties
- social and communication disorders (e.g., autistic spectrum disorder)

Different conditions tend to be detected at different ages (see Table 19.2).

Assessment and diagnosis

A comprehensive assessment is needed to assess where the main difficulties lie. This includes:

- physical health and mobility
- vision and coordination
- hearing, language and communication

Table 19.2 Age at which different conditions present

Age	Presentation
Neonatal period	Chromosomal abnormality or syndrome (e.g., Down syndrome, hypoxic-ischaemic encephalopathy)
Infancy	Cerebral palsy Severe visual or hearing impairment
Preschool	Speech and language delay Abnormal gait Global developmental delay Loss of skills from neurodegenerative disorder Autistic spectrum disorder
School age	Specific learning difficulties (e.g., dyslexia)

Table 19.3 Medical conditions in children with neurodisability

System	Conditions
Nervous system	Vision and hearing impairment Epilepsy Behavioural disorders and sleep disturbance
Skeleton	Postural deformities (e.g., scoliosis, contractures) Dislocation of hips
Gastrointestinal	Feeding difficulties Faltering growth Gastro-oesophageal reflux Constipation or faecal incontinence
Respiratory	Recurrent lower respiratory tract infection

- learning difficulties
- behaviour and emotions
- social interactions and self-care, including continence

Medical conditions commonly encountered in children with neurodisabilities are summarized in Table 19.3.

Diagnosis of a disability might be sudden and unexpected, or the culmination of protracted investigation. The news may provoke complex emotional reactions which can include grief accompanied by anger, guilt, despair or denial. The initial interview requires sensitive handling.

COMMUNICATION

Breaking news to parents/carers about a disability:
- They should be told as soon as possible.
- If there are two parents, they should be told together, not separately.

- Tell them in a quiet place with a colleague present (e.g., a nurse).
- Adopt an honest and direct approach.
- Arrange a period of privacy for the parents after the initial meeting.
- Arrange a second meeting to allow questions after the news has been assimilated.

Management: the multidisciplinary team

Management of a severe or complex disability requires a multidisciplinary clinical team, working with social services, local education authorities and voluntary agencies. The balance changes with age:

- Preschool children: community-led child development team, voluntary agencies
- School-age children: education authorities, community health services
- School leavers/young adults: social services, community disability teams

Members of the child development team will usually include:

- paediatricians
- physiotherapists
- occupational therapists
- speech and language therapists
- dieticians
- psychologists
- social workers
- nurses and health visitors

Education, health and care plan

Education authorities have a duty to identify children with special educational needs and disabilities and provide appropriate resources. A detailed assessment is undertaken with reports from the educational psychologist, members of the multidisciplinary team and the parents. Following this, an individualized education, health and care plan (previously known as a 'statement') sets out the child's educational and noneducational needs and the provision of services required to meet those needs. The education, health and care plan should be under regular review.

CHILD PROTECTION

The National Society for the Prevention of Cruelty to Children (NSPCC) estimates that there are over half a million children being abused in the UK per year. Child maltreatment can be

considered under four main categories but they often overlap: physical abuse, sexual abuse, emotional abuse and neglect.

Risk factors for child abuse and neglect include:

- parent/carer substance use
- parent/carer mental health problems
- domestic violence
- previous child maltreatment within the family
- known animal maltreatment within the family
- social deprivation and isolation
- disability or chronic illness in a child

Types of abuse

Physical abuse/nonaccidental injury

Any injury can be unintentional ('accidental') or inflicted but certain injuries are more likely to be due to abuse (e.g., burns or bites).

Potential indicators of physical abuse that can be elicited in the history:

- delay in seeking medical help
- differing or changing history from witnesses
- mechanism inconsistent with injury or developmental stage of child
- previous concerns about nonaccidental injury (NAI)
- parent/carer level of concern inappropriate

Features of physical abuse:

- signs of neglect
- unusual behaviour of child (e.g., withdrawn, overly affectionate with strangers, distress/recurrent nightmares)
- multiple injuries of differing ages
- injuries suggestive of an implement (e.g., belt marks, cigarette burns)

Specific injuries associated with physical abuse:

- Fractures in a nonambulant child.
- Rib fractures require considerable force and so in the absence of major trauma (e.g., road traffic accident), raise suspicions.
- Multiple bruises in unusual locations are worrying. Unintentional ('accidental') bruising usually occurs over bony prominences, bruising in other 'protected' areas should raise concern of physical abuse ('TEN-4' bruising; bruising to the torso, ears and neck in children less than 4 years old).
- Abusive Head Trauma is a severe, life-threatening form of abuse caused by violent shaking and/or impact trauma to the infant's head – this can cause intracranial (notably subdural) and retinal bleeding, apnoea and spinal cord injury.

Sexual abuse

Child sexual abuse is more common in girls but may be less commonly disclosed by boys. It has been defined as the involvement of dependent, immature children or adolescents in sexual activities that they do not fully understand and are unable to give informed consent to. This includes contact (which includes touching, kissing and oral sex) or noncontact (exposing or flashing, or forcing a child to make view or share sexual images). A child who is sexually abused may display unusual language/sexualized behaviours, self-harm or avoid/be frightened of being alone with people they know.

A normal physical examination does not exclude sexual abuse. The majority (80%) of abuse is conducted by someone known to the child.

- Child Sexual Exploitation (CSE) is a form of sexual abuse-exploiting a child with money/gifts/affection/status in exchange for sexual activities
- Female Genital Mutilation ('female circumcision' or 'cutting') is when a female's genitals are deliberately cut, removed or altered for nonmedical reasons

Emotional abuse

This includes rejection of a child, persistent criticism, belittling or threats. It can also occur when a parent fails to appreciate the developmental age of a child, for example, reversal of the parent–child role.

- Domestic abuse – any type of 'controlling, bullying threatening or violent behaviour between people in a relationship' – harms children, as a result of 'seeing or hearing the ill-treatment of another'. Domestic abuse is associated with neglect, poor physical health, physical injury and death.

Neglect

Neglect is persistently failing to provide the basic physical and psychological needs of a child. It can involve an unsafe living environment, poor hygiene, inadequate provision of food or not attending to health needs (e.g., missed appointments). It may manifest as a child who is unclean or not wearing appropriate clothes, has severe infestations of scabies or headlice, presents with faltering growth or developmental delay. The risk of fatality or morbidity can be as high as physical abuse.

Diagnosis

Suspicions of abuse or neglect may arise from a healthcare professional such as the general practitioner or health visitor, from the school or from a concerned neighbour or relative. Diagnosis is difficult and stressful for all concerned. Diligent note-keeping is vital as the records may be required for legal proceedings. Body map diagrams should be used to record findings and photographs taken with consent. Investigations are often indicated to exclude any organic cause for the signs and symptoms (e.g., a

bleeding diathesis in bruising). Further investigations may be directed at detecting occult injuries, for example, a skeletal survey to look for old/occult fractures, CT/MR imaging of the brain and ophthalmology review. Forensic samples must be taken in suspected sexual abuse and this examination should be conducted by a specialist in this field.

COMMUNICATION

If a child discloses abuse or neglect, they should be listened to immediately. Use open and nonleading questions, taking care not to prejudice potential criminal investigations. It is important to be open and honest with the child or young person, explaining with whom you will need to share the information.

ETHICS

If you are told about or you see physical signs of female genital mutilation, then you have a legal requirement to report this to the police.

Management

The first priority is to treat any injury or illness. Following this, a referral must be made to social care and the police, as well as to your local child protection team, and a decision should be taken to ensure a place of safety for the child (and other children in the home). If the parent/carer is the suspected perpetrator, an emergency foster care placement may need to be organized. If possible, this is done with parental consent but, if not, legal enforcement may be required. Senior staff should be involved from the beginning because experience is required in handling what is always a very difficult situation. Further management involves the evaluation of the family by social care. Multiagency working is key and a conference should be convened involving all the professionals involved in the child's life. A decision will be made on whether to make the child subject to a child protection plan, whether court proceedings are required and whether the child can be returned safely to the family. The child protection plan will define the kind of intervention and level of supervision required. Ongoing support for the child and young person may involve psychological intervention (e.g., cognitive behavioural therapy or individual psychotherapy). A high degree of vigilance is needed for the sequelae of abuse and neglect, which can involve depression, anxiety, post-traumatic stress disorder, self-harm, suicidality and eating disorders.

CHILDREN AND THE LAW

The principal legislation concerning children and health in the UK is contained in:

- The Children Act (England and Wales 1989, Scotland 1995)
- The Education Act (1993)
- The UN Convention on the Rights of the Child (1989)

The Children Act

This integrates the law relating to private individuals with the responsibilities of public authorities towards children. It aims to strike a balance between family independence and child protection. The essential components include:

- Parental responsibilities are defined. Responsibilities replace rights. Parents have the prime responsibility for their children and this is retained in all circumstances except adoption.
- The welfare of the child is paramount. The wishes and feelings of the child must be respected and courts should ensure any orders made positively benefit the child or children concerned.
- Professionals are encouraged to work in partnership with parents.
- Defines responsibilities for a 'child in need'. Local authorities are required to provide supportive services to assist parents in bringing up their children.
- The court must consider the child's race, religion, culture and language.
- A child should remain with his or her family whenever possible.
- Defines court orders in relation to custody and access and child protection. The latter includes Emergency Protection Order, Child Assessment Order, Care and Supervision Order and Police Protection Order.

Parental responsibility

Parental responsibility (PR) is held by:

- the biological mother (automatically)
- the biological father if:
  - married to mother at time of birth
  - named on birth certificate (for births since 1 December 2003)
  - PR agreement with mother
  - PR order from court
- same-sex parents if:
  - civil partners or married at time of fertility treatment/donor insemination, etc.
  - joint registration of birth
  - PR agreement
  - PR order from court
- legal guardian or step-parent with a PR order
- local authority may have joint responsibility in instances of emergency protection order or interim care orders.

Foster care

The purpose of foster care is to provide a safe, temporary placement for a child who is at physical, emotional or social risk. Common reasons for foster placement include:

- child abuse
- death or ill health of parents
- babies awaiting adoption

Foster care does not provide legal rights and these remain with the biological parents, local authority or courts. Attempts are made to place children with other family members where possible.

Adoption

The annual number of adoptions in the UK has fallen in recent years, thought to be due to wider use of contraception and abortion and also to the greater social acceptance of single parenthood.

Most children requiring adoption live with foster parents or in a children's home. Unfortunately, many are older, have disabilities or have suffered abuse or neglect and are less likely to be adopted.

Adoption is a legal procedure encompassing several important features:

- It is arranged by registered agencies.
- Adopters must be aged over 21 years.
- An adoption cannot be reversed except in exceptional circumstances.
- An adopted child loses all legal ties with his or her biological parents and the adoptive parents assume PR.
- The original parents have no right to access, although contact for older children is often maintained.
- The biological parents must give informed consent, unless they cannot be found or are judged unlikely to ever be able to look after the child adequately.
- The child lives with the adoptive parents for 3 months before the order is finalized.
- At age 18, an adopted child is entitled to his or her original birth certificate.

Consent to medical care

- A person older than 18 years can legally give his or her own consent (or refuse treatment) and this cannot be overridden.
- Between 16 and 18 years, consent for medical treatment can be given by the young person but refusal of treatment is not

permitted if those with PR give consent. In reality, this requires careful communication and negotiation, and may need to involve the courts.

Below 16 years, consent can either be from the young person themselves if the doctor considers that the child is of sufficient understanding to make an informed decision (i.e., they are Gillick competent) or from a person who holds PR. Ideally, the decision would be a shared one between the child or young person, their caregivers and the treating professionals. If the parent(s) of a child under 16 do not give consent for life-saving treatment (e.g., a blood transfusion in the child of parents who are Jehovah's Witnesses), a court can give consent. However, immediate life-saving treatment does not require consent. Children under 16 years of age are not legally allowed to refuse treatment.

ETHICS

Gillick competence is a judgement made by the healthcare professional that the young person is of sufficient maturity and understanding to give informed consent to medical treatment.

The Fraser guidelines were developed in relation to the prescription of contraception to a child under 16 without contraception, with the following criteria:

- The young person understands the advice given.
- They cannot be persuaded to inform their parents.
- They are likely to have unprotected sex with or without contraception.
- Their physical or mental health is likely to suffer without contraception.
- It is in their best interests to be given contraceptive advice/treatment without parental consent.

Note that children under 13 years do not have legal capacity to consent to sexual activity, and sexual intercourse with a child under 13 is statutory rape (Sexual Offences Act, 2003).

Confidentiality

Duties of confidentiality apply to young people who are competent and are not at risk of serious harm. This is vital to maintain trust in the doctor–patient relationship. There are times when there will be a duty to disclose information if abuse or neglect is suspected, or there is a risk of serious harm to another person.

If confidentiality needs to be broken, this should be explained to the child or young person, unless in exceptional circumstances where doing so will put them at risk of serious harm.

Chapter Summary

- Socioeconomic inequality underlies many major childhood health problems – public health measures should target groups at the highest risk.
- The Newborn Blood Spot Screening ('Guthrie) programme screens for important, treatable diseases in the newborn.
- Immunization is vital for the prevention of avoidable mortality and morbidity.
- Recognizing and acting on potential child abuse and neglect are the shared responsibility of all who work with children and young people; information sharing is key for safe outcomes.
- Types of abuse include physical, sexual, emotional/psychological and neglect.
- Children in whom (physical) abuse is suspected undergo a safeguarding medical, often including investigations such as skeletal survey, CT head and ophthalmological examination.
- Children <16 years of age may provide consent if deemed Gillick competent. They cannot lawfully refuse treatment.
- Understanding the law as it relates to children and young people is important, particularly with regard to consent and confidentiality.

UKMLA Conditions
Non-accidental injury
Subdural haemorrhage

UKMLA Presentations
Child abuse
Learning disability
Neonatal death or cot death
Vaccination

Accidents and emergencies | 20

EMERGENCIES

Children differ from adults in important ways that are relevant to emergency care (Box 20.1).

The seriously ill child

Cardiorespiratory arrest is rare in children and is usually a result of a progressive deterioration. This is why it is vital to recognize the critically ill child and intervene before they progress to what is called 'secondary cardiorespiratory arrest'. In infants and children the underlying cause is generally due to decompensated respiratory or circulatory failure. This is different to adults who often have underlying cardiovascular disease causing myocardial damage (resulting in a 'primary cardiorespiratory arrest').

BOX 20.1 ANATOMICAL AND PHYSIOLOGICAL CHARACTERISTICS OF YOUNG CHILDREN

Airway	Proportionately narrow airways and large tongue • Can cause obstruction particularly if reduced level of consciousness Obligate nasal breathers until 5 months old • Mucus/secretions can cause respiratory compromise Short neck, large occiput • Causes head to flex when supine
Breathing	Low oxygen reserve, high rate of consumption Compliant chest wall Weak respiratory muscles
Circulation	Small total circulating blood volume Low stroke volume • Cardiac output dependent on heart rate
Disability	Nonverbal, difficult to assess level of consciousness
Exposure	Large surface area-to-weight ratio • Susceptible to rapid heat loss

---

Assessment

Any child who is thought to be unwell should be assessed using a standardized approach (Fig. 20.1). This way any problems can be identified and interventions made before moving on to the next step.

Airway

Assess for signs of airway obstruction:

- coughing
- stridor
- snoring
- wheeze
- drooling
- lip swelling

If a child is crying or talking, their airway is patent.

If the level of consciousness is reduced, the child will need airway manoeuvres to keep their airway open, or they may tolerate airway adjuncts such as an oropharyngeal/Guedel or nasopharyngeal airway. A 'definitive' airway is obtained by intubation.

When assessing the airway if the child is thought to be sick, high-flow oxygen should be applied.

Breathing

Assess for signs of respiratory compromise.

Increased respiratory effort:

- nasal flare
- head bob
- accessory muscle use
- recession

Abnormal respiratory rate (Table 20.1):

- fast (tachypnoeic)
- slow (exhaustion or respiratory depression)
- apnoeic

Poor oxygenation:

- cyanosis
- low oxygen saturations

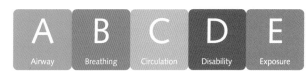

Fig. 20.1 Approach to assessing a sick child.

241

Table 20.1 Normal respiratory rate according to age

Age (years)	Respiratory rate (breaths/min)
<1	30–40
1–2	25–35
2–5	25–30
5–12	20–25
>12	12–20

Note: Adapted from "Paediatric Immediate Life Support (third edition)", published September 2016, produced by Resuscitation Council UK. Reproduced with the kind permission of Resuscitation Council UK

Abnormal breath sounds:

- unequal air entry
- dull or hyperresonant percussion notes
- wheeze
- crackles

Circulation

Assess for signs of circulatory compromise.
Abnormal perfusion:

- cool peripheries
- mottling
- capillary refill time over 2 seconds
- hypotension

Abnormal heart rate:

- tachycardia
- bradycardia
- weak or absent pulses

RED FLAG

Bradycardia and hypotension are late, preterminal signs of circulatory failure in children.

Other effects of circulatory failure may include a metabolic acidosis, altered mental state due to reduced cerebral perfusion and oliguria due to reduced renal perfusion.

Disability

Assess for signs of neurological compromise.
Reduced level of consciousness:

- Airway, Voice, Pain, Unresponsive (AVPU) or paediatric Glasgow Coma Scale (GCS)

Pupils:

- are they equal, reactive and responsive to light

Seizures:

- fontanelle (<18 months) – may be bulging or tense in raised intracranial pressure
- posture – most are hypotonic. Stiff posturing – decorticate (flexed arms, extended legs) and decerebrate (extended arm, extended legs) posturing are signs of serious brain dysfunction

Neurological failure can cause respiratory depression or irregular respiratory patterns.

RED FLAG

Hypertension, bradycardia and irregular respirations (Cushing triad) indicate herniation of the cerebellar tonsils through the foramen magnum and is a neurological emergency.

Cardiorespiratory arrest

Basic paediatric life support

Effective basic life support can improve morbidity and mortality in collapsed children (Fig. 20.2).

There are key differences between adult and paediatric basic life support, and even between infants (<1 year) and children (1 year to puberty).

Airway manoeuvres

- Infants <1 year: head in neutral position.
- Children >1 year: head tilt and chin lift.

Rescue breaths

The most common cause of cardiorespiratory arrest in children is respiratory insufficiency. With this in mind, resuscitation begins with five initial rescue breaths. They should be of 1-second duration and the chest must be observed to rise and fall after each breath before continuing.

Assessing for signs of life

This should take no longer than 10 seconds. Signs may include crying, coughing or talking. Health professionals may also feel the pulse at this time and the site for this depends on age:

- infants <1 year: brachial or femoral pulse
- children >1 year: carotid or femoral pulse

Chest compressions

Following the initial five rescue breaths, the ratio of cardiac compressions to breaths in children is 15:2. The rate of compressions should be 100–120/min. The landmark for chest compressions is one finger breadth above the xiphisternum and the desired depth is at least one-third of the chest. See Fig. 20.3 for the different chest compression techniques according to age.

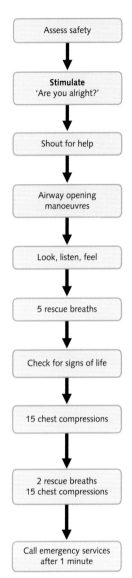

Fig. 20.2 Paediatric basic life support algorithm.

Assess safety

↓

Stimulate
'Are you alright?'

↓

Shout for help

↓

Airway opening
manoeuvres

↓

Look, listen, feel

↓

5 rescue breaths

↓

Check for signs of life

↓

15 chest compressions

↓

2 rescue breaths
15 chest compressions

↓

Call emergency services
after 1 minute

Advanced paediatric life support

After basic life support procedures, it might be necessary to proceed to:

- secure a definitive airway (i.e., intubation and ventilation)
- gain circulatory access (intravenous (IV) or intraosseous (IO))
- identify the cardiac rhythm as either:
  - nonshockable: asystole, pulseless electrical activity (PEA), bradycardia (<60/min) with inadequate perfusion despite respiratory support
  - shockable: ventricular fibrillation (VF) or pulseless ventricular tachycardia (VT)

Defibrillator pads should be applied below the right clavicle and over the left mid-axillary line. If the child's chest is too small, then one should be placed on the front and the other on the back of the chest. Figs. 20.4 and 20.5 outline the treatment algorithms for shockable and nonshockable rhythms.

> **HINTS AND TIPS**
>
> Nonshockable rythms; asystole, pulseless electrical activity and bradycardia are the most common cardiac arrhythmias seen in children.
>
> Shockable rhythms are less common, but most likely after witnessed, sudden collapse – on intensive care or cardiac units and in adolescents who had been playing sport

When performing cardiorespiratory resuscitation it is vital to consider whether the event could be due to a reversible cause. These are frequently referred to as the 'Four H's and four Ts' (Box 20.2).

Neurological emergencies

Reduced level of consciousness

There are many causes of a reduced conscious level due to a variety of causes including neurological, cardiac and respiratory. Evaluation is done by the GCS or AVPU (see Chapter 13). Some are self-evident, but others might be identified only after careful clinical evaluation and special investigations.

Assessment

A focused history should include information about:

- chronic medical conditions such as epilepsy and diabetes mellitus
- access to drugs and poisons
- normal or 'baseline' neurological state

A full clinical examination should be carried out starting with a full airway, breathing, circulation, disability, exposure (ABCDE) assessment. Ensure to also check for:

- fever
- rashes: especially purpura
- signs of head injury
- signs of meningism, focal neurology, abnormal posture, pupil size and reaction to light, papilloedema or retinal haemorrhages

Diagnosis

Investigations are determined by the clinical assessment. Blood glucose measurement in any child with a reduced level of consciousness is mandatory. Other investigations to consider include:

- blood gas (acid–base balance, electrolytes, lactate, glucose)

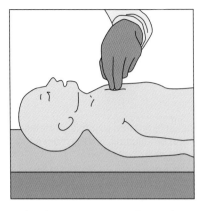

A Infant chest compression: Two-finger technique

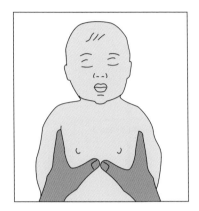

B Infant chest compression: Hand-encircling technique

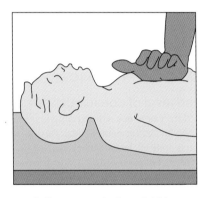

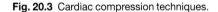

C Chest compression in small children

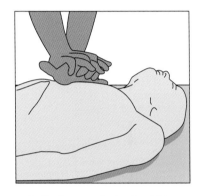

D Chest compression in older children

Fig. 20.3 Cardiac compression techniques.

- blood tests (full blood count, urea and electrolytes, liver function tests, bone profile, blood culture, ammonia)
- lumbar puncture (exclude raised intracranial pressure prior to lumbar puncture)
- brain imaging: CT or MRI
- urine for toxicology

HINTS AND TIPS

Check blood sugar in a comatose or convulsing child to identify treatable hypoglycaemia. Recognition and treatment are simple. If missed, brain damage can result. (ABC and DEFG (Don't Ever Forget Glucose))

Management

Initial management should be directed towards identifying and correcting problems with the airway, breathing and circulation. Further specific treatment depends on aetiology. All children with a GCS <8 or 'P' on the AVPU scale need early consideration whether airway protection with endotracheal intubation is required.

Maintaining oxygenation and perfusion minimizes secondary brain damage.

Seizures

There are many causes of seizures and some vary with age (Table 20.2). The most common cause in children aged 6 months to 6 years is a 'febrile seizure' (see Chapter 13).

A continuous seizure lasting more than 30 minutes, or clustered seizures without recovery of consciousness between attacks, is called 'status epilepticus'.

Prolonged seizures can result in brain damage or death from hypoxia. Cerebral blood flow and oxygen consumption increase fivefold to meet the extrametabolic demand. Oxygen delivery to the brain will be impaired if there is inadequate ventilation or hypotension.

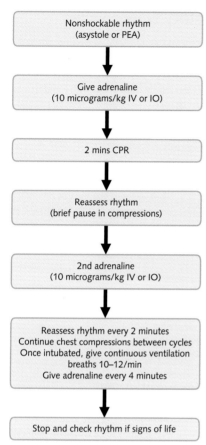

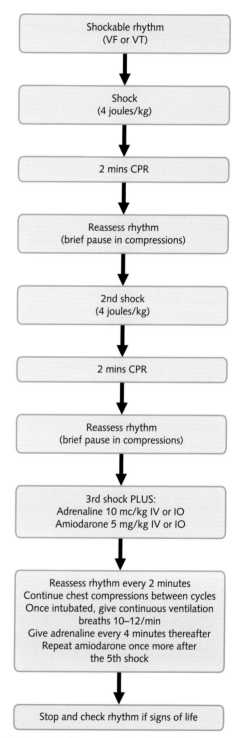

Fig. 20.4 Nonshockable life support algorithm. *CPR,* Cardiopulmonary resuscitation; *IO,* intraosseous; *IV,* intravenous; *PEA,* pulseless electrical activity.

History

- description of seizure (ideally from someone who witnessed the event)
- other features including tongue biting, eye rolling, incontinence
- duration of seizure
- any medications given
- history of recent trauma
- known epileptic? If so, medication regimen
- preceding illness or fever

Examination

A full clinical examination should be carried out starting with a full ABCDE assessment. Ensure to also check for:

- signs of head injury
- fever, petechial/purpuric rash, meningism

Fig. 20.5 Shockable life support algorithm. *CPR,* Cardiopulmonary resuscitation; *IO,* intraosseous; *IV,* intravenous; *mc,* micrograms.

BOX 20.2 REVERSIBLE CAUSES OF CARDIORESPIRATORY ARREST

Four Hs	Four Ts
Hypoxia	Thrombosis
Hypovolaemia	Tamponade (cardiac)
Hyperkalaemia/hypokalaemia	Toxins
Hypothermia	Tension pneumothorax

Table 20.2 Causes of seizures

System	Causes
Metabolic/endocrine	Hypoglycaemia Hypocalcaemia Inborn errors of metabolism
Infection	Meningitis Encephalitis Febrile seizure
Trauma	Head injury Nonaccidental injury
Other	Epilepsy Poisoning Reflex anoxic seizures

Management

All children with generalized tonic-clonic seizures should be given high-flow oxygen. If the seizure self-terminates in less than 5 minutes, then no other treatment is required; the child should be put into the recovery position. If the seizure lasts longer than 5 minutes, then the status epilepticus algorithm should be followed (Fig. 20.6). If seizures are recurrent, then antiepileptic medications may be commenced, and parents may be given 'rescue medication' in the form of a benzodiazepine to give at home in the event of a seizure.

HINTS AND TIPS

No more than two doses of benzodiazepine should be given due to the risk of respiratory depression.

Cardiac emergencies

Cardiac emergencies in children occur infrequently. They include cardiac failure and cardiac arrhythmias, which are discussed in Chapter 3.

Respiratory emergencies

The pattern of severe respiratory illness in children is determined by features of the anatomy and physiology of their respiratory system, including:

- small airways: easily obstructed with rapid increase in airways resistance
- compliant thoracic cage: reduced breathing efficiency
- respiratory muscles fatigue more quickly.
- susceptibility to infection

COMMON PITFALLS

Not all respiratory distress has a respiratory cause:
- Metabolic acidosis causes deep, rapid breathing.
- Heart failure causes tachypnoea.
- Sepsis causes tachypnoea.

The illnesses most commonly presenting as emergencies are:

- upper airway obstruction
- lower airway obstruction
- lower respiratory tract infection

Upper airways obstruction

The cardinal sign of upper airway obstruction is stridor. This is a noise associated with breathing and due to obstruction of the extrathoracic airway. It tends to be worse on inspiration but may also be biphasic.

The important common causes of acute stridor are:

- croup
- epiglottitis and bacterial tracheitis
- inhaled foreign body

HINTS AND TIPS

It is important not to cause further distress to a child with suspected upper airway obstruction as this may result in complete obstruction and rapid deterioration. Do NOT attempt to examine the throat, and wait for an anaesthetist to be present before undertaking procedures such as cannulation.

Croup

This is dealt with in detail in Chapter 4. The key principles of its acute management include:

- gentle handling
- monitoring of O_2 saturation and heart rate
- O_2 therapy

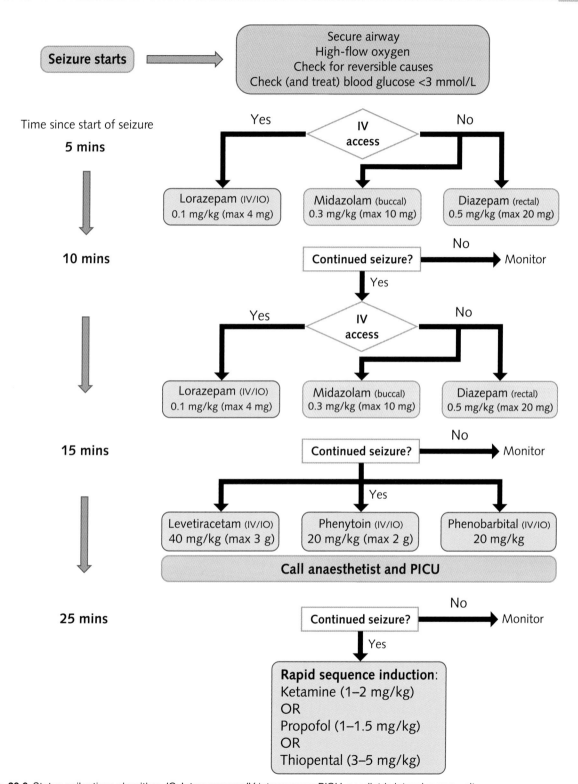

Fig. 20.6 Status epilepticus algorithm. *IO,* Intraosseous; *IV,* intravenous; *PICU,* paediatric intensive care unit.

- oral dexamethasone (less commonly nebulized budesonide)
- nebulized adrenaline (epinephrine): gives transient relief of severe obstruction and helps to buy time for the steroids to work or for intubation if needed

Acute epiglottitis

This is dealt with in Chapter 4. Epiglottitis has become uncommon since vaccination against *Haemophilus influenzae* was introduced; however, other organisms can still cause disease.

The principles of management of acute epiglottitis include:

- call for help (paediatrics, anaesthetics, ear, nose and throat (ENT) teams)
- minimize distress to the child
- arrange examination under anaesthesia
- secure the airway by endotracheal intubation
- IV antibiotics (e.g., ceftriaxone)

Foreign body inhalation

This presents with sudden-onset respiratory distress in an otherwise well child. This may be in the form of stridor, choking or coughing. Young toddlers and babies do not understand not to put small objects in their mouth and therefore are particularly at risk.

Management. The child may manage to clear their airway themselves by coughing. As long as they are alert and able to cough they should be encouraged to do so. If they begin to tire, their cough will become ineffective, and they are at risk of hypoxia and respiratory arrest. The algorithm for the choking child with an ineffective cough is shown in Fig. 20.7.

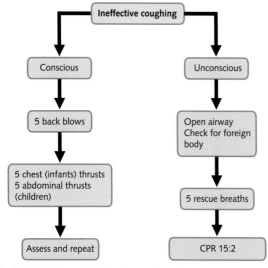

Fig. 20.7 Choking child algorithm. *CPR,* Cardiopulmonary resuscitation.

Lower airways obstruction
Acute asthma

Features of life-threatening asthma are shown in Box 20.3 and an algorithm for the management of acute asthma is shown in Fig. 20.8.

- β_2-Bronchodilators, steroids and oxygen are the mainstays of treatment of acute asthma. Inhaled bronchodilator therapy given by spacer is as effective as nebulized

---

BOX 20.3 CLINICAL FEATURES OF LIFE-THREATENING ASTHMA

Clinical features
Peak-expiratory flow <33% predicted value
    Oxygen saturations <92% in high-flow oxygen
    Silent chest
    Hypotension
    Fatigue
    Poor respiratory effort
    Reduced level of consciousness
    Agitation

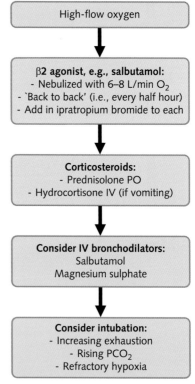

Fig. 20.8 Management of acute-severe asthma. *IV,* Intravenous; *PCO$_2$,* partial pressure of carbon dioxide; *PO,* per oral/oral route.

bronchodilators, although in severe cases it is given by nebulizer due to ease of giving oxygen.

- Short-course (3–5 days) oral steroids can reduce the severity of the attack and should be given early as they take up to 4 hours to act. If the child cannot take oral steroids or is vomiting, IV hydrocortisone can be given.
- If the child does not respond adequately to appropriate doses of nebulized bronchodilators, then magnesium sulphate (nebulized or IV) and IV salbutamol or IV aminophylline can be used.
- If IV fluids are required, it should be restricted to two-thirds of normal requirement as there is often excess antidiuretic hormone secretion.
- Do not routinely give antibiotics as the trigger is often allergic or viral.

COMMON PITFALLS

Worsening tachypnoea may indicate salbutamol toxicity rather than deteriorating asthma.
Other signs include:

- tremor
- vomiting
- rising lactate/metabolic acidosis
- severe hypokalaemia
- tachycardia/arrhythmias

Patients on intravenous salbutamol should be on a cardiac monitor.

Bronchiolitis

This is the commonest respiratory infection in infancy, and can result in a mild self-limiting illness through to requiring paediatric intensive care.

It is characterized by cough, tachypnoea, poor feeding and/or apnoea. Examination may find respiratory distress, crackles, wheeze and/or hypoxia. The management is mainly supportive and involves:

- Monitoring O_2 saturation, respiratory rate and heart rate.
- Respiratory support to maintain oxygen saturations above 90%–92%, facilitate carbon dioxide clearance and reduce work of breathing:
  - low-flow nasal oxygen
  - high-flow nasal oxygen (e.g., Vapotherm/Airvo)
  - continuous positive airway pressure (CPAP)
  - mechanical ventilation
  - maintaining adequate fluid and nutrition intake by giving nasogastric feeds or IV fluids at two-thirds maintenance rate
- antibiotics may be warranted if there is clinical evidence of infection

Circulatory failure (shock)

Fundamentally shock is inadequate cellular respiration, in paediatrics most commonly resulting from acute failure of circulatory function leading to poor tissue perfusion. It tends to progress through three phases (Table 20.3):

- compensated
- uncompensated
- irreversible

There are many causes of shock; the most common causes in paediatrics are hypovolaemia due to diarrhoea or vomiting, septicaemia and anaphylaxis (Table 20.4).

Clinical features

A brief history might identify the cause. The early physical signs of shock include:

- pallor (due to vasoconstriction)
- tachycardia with reduced pulse volume (compensatory mechanism to maintain cardiac output)

Table 20.3 Three phases of shock

Phase	Description
Compensated shock	Vital organ function (brain and heart) is preserved by sympathetic response. Pallor, tachycardia, cold periphery, poor capillary return but systolic blood pressure is maintained.
Uncompensated shock	Inadequate perfusion leads to anaerobic metabolism, metabolic acidosis, and, on occasion, a bleeding diathesis. Blood pressure falls, acidotic breathing, very slow capillary return, altered consciousness, anuria.
Irreversible shock	A retrospective diagnosis. Damage to heart and brain irreversible, with no improvement even if circulation is restored.

Table 20.4 Causes of shock

Mechanism	Causes
Hypovolaemia	Diarrhoea and vomiting Haemorrhage Intussusception/volvulus Peritonitis Burns
Distributive	Septicaemia Anaphylaxis Diabetic ketoacidosis
Cardiogenic	Arrhythmias Heart failure

- capillary refill time >2 seconds, core/toe temperature difference of >2°C (due to poor skin perfusion)

The late physical signs include:

- rapid deep breathing (response to metabolic acidosis)
- agitation, confusion (due to brain hypoperfusion)
- oliguria (urine flow <2 mL/kg per hour in infants and <1 mL/kg per hour in children)
- hypotension

Management

This is a medical emergency and children should be assessed and treatment initiated immediately. In an ABCDE approach, the general management principles of shock are:

- high-flow oxygen
- airway protection if child is obtunded
- continuous monitoring of respiratory rate, oxygen saturations, heart rate and blood pressure
- IV access (two large bore cannulas or intraosseous if difficult access – taking more than two attempts or 5 minutes)
- fluid resuscitation 10 mL/kg bolus (preferably isotonic crystalloid, 0.9% sodium chloride is an acceptable alternative)
- reassess for signs of improvement after each bolus; repeat up to total of 40–60 mL/kg in the first hour
- consider need for intubation if signs of fluid overload or deteriorating GCS
- consider need for inotropes if blood pressure refractory to fluid boluses

Specific shock syndromes

Three important specific syndromes in which shock occurs are:

- anaphylactic shock
- septic shock
- diabetic ketoacidosis (DKA)

Anaphylactic shock

See Chapter 11 for the features of anaphylaxis. The major life-threatening problems are airway oedema leading to obstruction, bronchospasm causing hypoxia and vasodilatation and capillary leak causing shock due to fluid shifts. Children with anaphylactic shock have the potential to deteriorate rapidly with circulatory and respiratory failure.

A summary of treatment is shown in Chapter 11, Allergy and anaphylaxis.

Septic shock

Septicaemia is an important cause of shock in children. The main pathogens include:

- gram-positive bacteria: staphylococci, pneumococci, streptococci

- gram-negative bacteria: *Neisseria meningitidis*, *Escherichia coli*, *H. influenzae* (rare if *H. influenzae* type b (Hib) immunized)

Meningococcal septicaemia is the most fulminant variety. Death can occur within hours of the first symptom; early diagnosis is vital.

Bacterial toxins trigger the release of various mediators and activators, which can:

- cause vasodilatation or vasoconstriction
- depress cardiac function
- disturb cellular oxygen consumption
- cause 'capillary leak' with hypovolaemia
- promote disseminated intravascular coagulation

Clinical features

The clinical features are that of early (compensated) or late (decompensated) shock as described in Table 20.3.

> **RED FLAG**
>
> Fever and petechial = meningococcal septicaemia until proven otherwise. Always examine for signs of shock. Antibiotics within the first hour are crucial for survival.

The cardinal sign of meningococcal septicaemia is a petechial or purpuric rash (Fig. 20.9). This might be subtle in the early stages and a careful search for petechiae is required (in 10% of cases a blanching erythematous rash might occur first). Systemic antibiotics should be given immediately if a diagnosis of meningococcal septicaemia or meningitis is suspected.

Management

Key points in initial management include calling for senior help and anaesthetic support early. Use an ABCDE approach and treat as per shock management described above.

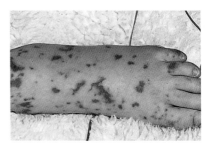

Fig. 20.9 Rash of meningococcal infection. (A) Characteristic purpuric skin lesions, irregular in size and outline and with a necrotic centre; and (B) the lesions may be extensive, when it is called 'purpura fulminans'.

Specifically, in septic shock remember:

- high-flow oxygen
- airway protection if child is obtunded
- continuous monitoring of respiratory rate, oxygen saturations, heart rate and blood pressure
- IV access (two large bore cannulas or intraosseous if difficult access – taking more than two attempts or 5 minutes)
- fluid resuscitation 10 mL/kg bolus (preferably isotonic crystalloid, 0.9% sodium chloride is an acceptable alternative)
- reassess for signs of improvement after each bolus; repeat up to total of 40–60 mL/kg in the first hour
- consider need for intubation if signs of fluid overload or deteriorating GCS
- consider need for inotropes if blood pressure refractory to fluid boluses
- investigations (Table 20.5)
- antibiotics: broad-spectrum IV antibiotics (depending upon local policy; e.g., IV ceftriaxone)

In severe illness, intensive care facilities are required to allow continuous monitoring of circulatory parameters (including central venous pressure), urine output and pulse oximetry. Assisted ventilation, inotropic agents and renal replacement therapy might be required.

Diabetic ketoacidosis

This is an important and life-threatening complication of insulin-dependent diabetes mellitus. This is seen in patients who are known to have type 1 diabetes mellitus but can also be a presenting feature.

DKA represents the end stage of insulin deficiency. Deficiency of insulin causes increased glycogenolysis and gluconeogenesis, reduced glucose uptake in skeletal muscle and adipose cells and impaired glucose utilization – culminating in hyperglycaemia. As glucose levels exceed the renal threshold, an osmotic diuresis ensues with severe dehydration and electrolyte losses. Without insulin, fat is used as a source of energy (lipolysis), leading to the generation of ketones and metabolic acidosis.

To diagnose DKA, the following biochemical criteria has been adopted:

pH <7.30 or HCO_3^- <15 mmol/L
and
Ketonaemia; blood ketones >3 mmol/L

Clinical features

The clinical features evolve as the severity of dehydration and acidosis worsens:

- Vomiting.
- Lethargy.
- Abdominal pain.

- The new diabetic may have a history of polyuria, polydipsia and weight loss.
- The known diabetic may have an intercurrent illness which has led to poor glucose control.

Characteristic physical signs are listed in Table 20.6.

Diagnosis

Essential initial investigations include:

- blood glucose and ketones (hyperglycaemia, ketonaemia)
- urea and electrolytes (raised urea, hyponatraemia, hypokalaemia)
- blood gas analysis (metabolic acidosis)
- urine glucose and ketones (glycosuria, ketonuria)

HINTS AND TIPS

In DKA:

- Total body potassium depletion is always present (even if serum potassium seems normal).
- Current guidelines emphasize treating shock and restoring adequate circulation first, then carefully managing fluid administration to reduce the risk of cerebral oedema.
- Cerebral oedema is rare but associated with a high mortality. If headache, agitation/irritability, unexpected fall in heart rate or rise in blood pressure develops, suspect cerebral oedema and discuss urgently with a senior paediatrician.

Management

The mainstays of management are, having treated shock, the slow and careful restoration of fluid and electrolyte status, and insulin. There may be other comorbidities such as infection/sepsis.

DKA can be classified by severity:

- mild/moderate: pH >7.1, dry mucus membranes, reduced skin turgor (assume 5% dehydration)
- severe: pH <7.1, dry mucus membranes, reduced skin turgor, sunken eyes (assume 10% dehydration)

Mild DKA can be treated with oral fluids and subcutaneous insulin ONLY if the child is alert, not vomiting and is not clinically dehydrated.

Fluids

- If using IV fluids and insulin, the child should be made nil by mouth.
- All children requiring IV fluids in DKA should be given 10 mL/kg (preferably isotonic crystalloid, 0.9% sodium chloride is an acceptable alternative) over 30 minutes.
- Further resuscitation fluid boluses up to a total of 40 mL/kg (then consider inotropes) should only be given to children with signs of shock (= tachycardia and other features) acidosis and hypercapnia will cause peripheral

Table 20.5 Investigations in suspected septic shock

Investigations to assess severity	• Full blood count • Electrolytes and liver function • Blood gas • Lactate • Glucose • Coagulation screen • C-reactive protein
Investigations to identify focus	• Blood culture • Urine culture • Throat swab • PCR (meningococcus, pneumococcus) • Chest X-ray • • Abdominal ultrasound (looking for abscesses, collections, etc.)

Table 20.6 Physical signs in diabetic ketoacidosis

Dehydration	Dry mucous membranes Loss of skin turgor Tachycardia Hypotension (if severe)
Acidosis	Ketotic breath (fruity) Kussmaul breathing: rapid, deep, sighing respiration
Cerebral oedema	Headache Confusion Decreased conscious level Seizures and focal neurological signs Cushing triad (bradycardia, hypertension, irregular respiration)

vasoconstriction (prolonged capillary refill time, mottling) in all children with DKA.

• For fluid replacement use 0.9% sodium chloride + 20 mmol potassium chloride/500 mL.

Fluid replacement is calculated using the following four-stage calculation:

1. Fluid deficit (mL) = weight (kg-to a maximum of 75 kg) × dehydration × 10
2. Replacement (mL) = fluid deficit-10x weight (to account for no more than a single fluid bolus given, do not subtract more)
3. Maintenance fluid rate is calculated as standard – to a 75 kg maximum weight (Chapter 21)
4. Hourly rate = (replacement/48 hours) + maintenance/hours
   • Do not give sodium bicarbonate.

Insulin

• There is some evidence that early use of insulin increases the risk of cerebral oedema.

• Start insulin infusion 1 to 2 hours hour after starting IV fluids.
• Start insulin infusion at 0.05–0.1 units/kg per hour.
• Aim to reduce blood glucose by no more than 5 mmol/hour.
• Once blood glucose <14 mmol change to 5% glucose (dextrose) with 0.9% sodium chloride.
• Once ketones are <1.0 mmol/L consider switching from IV to subcutaneous insulin.

Careful monitoring is required of:

• blood glucose: monitor hourly
• acid–base status: 2 hours initially
• electrolytes: 4 hours initially
• fluid status: input and output, weight
• vital signs and neurological observations
• cardiac rhythm: electrocardiogram monitoring allows early identification of dysrhythmias secondary to electrolyte imbalances

Complications

Major complications include:

• Cerebral oedema: manifested by reduced conscious level, headache, irritability and fits. Attempt to prevent this by avoiding *rapid* falls in blood glucose or serum sodium concentrations by giving too much fluid or insulin.
• Cardiac dysrhythmias: usually secondary to electrolyte (potassium) disturbances. Acute renal failure is uncommon.

Once the biochemical markers have stabilized and the child can tolerate oral fluids, subcutaneous insulin can be restarted. It is important to take this opportunity to review the family's understanding of diabetes and ensure concordance with therapy.

UNINTENTIONAL INJURIES

Unintentional injuries are not 'accidents' in that most are, potentially, preventable – under 5s are at particular risk; these injuries are a leading cause of death and disability to children in the UK. The World Health Organization estimates 950,000 deaths globally in children and young people under the age of 18. The pattern of injury varies with age (Box 20.4); however, road traffic

BOX 20.4 PATTERNS OF INJURY IN CHILDREN

Toddlers	School age	Adolescents
Falls Scalds Drowning Accidental ingestion Choking	Falls from heights Road traffic collision	Road traffic collision Alcohol or drug related

collision accounts for the majority of fatal injury. Child abuse needs to be considered in any child presenting with injury.

Trauma

Physical trauma causing multiple serious injuries is an important cause of death. Early, appropriate management of the child with multiple injuries is vital to reduce mortality and long-term morbidity.

Major trauma

These are best dealt with in hospitals with major trauma centres where a trauma team leads the resuscitation. Initial assessment is summarized in Fig. 20.10.

Management

Immediate.
- Primary survey.
- A quick assessment to identify immediate life threats.
- Resuscitation.

Events during the first 'golden hour' determine the outcome. Similar to the seriously ill child, an ABCDE approach is taken; however, the key difference in trauma is to deal with catastrophic (i.e., life-threatening) haemorrhage first. In addition to this, when dealing with the airway in trauma, C-spine injury should always be suspected. In this instance jaw thrust is recommended rather than head-tilt chin-lift.

Focused. Once the initial steps of immediate resuscitation have been carried out, a comprehensive secondary survey to identify occult injuries is completed (Table 20.7). This would also involve a full history and radiological investigations as indicated.

Detailed review. This includes reassessment of the child using an ABCDE approach, stabilization and transfer to a ward or intensive care.

Head injury

Minor head injuries in children are very common and most children recover without ill effect. A small minority, about 1 in 800 of those admitted, develops serious complications such as intracranial haemorrhage. Causes of head injury include:
- road traffic accidents
- falls from trees, windows, bicycles, etc.

Table 20.7 Secondary survey and treatment of major trauma

Head	Bruising/haematomas Lacerations Cerebrospinal fluid leak from ears or nose Mini-neurological examination
Face	Bruising Lacerations Loose teeth
Neck	Cervical spine injury: • bony tenderness • bruising or wounds Tracheal deviation (tension pneumothorax)
Chest	Bruising or wounds Auscultate heart and breath sounds
Abdomen	Bruising or wounds Tenderness or signs of peritonism (Per rectal examination (PR) not routinely indicated in children)
Pelvis	Deformity
Spine	Log roll: • bony deformity • bony tenderness • bruising or wounds Assess motor and sensory function
Extremities	Deformity Observe movement Peripheral circulation

- child abuse (nonaccidental injury – NAI): especially, abusive head injury

Damage to the brain might be primary or secondary (Table 20.8).

The history should establish:
- the mechanism of injury
- history of loss of consciousness
- subsequent symptoms: vomiting, drowsiness, seizures, bleeding from nose or ears
- amnesia (if yes, duration)

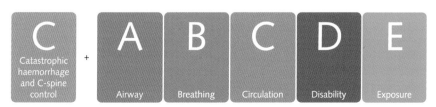

Fig. 20.10 Approach to major trauma.

Table 20.8 Brain damage in head injury

Primary damage	Cerebral laceration and contusion Diffuse axonal injury Dural sac tears Intracranial haemorrhage
Secondary damage	Ischaemia from shock, hypoxia or raised intracranial pressure Hypoglycaemia Central nervous system infection Seizures Hyperthermia

Clinical features

Clinical examination should look for the following signs:

- Head: external injury including haematoma, laceration, depressed fracture. In babies, the anterior fontanelle tension provides a useful indicator of intracranial pressure. Look for blood or cerebrospinal fluid leak from the ears or nose.
- Central nervous system: assess GCS/AVPU scale, fundi and pupillary reflexes. Examine for focal neurological signs.

Diagnosis

Investigations include:

- cranial CT:
- see Box 20.5 for National Institute for Health and Care Excellence (NICE) guidance for indications for CT head
- if the CT scan is normal but the infant or child remains unwell or symptomatic, then admit for observation

Management

In minor head injuries the child may be assessed and discharged home after a period of observation. Parents should be given written information and safety netting advice. This should include instructions to bring the child back if there is severe headache, recurrent vomiting or a declining level of consciousness.

Moderate head injuries in which the child did not meet criteria for CT head but is symptomatic should be admitted for observation. Children who have a bleeding tendency should also be closely observed. Any suspicion of NAI requires admission and discussion with senior staff and social workers.

If admitted, neurological observations should be made at intervals dictated by the child's clinical state and existing guidelines. In all cases of head injury particular attention should be paid to analgesic control and titrated according to the child's response.

BOX 20.5 NICE GUIDELINES: INDICATIONS FOR CT IN HEAD INJURIES

CT head within 1 hour if any ONE of the following:	CT head within 1 hour if more than one of the following:
• Suspicion of nonaccidental injury, Posttraumatic seizure (nonepileptic), GCS less than 14 (<15 in under 1 year olds) on admission, GCS less than 15 2 hours after the injury, Suspected open or depressed skull fracture, Suspected basal skull fracture (haemotympanum, 'panda' eyes, cerebrospinal fluid leakage from the ear or nose, Battle sign), Presence of bruise, swelling or laceration of more than 5 cm on the head in under 1 year olds, Tense fontanelle, Focal neurological deficit	• Loss of consciousness lasting more than 5 minutes (witnessed), Abnormal drowsiness, Three or more discrete episodes of vomiting, Dangerous mechanism of injury (high-speed road traffic collision or other injury, fall from a height >3 m), Amnesia (antegrade or retrograde) lasting >5 minutes (unable to assess in <5 year olds)

CT, Computed tomography; GCS, Glasgow Coma Scale; NICE, National Institute for Health and Care Excellence.

RED FLAG

Nonaccidental injury (NAI) should be suspected if:

- The mechanism of injury or history is incompatible with the infant's or child's stage of development.
- The injury does not fit with the mechanism offered.
- Inappropriate care or concern by the parent/carer or delay in presentation.

Severe head injuries usually occur in the context of multiple major trauma requiring intensive care. Urgent referral to a neurosurgeon is indicated if there is any evidence of an expanding haematoma, such as:

- declining level of consciousness
- focal neurological signs
- depressed skull fracture

- Cushing triad: bradycardia, rise in systolic blood pressure and irregular respirations

In severe head injuries neuroprotective measures are used on intensive care units to minimize further rises in intracranial pressure. These include:

- nursing head up (15°–30°)
- adequate oxygenation
- avoid hypercarbia (partial pressure of carbon dioxide (PCO_2) 4.5–5 kPa)
- tight blood pressure control
- adequate sedation and analgesia
- avoid hyperglycaemia

Burns and scalds

Scalds from contact with hot liquids are the most common form of thermal trauma in childhood (most of the fatalities are from house fires but those are due to gas and smoke inhalation rather than burns). Burns and scalds can be nonaccidental. Toddlers are most at risk of unintentional scald injury.

Assessment
The extent, depth and distribution of the injury should be estimated (see Box 20.6 and Fig. 20.11).

HINTS AND TIPS

Location of the burn is important, as well as extent:

- face – potential airway involvement, scarring
- hands – contractures and functional loss
- genitalia – difficult to nurse, risk of infection

Area indicated	Surface area at				
	0 years	1 year	5 years	10 years	15 years
A	9.5	8.5	6.5	5.5	4.5
B	2.75	3.25	4.0	4.5	4.5
C	2.5	2.5	2.75	3.0	3.25

Fig. 20.11 Assessing depth of a burn.

BOX 20.6 ASSESSING DEPTH OF A BURN

Depth of burn	Layers of skin affected	Skin examination
Superficial epidermal (sunburn)	The epidermis is affected, but the dermis is intact	Red and painful, but not blistered. Capillary refill: blanches then rapidly refills
Superficial dermal (partial thickness)	The epidermis and upper layers of dermis are involved	Red or pale pink and painful with blistering. Capillary refill: blanches but regains colour slowly
Deep dermal (partial thickness)	The epidermis, upper and deeper layers of dermis are involved, but not underlying subcutaneous tissues	Dry, mottled, red, painful, may be blisters. Capillary refill: does not blanch
Full thickness	The burn extends through all the layers of skin to subcutaneous tissues. If severe, extends into muscle and bone	White/brown/black in colour with no blisters. Dry, leathery/waxy – painless. Capillary refill: does not blanch

Assess capillary refill by pressing with a sterile cotton bud (e.g., bacteriology swab)

Management

The recommended advice to the general public and first-aid providers is to run cold water over the affected anatomy for 20 minutes.

When managing a child with a burn injury you should take an ABCDE approach. The key aspects specific to emergency management of burns include:

- Fluid resuscitation: if shocked, give 10 mL/kg boluses (preferably isotonic crystalloid, 0.9% sodium chloride is an acceptable alternative), titrated to cardiovascular response. Then:
  - Use a burn chart to calculate total burn surface area (TBSA)
  - Give replacement IV fluid to any child with >10% TBSA in addition to normal maintenance fluid. This is calculated using the Parkland formula in three steps:
    1. % Burn × Weight (kg) × 4 = Fluid replacement
    2. Give 50% of this volume in the 8 hours from the burn occurrence (not arrival in hospital) + maintenance rate (see Chapter 21)_____
    3. Give remaining 50% over 16 hours + maintenance rate (see Chapter 21)
- Adequate analgesia: intranasal diamorphine/fentanyl or IV/oral morphine is often required.
- Maintain normothermia (risk of hypothermia – cool the burn, warm the child).
- Wound care: ensure burn cooled for 20 minutes (effective upto 3 hours after injury), use cling film in the first instance. Minimal handling.

Carbon monoxide poisoning occurs when the victim inhales the fumes in a fire. It results in cellular hypoxia as carboxyhaemoglobin has a greater affinity for oxygen than haemoglobin. Carboxyhaemoglobin levels should be measured and the mainstay of treatment is oxygen. In severe cases a hyperbaric oxygen chamber is used.

Following emergency management, refer to local tertiary burns unit in any of the below circumstances:

- partial thickness burns >2%
- full thickness burns >1%
- inhalation injury
- burns to difficult areas including face, neck, hands, feet, perineum
- burns over a joint
- electrical or chemical burns
- suspicion of nonaccidental injury (urgent assessment required within 24 hours)
- circumferential burns to trunk/limbs
- burns associated with major trauma or significant comorbidities

Nonaccidental injury consideration in burns and scalds

Nonaccidental injury should be suspected when dealing with cases of burns and scalds if any of the following are present:

- a 'glove and sock' distribution of burns (suggestive of an immersion injury)
- delay in presentation
- burns or scalds to the buttocks or perineum
- other social concerns in the family

Drowning

Drowning is respiratory impairment following immersion in a liquid (terms 'near drowning' and 'wet'/'dry' drowning are no longer used). It is more common in boys than girls. Since 2012 there have been over 40 deaths from drowning in children under 5. In the UK, drowning incidents are more common in freshwater canals and lakes, swimming pools and domestic baths than in the sea.

The two principal problems in drowning are:

- Hypoxia: laryngospasm results in asphyxia. Only a small amount of water initially enters the lungs.
- Hypothermia: this leads to bradycardia and asystole (extreme hypothermia can be protective).

Haemolysis or electrolyte problems caused by the ingestion or inhalation of large amounts of water can occur.

Management

Skilled resuscitation and warming are vital. Cervical injury should be assumed. All children should be hospitalized for at least 24 hours. Patients admitted in asystole or respiratory arrest are managed with cardiopulmonary resuscitation – and if hypothermic (<30°C) aggressive rewarming because many arrhythmias are refractory at temperatures below 30°C.

Prognostic indicators of drowning

The prognostic indicators are shown in Table 20.9.

Late respiratory sequelae can occur in the 72-hour period after drowning. These include pneumonia and pulmonary oedema.

Poisoning

Most cases of poisoning in young children follow ingestion by an inquisitive toddler; in adolescents most poisoning is self-harm. Children can also be poisoned deliberately by their parents (or inadvertently by their doctors). Although many thousands of children attend hospital each year, very few die as a result of accidental ingestion.

The history should establish:

- what was ingested: identify from carton or bottle

Table 20.9 Prognostic indications for near drowning

Prognostic indicators	Poor if:
Immersion time	Submerged for >5 minutes
Age	<3 years
Effective basic life support	Commenced >10 minutes after drowning
Advanced life support	Asystole at scene, cardiac arrest >30 minutes
Type of water	No difference on prognosis

- amount ingested: usually an approximation
- time ingested: important in relation to management

The toxicity of the ingested substance can then be assessed and treatment can be started (Table 20.10). The National Poisons Information Service hosts the TOXBASE database, and provides 24-hour access to toxicologists for further advice and guidance.

Clinical features

Examination should include the following:

- Inspect oropharynx and any vomitus.
- Assess level of consciousness.
- Look for features specific to various poisons, for example, small pupils (opiates or barbiturates), tachypnoea (salicylate poisoning) or cardiac arrhythmias (tricyclic antidepressants or digoxin).

Diagnosis

Relevant investigations include:

- Blood levels (at optimum time after ingestion) can be measured for salicylates, paracetamol, digoxin, iron, lithium and tricyclic antidepressants.
- Take a urine specimen for analysis.
- Other blood tests may be relevant; for example – blood gas in salicylate poisoning, liver function and coagulation studies in paracetamol overdose.

Management

Following the guidance hosted on TOXBASE, if the agent ingested was relatively innocuous, the patient can be allowed home after a period of observation. Advice regarding safe storage of medicines should be given to parents of young children, referring for follow-up with Health visiting teams.

Efforts should be made to remove the poison if there has been a large ingestion of a highly toxic substance. These include:

- Activated charcoal: give 1 g/kg, if necessary by nasogastric tube. It binds a wide range of toxic drugs, with the exception of iron and lithium. It is most efficacious if used within 1 hour of ingestion.

Specific treatment is indicated for certain drugs and toxins (Table 20.10).

Self-harm (overdosing and excessive use of drugs and alcohol)

Self-harm (and self-injury) often are a response by a young person to distressing feelings they are experiencing. Equally, young people may experiment with drugs and alcohol – distinguishing between an act motivated by negative thoughts is important – to facilitate engagement with appropriate support.

In most cases self-harm does not represent a concrete desire to end life, although the young person may have conflicting thoughts and feelings about this, but this behaviour can involve very dangerous acts – running the risk of inadvertent death.

Self-harm by overdose is a significant matter, for which children and young people need a place of safety (hospital) and, at an appropriate point – often following 'cooling off', discussion with mental health professionals.

Table 20.10 Poison-specific adverse effects and treatments

Poison	Adverse effects	Specific treatment
Iron	Shock, gut haemorrhage	Intravenous (IV) desferrioxamine
Paracetamol	Liver failure	IV N-acetylcysteine
Salicylates	Metabolic acidosis	Gastric lavage if <4 hours Activated charcoal Alkalinization of urine with bicarbonate
Ethylene glycol (antifreeze)	Widespread cellular damage	Ethanol, dialysis if severe
Tricyclic antidepressants	Cardiac dysrhythmias	Alkalinization of urine with bicarbonate Antiarrhythmics as guided by poisons centre
Opiates (including methadone)	Respiratory depression	Naloxone
Ecstasy	Hyperpyrexia and rhabdomyolysis Dysrhythmias	Active cooling benzodiazepines (e.g., diazepam) to control anxiety

Chapter Summary

- The seriously ill child should be assessed using the structured airway, breathing, circulation, disability, exposure (ABCDE) approach.
- Cardiorespiratory arrest in children is usually a secondary occurrence, and the focus should be on recognizing sick children and preventing deterioration.
- There are key differences in paediatric basic life support compared to in adults. Paediatric basic life support begins with five rescue breaths and follows a ratio of 15:2, compared with adults who begin with two rescue breaths and a ratio of 30:2.
- There are many forms of respiratory emergencies in children, which are divided into upper airway and lower airway obstruction.
- Childhood injury is the most common cause of death in over 1 year olds, the majority of which are caused by road traffic collisions which cause major trauma.

UKMLA Conditions	UKMLA presentations
Anaphylaxis	Breathlessness
Cardiac arrest	Decreased/loss of consciousness
Dehydration	Dehydration
Diabetic ketoacidosis	Deteriorating patient
Drug overdose	Fits/seizures
Raised intracranial pressure	Overdose
Respiratory arrest	Poisoning
	Shock
	The sick child
	Trauma
	Vomiting

Infants and children are more vulnerable than adults to inadequate nutrition or the derangement of fluid and electrolyte balance. A higher surface area-to-volume ratio is associated with a higher metabolic rate, larger calorific requirements and corresponding rapid fluid turnover.

Globally, malnutrition is directly or indirectly responsible for a third of all deaths of children. Conversely, in the developed world obesity is increasing in children and likely to shorten life expectancy in the long term.

HINTS AND TIPS

Breastfeeding in early infancy saves lives in developing countries due to the risk of waterborne diseases for formula-fed infants.

Dehydration associated with diarrhoeal diseases is a major killer worldwide and its treatment with oral rehydration solution represented a major advance. However, attention to fluid and electrolyte status is an important aspect of many childhood illnesses.

Prescribing for infants and children involves many considerations unique to this age group. The route and frequency of administration must be adapted to the age, and dosage must take into account bodyweight, surface area and age-dependent changes in drug metabolism and excretion.

NUTRITION

Normal nutritional requirements

A satisfactory dietary intake should meet the normal requirements for energy and protein, together with providing an adequate supply of vitamins and trace elements. A neonate requires 115 kcal/kg day which falls during childhood to 50 kcal/kg day by the age of 18 years.

Infants and children are vulnerable to undernutrition because of:

- Low stores of fat and protein.
- Nutritional demands of growth (at 4 months of age, 30% of an infant's energy intake is used for growth; by 3 years of age this has fallen to 2%).

- Brain growth: the brain is proportionally larger in infants and is growing rapidly during the last trimester and first 2 years of life. It is vulnerable to energy deprivation during this period.

Infant feeding

An infant's primary source of nutrition is milk, either human breast milk or so-called formula milk, usually based on modified cow's milk.

Common and important issues that may affect infant feeding are displayed in Table 21.1.

Breastfeeding

This is the preferred method for most infants. Galactosaemia is the only absolute contraindication. Human immunodeficiency virus (HIV)-positive mothers should not breastfeed in the developed world due to risk of transmission. The many advantages, and few disadvantages, of breastfeeding are listed in Box 21.1.

Table 21.1 Issues that can lead to reduced feeding in an infant

	Mother	Baby/infant
Infection/ inflammation	Thrush, abscess, mastitis	Thrush, peri-oral skin[a] infection
Structural	Breast and nipple size/shape, sore/ cracked nipples	Tongue tie, cleft lip/palate, neonatal tooth, reflux
Neurological		Syndromes associated with reduced tone, poor swallow coordination, IVH and PVL[b]
Metabolic/allergy/ intolerance		CMPA[c], galactosaemia, lactose intolerance, neonatal jaundice
Miscellaneous	Low milk supply	Colic, prematurity

[a]Herpes simplex, cellulitis/erysipelas, secondary bacterial infection
[b]Intraventricular haemorrhage, periventricular leukomalacia
[c]Cow's milk protein allergy

BOX 21.1 ADVANTAGES AND DISADVANTAGES OF BREASTFEEDING

Advantages	Disadvantages
Health benefits- reduced risk of: • Infection, constipation, sudden infant death syndrome (SIDS), atopic conditions, maternal breast cancer	Volume of intake uncertain. Need for vitamin D and vitamin K supplementation. Transmission of drugs: illicit and prescribed.
Convenient, affordable: • No need to heat up or sterilize equipment	
Emotional • Promotes bonding	• Failure to establish breastfeeding results in emotional upset and guilt

HINTS AND TIPS

Establishing breastfeeding:

- The baby should be put to the breast as soon as possible after birth.
- Frequent suckling promotes lactation.
- Advice with positioning helps to establish feeding.
- Colostrum (high content of protein and immunoglobulin) rather than milk is produced in first few days.
- The interval between feeds gradually lengthens from 2–3 hours to approximately a 4-hourly schedule.

The composition of breast milk, cow's milk and infant formula differs significantly (Table 21.2). Unmodified, whole,

Table 21.2 Composition of different milks (per 100 mL)

	Breast milk	Cow's milk	Infant formula
Protein (g)	1.3	3.3	1.5
Casein:whey	40:60	60:40	Variable
Carbohydrate (g)	7.0	4.5	7.0–8.0
Fat (g)	4.2	3.6	2.6–3.8
Energy (kcal)	70	65	65
Sodium (mmol)	0.65	2.3	0.65–1.1
Calcium (mmol)	0.87	3.0	1.4
Iron (µmol)	1.36	0.9	10
Vitamin D (pg)	0.6	0.03	1.0

pasteurized cow's milk is unsuitable as a main diet for infants under the age of 1 year because:

- It contains too much protein and sodium.
- It is deficient in iron and vitamins.

Modified cow's milk formulas have a modified casein-to-whey ratio, reduced mineral content and are fortified with iron and vitamins.

HINTS AND TIPS

Breastfeeding mothers might be concerned about whether their baby has had an adequate milk intake. This is best measured by the baby's weight gain and wet nappies.

Weaning

The World Health Organization (WHO) advise the introduction of solid foods (weaning) at 6 months but it can be safely done from 4 months. At this age the infant can coordinate swallowing and has reasonable head control.

A typical scheme for the introduction of solids is shown in Table 21.3.

Special milks

A variety of specialized milks exist that are used in infants who are intolerant of specific constituents. Examples include:

- lactose-free milk: lactose intolerance
- hydrolyzed milk: cow's milk protein allergy
- low phenylalanine milk: phenylketonuria

Soya was used previously in cow's milk protein allergy but there is cross-reactivity in up to 40% of children and so it is not advised.

Malnutrition

Worldwide, malnutrition due to inadequate intake (starvation) is responsible for millions of childhood deaths. However,

Table 21.3 Introduction of solids

Age	Feeding
4–6 months	Smooth purees (fruit, vegetables, rice, meat, dairy products – avoid gluten)
6–9 months	Thicker consistencies and finger foods (fruit, vegetables, rice, meat, dairy products, cereals)
9–12 months	Mashed, chopped and minced consistencies (encourage variety of tastes and textures)
12 months	Mashed and chopped foods (encourage finger foods, can introduce whole cow's milk)

Table 21.4 Causes of malnutrition in childhood

Inadequate intake	Malabsorption	Increased energy requirements
Starvation (poverty)	Pancreatic insufficiency (cystic fibrosis)	Cystic fibrosis
Anorexia nervosa	Coeliac disease	Malignancy
Restrictive diets (parental, iatrogenic, self-inflicted)	Short gut (postoperative)	Chronic disease
		Burns
Loss of appetite (chronic disease)	Inflammatory bowel disease	

malnutrition can also exacerbate many childhood diseases resulting in impaired immunity, slower recovery time and developmental delay. Causes of malnutrition are listed in Table 21.4.

Assessment of nutritional status

Evaluation involves:

- dietary history
- anthropometry and clinical examination
- laboratory investigations

Dietary history

The food intake, as recalled by the parents or recorded in a diary, is determined over a period of several days.

Anthropometry

This involves measurement of:

- Height: height for age is reduced (stunted growth) in chronic malnutrition.
- Weight: reduced weight with normal height (wasting) is an index of acute malnutrition.
- Mid-upper arm circumference: an indication of skeletal muscle mass.
- Skinfold thickness: triceps skinfold thickness is a measure of subcutaneous fat stores.

Clinical syndromes of protein-energy malnutrition include:

- Marasmus: wasted (weight less than 60% of mean for age), wizened appearance, withdrawn and apathetic.
- Kwashiorkor: occurs in children weaned late from the breast and fed on a relatively high-starch diet. It can be precipitated by an acute intercurrent infection. Features include wasting, oedema, sparse hair, depigmented skin, angular stomatitis and hepatomegaly.

Laboratory investigations

Useful laboratory tests include:

- serum albumin: reduced in severe malnutrition
- full blood count: low haemoglobin and lymphocyte count
- blood glucose
- calcium, phosphate and vitamin D levels
- serum potassium and magnesium levels

Management

Nutrition can be supplied:

- Enterally, via the gastrointestinal tract: this route is preferred wherever possible.
- Parenterally, directly into the circulation.

In many cases, malnutrition is due to inadequate intake and can be managed by the provision of supplementary enteral feeds given via a nasogastric or gastrostomy tube.

Examples of chronic diseases requiring such supplemental feeding include:

- cystic fibrosis
- congenital heart disease
- cerebral palsy
- chronic renal failure
- malignancy
- inflammatory bowel disease
- anorexia nervosa

Vitamin deficiencies

Several important vitamin deficiency diseases still occur in childhood. These include in particular:

- vitamin D deficiency: rickets
- vitamin A deficiency: blindness
- vitamin K deficiency: haemorrhagic disease of the newborn

HINTS AND TIPS

The most common dietary deficiencies in the UK are of iron and vitamin D. Scurvy due to vitamin C deficiency is now extremely rare in developed countries.

Vitamin D deficiency: rickets

The effects of vitamin D deficiency on growing bone cause rickets. The bone matrix (osteoid) of the growing bone is inadequately mineralized, giving rise to the clinical features described in Box 21.2. The undermineralized bone is less rigid, resulting in the classic bowed legs.

The normal pathways of vitamin D absorption and metabolism are shown in Fig. 21.1.

The most important source of vitamin D is sunshine. It is difficult to correct deficiency by dietary manipulation alone. The minimum daily requirement of vitamin D is 400 to 600 international units (IU) and this might not be attained in infants who are

BOX 21.2 CLINICAL FEATURES OF RICKETS

General	Skeletal
Misery	Craniotabes
Hypotonia	Enlarged metaphyses
Developmental delay	(wrists, knees)
(especially walking)	Enlarged costochondral
Growth failure	junction (rachitic rosary)
Late eruption of teeth	Leg bowing

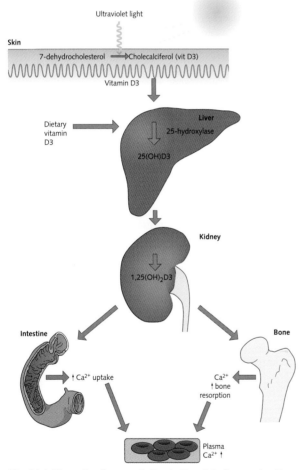

Fig. 21.1 Normal pathways of vitamin D metabolism and action.

breastfed for a protracted period. Decreased sun exposure is exacerbated by:

- infants with pigmented skin
- full coverage with religious garments

- urban living conditions
- winter

Much less common causes of rickets include:

- inherited abnormalities of vitamin D metabolism or of the vitamin D receptor
- mineral deficiency (e.g., X-linked hypophosphatemia)
- chronic renal disease
- decreased activity of 1α-hydroxylase in the kidneys leads to rickets as one component of renal osteodystrophy

Rickets of prematurity is a metabolic bone disease in the premature infant that occurs if the milk used contains inadequate calcium and phosphate (1α-dihydroxycholecalciferol levels are elevated because of the hypophosphatemic stimulus, but there is osteopenia and inadequate mineralization of growing bone).

Diagnosis

This is confirmed by X-ray imaging and blood biochemistry. X-ray of the wrist shows cupping and fraying of the metaphysis and a widened metaphyseal plate (Fig. 21.2).

The biochemical changes in classic nutritional rickets include:

- serum calcium: low or normal (may be normalized by secondary hyperparathyroidism)
- serum phosphate: low
- serum alkaline phosphatase: elevated
- serum parathormone: elevated
- serum 1,25-dihydroxycholecalciferol: low

Treatment

Prevention is obviously preferred and this is achieved by health education, exposure to sunlight and supplementation of the diet with minerals and vitamin D when indicated.

Treatment of nutritional rickets is with vitamin D3 (1,25-dihydroxycholecalciferol) 6000 to 10,000 IU/day initially for several weeks, followed by provision of 600 IU/day in the diet.

Higher doses might be required in inherited forms. Biochemistry and radiography monitor the effect of therapy.

Vitamin A (retinol) deficiency

Vitamin A is necessary for membrane stability and it plays a role in vision, keratinization, cornification and placental development. The body's need for vitamin A can be met by milk, butter, eggs, liver and dark green or orange-coloured (e.g., carrots) vegetables.

Worldwide, about 150 million children are at risk of vitamin A deficiency, and it has been calculated that up to a third of a million children go blind each year from vitamin A deficiency. In addition, vitamin A deficiency carries increased mortality from infection and poor growth.

The eye disease develops insidiously with impaired dark adaptation followed by drying of the conjunctiva and cornea (xerophthalmia).

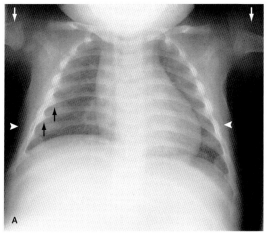

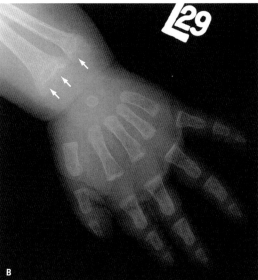

Fig. 21.2 X-ray appearance of rickets. (A) Rachitic rosary, bulging of the anterior ends (*black arrows*); (B) Metaphyseal cupping with loss of bone density (*white arrows*).

Disease is treated with dietary advice and/or with supplementation.

Obesity

The WHO describes obesity as a global epidemic, and in 2015 the Royal College of Paediatrics and Child Heath reported that a third of children aged 2 to 15 years are obese. It results from numerous social and environmental factors that are difficult to alter. Obesity in children is increasing in prevalence and treatment is often disappointing. Prevention of obesity remains the optimal solution.

The body mass index (BMI) is a useful measurement of obesity and should be plotted on a BMI chart to assess if a child is obese. Aetiological factors include:

- excess caloric intake
- reduced activity levels
- prevalence of obesity in family

Rarely, an endocrine or chromosomal cause is present such as Cushing syndrome, hypothyroidism or Prader-Willi syndrome.
Obesity has several deleterious consequences including:

- long-term health risks (diabetes, hypertension, ischaemic heart disease)
- emotional disturbance: many psychological problems are associated with obesity
- obstructive sleep apnoea leading to poor school performance

Management

A large number of interventions have been tried and involvement of the family as a whole is necessary. An aim to maintain the same weight while linear growth occurs may be more successful than attempting weight loss. Psychological support should be offered. For a small number of morbidly obese adolescents, bariatric surgery may be required. The government is implementing changes too, including placing a tax on sugary drinks.

FLUIDS AND ELECTROLYTES

Basic physiology

It is useful to know how fluid is distributed between the different compartments of the body and what the normal requirements for fluid and electrolytes are. Important changes occur with age as the ratio of surface area to volume alters.

Fluid compartments

These are shown in Table 21.5. Infants have greater water content than adults with a higher proportion of fluid in the extracellular space. The percentages can be expressed as volumes: for example, 70% is equivalent to 700 mL/kg bodyweight.
Blood volume is about 80 mL/kg at birth and falls to about 60 mL/kg by adulthood.

Table 21.5 Body fluid compartments (as a percentage of bodyweight)

Age	Total body water	Extracellular fluid	Intracellular fluid
Newborn	70	35	35
12 months	65	25	40
Adult	60	20	40

HINTS AND TIPS

- As body density is close to that of water, and 1 L of water weighs close to 1 kg, weights and volumes are freely interchangeable. For example, 1000 mL = 1000 g (1 L = 1 kg).
- Changes in bodyweight are the best guide to short-term changes in fluid balance (e.g., a weight loss of 500 g indicates a fluid deficit of 500 mL).

Normal requirements

Fluid requirement is that needed to make up for normal fluid losses, which include essential urine output and 'insensible' losses through sweat, respiration and the gastrointestinal tract. In pathological states there will be additional abnormal losses, such as those associated with diarrhoea or vomiting.

A simple formula for calculating normal fluid requirements according to bodyweight is shown in Table 21.6.

There are obligatory electrolyte losses in the stools, urine and sweat, and these require replacement. The maintenance requirement for sodium is about 3 mmol/kg per day and for potassium is 2 mmol/kg per day.

Intravenous fluids

These can be divided into colloids, which include large molecules such as proteins, and crystalloids, which usually contain dextrose (glucose) and electrolytes. Colloids are rarely used outside of intensive care settings.

The compositions of commonly available crystalloid fluids for intravenous (IV) use are shown in Table 21.7.

Important features of intravenous solutions

- Deaths and neurological damage occur due to erroneous fluid prescriptions in children.
- Regular measurement of urea and electrolytes is required for children on IV fluids (not less than 24 hourly).
- Balanced crystalloids or 0.9% sodium chloride (saline) should be used for initial volume resuscitation – in serious injury blood products may be indicated.
- Isotonic solutions (0.9% sodium chloride or 0.9% sodium chloride with 5% glucose) are the safest solutions to use for replacement and maintenance fluids. They can be given in hyponatraemia and hypernatraemia.
- 0.45% sodium chloride with 5% glucose can be used as maintenance fluid but only if the electrolytes are normal.
- Neonates require 10% glucose with electrolytes added, usually on day 3 of life.
- 0.18% sodium chloride should never be used in paediatric medicine due to its hypotonicity.

Specific fluid and electrolyte problems

Electrolyte disturbances are common particularly in pathological states, children treated with IV fluids or as a result of prematurity. Abnormalities of sodium and potassium can have serious consequences including cardiac arrhythmias and cerebral oedema. The causes of hypo/hypernatraemia and hypo/hyperkalaemia are shown below in Tables 21.8 to 21.11.

The normal regime for fluid replacement is described in Table 21.6. There are a few conditions, however, that have different fluid calculations to be aware of:

- dehydration (see Chapter 20)
- diabetic ketoacidosis (DKA – see Chapter 20)
- burns (see Chapter 20)

Important features concerning certain electrolyte disturbances are considered here.

Table 21.6 Normal fluid requirements

Body weight	Fluid requirement per 24 hours
First 10 kg	100 mL/kg
Second 10 kg	50 mL/kg
Further kg	20 mL/kg
Example: 24-hour requirement for child weighing 25 kg	
10 kg at 100 mL/kg	= 1000 mL
10 kg at 50 mL/kg	= 500 mL
5 kg at 20 mL/kg	= 100 mL
Total	= 1600 mL

Table 21.7 Isotonic crystalloid fluids composition

Fluid	Sodium (mmol/L)	Potassium (mmol/L)	Chloride (mmol/L)	Energy (kcal/L)
0.9% sodium chloride	150	0	150	0
0.9% sodium chloride/5% glucose (maintenance and suitable in electrolyte abnormalities)	150	0	150	200
0.45% sodium chloride/5% glucose (maintenance if electrolytes in normal range)	75	0	75	200

Table 21.8 Causes of hyponatraemia (Na$^+$ <135 mmol/L)

Mechanism	Cause
Water excess	Iatrogenic (e.g., hypotonic fluids) SIADH Underlying causes include head injury, meningitis, bronchiolitis, malignancy and drugs Polydipsia (e.g., psychogenic) Renal failure Cardiac failure
Sodium depletion	Iatrogenic (e.g., diuretics) Diarrhoea Fistulas Burns Cystic fibrosis (sweating) Adrenal insufficiency Diabetic ketoacidosis (DKA)[a]

[a]Sodium levels in DKA are falsely low due to excessive glucose in the extracellular fluid causing fluid shifts. An equation exists for 'Corrected Na': Na$^+$ 0.4 ([glucose] – 5.5).

Table 21.9 Causes of hypernatraemia (Na$^+$ >145 mmol/L)

Mechanism	Cause
Water deficit	Diarrhoea Reduced intake (e.g., poor feeding in neonate) Diabetes insipidus Increased insensible losses (e.g., overhead heater, fever, tachypnoea)
Sodium excess	Iatrogenic (e.g., excess hypertonic fluids) Salt poisoning (nonaccidental injury)

Sodium

Changes in the plasma sodium concentration can reflect changes in either the sodium or water balance. When interpreting a serum sodium result it is also important to assess the child's hydration status. Causes of sodium imbalance are shown in Tables 21.8 and 21.9.

Management is dependent on the cause. For example:

- Syndrome of inappropriate antidiuretic hormone (SIADH) secretion is treated with fluid restriction.
- Severe and symptomatic hyponatraemia is treated with oral or IV supplementation.
- Hypernatraemia relating to dehydration is treated with optimizing hydration through either enteral, parenteral or IV routes.

Potassium

This is a predominantly intracellular cation. Plasma concentration is therefore influenced by exchange with the intracellular compartment as well as the whole-body potassium status. The

Table 21.10 Causes of hypokalaemia (K$^+$ <3.4 mmol/L)

Mechanism	Cause
Potassium depletion	Diarrhoea Vomiting (e.g., pyloric stenosis) Iatrogenic (e.g., diuretics, insulin, β_2 agonists) Renal tubular acidosis
Inadequate intake	Anorexia Inadequate total parenteral nutrition constitution
Other	Metabolic alkalosis DKA[a]

[a]Total body potassium is always low in DKA despite plasma levels being low, normal or even high. It will fall further with insulin therapy.

Table 21.11 Causes of hyperkalaemia (K$^+$ >5.5 mmol/L)

Mechanism	Cause
Potassium excess	Iatrogenic (intravenous or oral supplements)
Inadequate excretion	Renal failure Adrenocortical insufficiency
Other	Metabolic acidosis DKA[a] Hypoxia Tumour lysis syndrome Artefact (e.g., haemolyzed sample)

[a]Total body potassium is always low in DKA despite plasma levels being low, normal or even high. It will fall further with insulin therapy.

causes of changes in plasma potassium are shown in Tables 21.10 and 21.11.

True hyperkalaemia is a medical emergency. Immediate management involves:

- Electrocardiogram monitoring.
- Calcium gluconate to stabilize myocardium: this does not remove potassium.
- Promotion of cellular potassium uptake by nebulized or IV salbutamol. An alternative is IV insulin and glucose (dextrose).
- Ion-exchange resins (e.g., oral or per rectum (PR) calcium resonium).
- Dialysis or haemofiltration if the above measures fail.

PAEDIATRIC PHARMACOLOGY AND PRESCRIBING

Great variability exists between children and adults in the pharmacology of drugs; differences also exist between the preterm neonate, neonate and older children. It is therefore important that clinicians recognize that much of the information that applies to adults is not always applicable to children, and must be

Table 21.12 Bodyweight and body surface area (BSA)

Age	Weight (kg)	BSA (m²)
Newborn	3.5	0.25
6 months	7.7	0.40
1 year	10	0.50
5 years	18	0.75
12 years	36	1.25
Adult	70	1.80

cautious in extrapolating adult data into paediatric practice. Most paediatric doses are calculated based on the child's weight or body surface area (Table 21.12).

HINTS AND TIPS

Water-soluble drugs (e.g., most antibiotics) require a larger initial dose in neonates because they have the greatest amount of total body water. The large volume also means delayed excretion, so doses are less frequent.

Many drugs currently used in paediatric practice remain unlicensed. Thus, pharmacokinetic and pharmacodynamic data are rarely available. A paediatric version of the British National Formulary (BNFc) is available.

Absorption and administration

The oral route is most commonly used for administering medication because it is easy, safe and cheap. Its limitations are that many children find certain drugs unpalatable and tablets need to be crushed.

The IV route is reliable and effective but requires venepuncture. The PR route is useful in emergencies, and diazepam and paracetamol can be given this way. Intramuscular injections are rarely used except for immunizations.

In neonates and infants, gastric absorption is altered as normal gastric acid secretion is reduced until 3 years of age; gastric motility is also delayed.

Metabolism and excretion

Hepatic metabolism differs from that in adults in that it is slow at birth but increases rapidly with age; the metabolic processes also differ. For example, paracetamol is metabolised by sulphation, whereas adults use the glucuronidation pathway- in children under 6 paracetamol toxicity is unlikely if less than 150 mg/kg is ingested; in adults or older children this number if lower- 75 mg/kg.

The renal handling of drugs also differs because the glomerular filtration rate in children does not approach adult levels until 9 to 12 months age.

● Chapter Summary

- Breastfeeding has many health advantages including protective health properties for the infant and promotes bonding.
- Malnutrition is often associated with starvation and poverty. Causes other than famine include malabsorption syndromes and disease associated with increased energy requirements such as malignancy.
- There is a calculation for normal maintenance fluids in children. Fluid is calculated differently in diabetic ketoacidosis, burns and dehydration.
- Absorption, metabolism and excretion are different in children compared to adults. Most paediatric prescribing is based on weight.

UKMLA Conditions
Malnutrition
Obesity

UKMLA Presentations
Difficulty with breast feeding
Infant feeding problems

SELF-ASSESSMENT

UKMLA High Yield Association Table

Key findings	Diagnoses
Hypochloraemic, hypokalaemic, metabolic alkalosis, projectile vomiting	Pyloric stenosis
Stridor, drooling	Epiglottitis
Distended abdomen, mass in flank does not cross midline	Nephroblastoma/Wilms
Overlapping fingers	Edward's
Newborn, continuous machine-like murmur	PDA (patent ductus arteriosus)
Newborn, harsh pansystolic murmur, radiating all over but loudest at LLSE	VSD (ventricular septal defect)
Newborn, ejection systolic, wide fixed and split 2nd HS, loudest pulmonary area	ASD (atrial septal defect)
Drawing legs up, mass in RUQ, redcurrant jelly stools	Intussusception
Boot shaped heart	ToF (tetralogy of Fallot)
Absent femoral pulses	Coarctation of the aorta
Golden/yellow crusted lesion	Impetigo
Port wine stain and new onset seizures	Sturge Weber
Skin lesion on shoulder/upper arm, i.e., Herald patch	Pityriasis rosea
21-Hydroxylase deficiency, hence, raised 17-hydroxy progesterone	Congenital adrenal hyperplasia
Teen, changed behaviour, liver change	Wilson disease
Reed Sternberg cells	Hodgkin lymphoma
Auer rods	Acute myeloid leukaemia (AML)
Heinz bodies	G6PD deficiency
Worsening school performance, abdominal pain, basophilic stippling	Lead poisoning
Young boy, difficulty standing (Gower sign), calf hypertrophy	Muscular dystrophy
Symmetrical, ascending paralysis post infection	Guillain-Barré
Tired with repetitive movement	Myasthenia gravis
Sudden severe headache, known polycystic kidney disease	Subarachnoid haemorrhage
Child, generalized pink rash, swollen knees	Systemic juvenile idiopathic arthritis (JIA)/Still's
Overweight boy, pain in hip	SUFE (slipped upper femoral epiphysis)
Young, knee pain, periosteal elevation, calcification	Osteosarcoma
Young boy, hip pain, gradual onset, X-ray = collapsed femoral head	Perthe disease
Failure to pass meconium <48 hours of birth and subsequent constipation	Hirschsprung disease
Bilious vomits in neonate	Malrotation volvulus
Day 2 neonates, collapse, cyanosis not improved with oxygen	Transposition of the great arteries (TGA)
Painless PR bleeding	Meckel diverticulum
Failure to thrive, greasy stools, cough	Cystic fibrosis
Barking cough	Croup
Testicular pain, absent cremasteric reflex	Testicular torsion

Continued

Key findings	Diagnoses
Testicular pain, blue dot sign	Torsion of testicular appendage
Scrotal mass, can get above it, transilluminates	Hydrocele
Non-blanching rash +/- fever	Meningococcal sepsis
Hot swollen joint	Septic arthritis
Rash on flexor surfaces	Atopic dermatitis (eczema)
Fever in patient receiving chemotherapy	Neutropenic sepsis
Fever for ≥5 days with no focus	Kawasaki disease
Child <1 year with fits and developmental regression and hypsarrhythmia on EEG	West syndrome
Child with unilateral weakness of face including forehead	Erb palsy
Pain in knees, dysuria and red eye	Reactive arthritis
Child with impaired speech development and restrictive or repetitive behaviours or interests	Autistic spectrum disorder
Child presenting with abdominal pain, vomiting, and a blood sugar >11	Diabetic ketoacidosis
High fever followed by a rash days later	Roseola infantum

UKMLA Single Best Answer (SBA) Questions

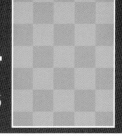

Chapter 3 Cardiovascular system

1. A paediatrician is called to urgently review a 2-day-old baby on the postnatal ward. On arrival, the baby is profoundly cyanotic and saturations do not improve with high-flow oxygen therapy. Examination reveals a single loud second heart sound but no murmur. Intravenous access is secured and the blood gas shows severe metabolic acidosis. A chest X-ray performed shows increased pulmonary vasculature and 'egg-on-side' appearance of the heart. What is the most likely diagnosis?
   A Atrial septal defect
   B Transposition of the great arteries
   C Patent ductus arteriosus
   D Tetralogy of Fallot
   E Ventricular septal defect

2. A 4-year-old girl has been admitted to the ward with 2 days of fever and cough. A diagnosis of a lower respiratory chest infection has been made and intravenous antibiotics have been commenced. The following morning on the ward round, the medical team note that she has a soft ejection systolic murmur with normal heart sounds and no radiation. She appears clinically well in herself. What would be the single most appropriate management plan?
   A Arrange a chest X-ray
   B Discuss with the local paediatric cardiology centre for advice
   C Once medically fit for discharge, arrange an outpatient ECHO
   D Explain that this is an innocent murmur and inform the general practitioner (GP) to reevaluate the child once she has recovered from illness
   E Change the present antibiotic regime

3. A paediatrician is asked to review a heart murmur of a 2-day-old baby born by vaginal delivery following an uneventful pregnancy to a primiparous mother, aged 38 years. The perinatal period was normal and baby has been feeding well. On examination, he is hypotonic, has single palmar creases and epicanthic folds. What is the most likely heart lesion?
   A Atrioventricular septal defect
   B Atrial septal defect
   C Aortic stenosis
   D Coarctation of the aorta
   E Patent ductus arteriosus

4. A mother on the postnatal ward has called for help as her 2-day-old baby appears blue. On arrival, the baby is deeply cyanosed with cool peripheries and saturations do not improve despite maximum oxygen therapy. Femoral pulses are palpable and a single, loud second heart sound can be heard but no murmur. The baby is brought to the neonatal unit for further care. What is the next most important intervention?
   A Intravenous (IV) furosemide
   B IV antibiotics
   C IV bolus of normal saline
   D IV bolus of dextrose
   E IV infusion of prostaglandin E

5. A 3-year-old girl with complex congenital heart disease is admitted with fever. On examination, her temperature is 39.5°C and there is a loud ejection systolic murmur. Her C-reactive protein is 250 mg/L and a transthoracic echocardiogram confirms vegetations. What is the most likely causative pathogen?
   A Streptococcal pneumonia
   B *Streptococcus pyogenes*
   C *Streptococcus viridans*
   D Group A haemolytic streptococcus
   E Group B haemolytic streptococcus

6. A 36-hour-old baby is due to have his newborn check prior to discharge. The paediatrician notes that the antenatal serology is missing because the pregnancy was unbooked. The baby is symmetrically growth restricted, red reflexes are bilaterally absent and a heart murmur is noted. Femoral pulses can be palpated, the baby is pink and otherwise well. What is an echocardiogram most likely to show?
   A Ventricular septal defect
   B Coarctation of the aorta
   C Atrial septal defect
   D Tetralogy of Fallot
   E Patent ductus arteriosus

7. It can be possible to differentiate an innocent murmur from a pathological murmur by its character and associated features. Which of the following suggests a pathological murmur?
   A No radiation
   B Varies with posture

C Systolic

D Third heart sound

E No symptoms

8. A 3-day-old male infant is noted to have a cardiac murmur. Four-limb blood pressures are normal but the oxygen saturation is 78% and does not improve with oxygen therapy. Which of the following congenital heart defects is the most likely diagnosis?

A Patent ductus arteriosus

B Tetralogy of Fallot

C Ventricular septal defect

D Atrial septal defect

E Coarctation of the aorta

9. A 3-year-old boy is brought into accident and emergency crying and distressed. He has a heart rate of 225 beats/min but his blood pressure is within normal limits and oxygen saturations are 99% in air. His electrocardiogram shows a regular, narrow complex tachycardia with P waves not easily visible. What would your initial management plan be?

A Direct current (DC) cardioversion at 4 J/kg

B Trial of β-blocker

C 20 mL/kg bolus of normal saline

D Intravenous (IV) adenosine

E IV antibiotics

10. A 6-year-old boy is on the ward with polyarthritis and fever. On the ward round today, he was noted to have a pericardial rub on auscultation. His blood tests show a C-reactive protein (CRP) of 110 mg/L and erythrocyte sedimentation rate of 99 mm/hr. Which of the following statements is true regarding the Jones criteria for diagnosing rheumatic fever?

A Arthralgia is a major criterion

B History suggestive of a throat infection is sufficient

C A raised antistreptolysin O titre, pericarditis and a CRP of 110 mg/L are diagnostic

D A raised antistreptolysin O titre, pericarditis and polyarthritis are diagnostic

E Chorea is a common presenting feature

Chapter 4 Respiratory system

1. An 18-month-old girl presents with a sudden onset of cough associated with difficulty in breathing. Her mother says she was playing alone in the playroom when it started. On examination, she has a heart rate of 160 beats/min, respiratory rate of 50 breaths/min and saturations of 92% in air. She has respiratory distress and a high-pitched inspiratory noise. What would be the most important investigation to guide your management?

A A full family history, asking about atopy

B A sputum sample for bacteria microscopy, culture and sensitivity testing

C A nasopharyngeal aspirate for respiratory syncytial virus immunofluorescence

D An urgent chest X-ray

E A V/Q scan

2. A 5-year-old boy is brought in by his father who reports that his teachers have said he does not pay attention in class and that his speech has not been developing as fast as his older brother. He is able to run and play football, can do jigsaw puzzles and likes colouring in. He is very loving towards his parents and plays well with his brother. He is otherwise well in himself and is growing well along the 50th centile. Which of the following would be an appropriate next step in management?

A Assess for attention deficit hyperactivity disorder

B Refer to a community paediatrician for a full developmental assessment

C Refer for pure-tone audiometry testing

D Assess for an autistic spectrum disorder

E Take a full set of screening blood tests

3. A 3-year-old girl is admitted with a 3-day history of coryzal symptoms followed by an acute history of breathing difficulty. She is previously fit and the parents are nonsmokers. She is thriving and on examination she has widespread wheeze with no crepitations. What is the most likely diagnosis?

A Viral wheeze

B Asthma

C Heart failure

D Bronchiolitis

E Recurrent aspiration

4. A 6-year-old boy with known asthma has been brought in by ambulance to the local emergency department with an acute severe exacerbation. He has already received salbutamol and ipratropium nebulizers together with intravenous (IV) steroid. Upon reassessment, he appears exhausted with varying responsiveness. Oxygen (15 L) is needed to maintain his saturations and auscultation of his chest reveals reduced air entry bilaterally. What is the next most important step in this child's care?

A Reassess 30 minutes later

B Give IV antibiotics

C Start noninvasive ventilation

D Give IV magnesium sulphate

E Admit to the high-dependency unit

5. A 5-year-old boy is under outpatient review for asthma. His chest X-ray shows hyperexpansion but his symptoms remain unresponsive despite stepwise increase in asthma therapy. Further questioning reveals delayed passage of meconium at birth and finger clubbing is evident on examination. What is the most appropriate next step in the management of this child?
    A Arrange a computed tomography chest scan
    B Organize a sweat test
    C Test lung function using spirometry
    D Take a per-nasal swab
    E Send sputum cultures

6. A 2-year-old boy is brought into the emergency department by ambulance at night with an acute history of cough and stridor following a 2-day history of coryzal symptoms. On examination, he is afebrile but has marked intercostal recession with stridor and a 'barking cough' is heard. What is the most likely causative organism?
    A Adenovirus
    B Respiratory syncytial virus (RSV)
    C Parainfluenza virus
    D Rhinovirus
    E Influenza virus

7. A previously well 5-year-old boy is brought in by ambulance to the emergency department with an acute onset of breathing difficulty. On arrival, he appears unwell, pale with audible stridor and is sitting upright unable to speak. His temperature is 40°C. What is the first priority in this child's management?
    A Lie the child down
    B Take a throat swab
    C Obtain intravenous access
    D Give oral dexamethasone
    E Summon immediate anaesthetic help

8. A 3-month-old female infant presents with a 2-day history of coryzal symptoms and increased work of breathing. Her mother reports that she had two wet nappies over the last 24 hours and is taking half of her bottle feeds. Her heart rate is 150 beats/min, and she has a respiratory rate of 60 breaths/min with saturations of 96% in air. On examination she is alert, well perfused and with slight recession. Clinical findings are consistent with bronchiolitis. What is the most appropriate management?
    A Admit and give supplemental oxygen
    B Admit and start continuous positive airway pressure
    C Admit and give nasogastric feeds
    D Admit for regular nebulizers
    E Admit for intravenous antibiotics

9. A 4-year-old girl is under outpatient review for asthma. Her regular treatment consists of a preventative steroid inhaler (200 µg BD) and a reliever inhaler when required (about fortnightly). However, over the last 3 months she has had to use her reliever inhaler every other day. Her nocturnal coughing has increased resulting in disturbed sleep. What is the appropriate next step in care for this child?
    A Continue on the same dose of steroid inhaler
    B Increase the steroid inhaler dose to 400 µg BD
    C Start a course of oral steroids
    D Start oral theophylline
    E Add a long-acting β agonist

10. A 4-year-old girl is admitted with fever, difficulty breathing and cough. A diagnosis of left lower lobe pneumonia is made and intravenous antibiotics are commenced. What is the most likely pathogen?
    A *Streptococcus pneumoniae*
    B *Haemophilus influenza*
    C *Mycoplasma pneumoniae*
    D *Chlamydia trachomatis*
    E *Escherichia coli*

11. A 6-month-old female infant with respiratory syncytial virus-positive bronchiolitis is requiring 1 L of nasal prong humidified oxygen and nasogastric feeding. Over the last 8 hours her work of breathing has increased and is showing signs of recession. Her oxygen requirement has also increased to 2 L and she appears tired. A blood gas is performed, which shows a pH of 7.30 and partial pressure of carbon dioxide (pCO_2) of 7.8 kPa. What is the most appropriate next step in management?
    A Salbutamol nebulizer
    B Intravenous antibiotics
    C High-flow oxygen therapy
    D Intubate and ventilate
    E Steroids

12. A 10-year-old boy is admitted with left lower lobe pneumonia. On day 3 of admission, he develops gradually increased work of breathing and a fever of 40°C. On assessment, he has a respiratory rate of 40 breaths/min, and auscultation reveals a clear right lung field but reduced breath sounds throughout his left lung. The percussion note is 'stony dull' and chest expansion is reduced on his left side. What is the most likely diagnosis?
    A Empyema
    B Lobar collapse
    C Lung abscess
    D Pneumothorax
    E Cor pulmonale

Chapter 5 Gastrointestinal and hepatobiliary systems

1. A 5-week-old baby boy is brought into the emergency department with a 48-hour history of projectile vomiting. The infant is hungry after vomiting and has not opened his bowels in 3 days. Clinical examination reveals a mass in the left upper quadrant region. A blood gas is performed – what would you expect it to show?
   A pH 7.40, pCO_2 5.0 kPa and bicarbonate 26 mmol/L
   B pH 7.25, pCO_2 4.0 kPa and bicarbonate 12 mmol/L
   C pH 7.50, pCO_2 5.5 kPa and bicarbonate 30 mmol/L
   D pH 7.25, pCO_2 8.0 kPa and bicarbonate 24 mmol/L
   E pH 7.50, pCO_2 2.5 kPa and bicarbonate 22 mmol/L

2. An 11-year-old girl presents following 6 days of fever, abdominal pain and bloody diarrhoea. She has become increasingly irritable and lethargic. Blood tests reveal: haemoglobin 75 g/L, white cell count 15×10^9/L, platelets 40×10^9/L, urea 9.0 mmol/L, creatinine 200 µmol/L, blood film shows red blood cell fragments. The most likely diagnosis is which of the following?
   A Ulcerative colitis
   B Haemolytic-uraemic syndrome
   C Viral gastroenteritis
   D Glucose-6-phosphate dehydrogenase deficiency
   E Crohn disease

3. A 15-year-old girl attends her general practitioner with lethargy and irregular menstruation. She has previously had regular periods and has developed secondary sexual characteristics. She has also been experiencing intermittent palpitations. On examination, she has a body mass index (BMI) of 20 kg/m^2 and has firm parotid swelling bilaterally. Blood tests are arranged which show: sodium 134 mmol/L, potassium 3.0 mmol/L, chloride 90 mmol/L. What is the most likely diagnosis?
   A Mumps
   B Polycystic ovarian syndrome
   C Anorexia nervosa
   D Bulimia nervosa
   E Hypothyroidism

4. A 3-month-old infant is brought to the general practitioner by his mother. She is concerned that he has been constipated since birth and only opens his bowels every 4 days. She remembers that after birth, he did not open his bowels for 3 days. His abdomen has become distended and he vomits after feeds. Which of the following investigations would confirm the diagnosis?
   A Thyroid function tests
   B Barium enema
   C Abdominal ultrasound scan
   D Abdominal X-ray
   E Suction biopsy of the rectum

5. A 9-year-old presents with a 6-month history of nonbloody diarrhoea associated with 4 kg of weight loss. His mother says he is less energetic than before and looks paler than normal. There is no history of foreign travel. Blood tests show a microcytic anaemia (haemoglobin 85 g/L, mean corpuscular volume 72) but normal inflammatory markers. What is the best treatment for this condition?
   A A course of high-dose oral steroids
   B A short course of oral antibiotics
   C Excluding gluten from the diet
   D Excluding cow's milk from the diet
   E Total colectomy with stoma

6. A 13-year-old boy with a 3-month history of bloody diarrhoea, abdominal pain and 4-kg weight loss undergoes an endoscopy and colonoscopy. The results show patchy inflammation affecting the ileum and colon. What is the most likely diagnosis?
   A Crohn disease
   B Coeliac disease
   C Ulcerative colitis
   D Infective colitis
   E Cow's milk protein allergy

7. A 7-month-old infant presents with a 12-hour history of intermittent inconsolable crying, has vomited several times and has had an episode of loose stool with blood and mucus. On examination, he has cool peripheries and there is a palpable mass in the right upper quadrant of the abdomen. What is the most useful investigation?
   A pH study
   B Endoscopy
   C Stool culture
   D Abdominal ultrasound scan
   E Exploratory laparoscopy

8. An 8-year-old girl presents with a 2-month history of pain most days around the umbilicus which lasts for an hour and responds to paracetamol syrup. It does not occur at weekends usually. She opens her bowels daily and passes a soft stool. On examination, there are no abnormal findings. She is growing well with her weight and height on the 50th centile. Which of the following options is the appropriate next step?
   A Abdominal ultrasound scan
   B Routine referral to a paediatric gastroenterologist
   C Inflammatory markers and liver function tests

D Reassurance and encouragement to continue normal activities

E Stool culture

9. A 15-year-old boy attends accident and emergency with a 2-day history of bloody diarrhoea associated with abdominal cramps and lethargy. He has a fever of 39°C. His parents have similar symptoms, and they all ate at the same takeaway chicken shop 3 days before. He has not travelled abroad recently. Which organism is most likely responsible for his symptoms?

A Rotavirus

B *Shigella*

C *Escherichia coli*

D Norovirus

E *Campylobacter*

10. A 9-year-old boy attends hospital with a 24-hour history of abdominal pain. He has not eaten and is finding it difficult to stand up. On palpation of the abdomen, there is tenderness and he is not distractible. What is the next step in management?

A Referral to surgical team

B Computed tomography of the abdomen

C Intravenous antibiotics

D Abdominal ultrasound scan

E Admit for monitoring

11. A 4-week-old formula-fed girl presents with jaundice. Her mother reports that her urine looks dark and her stools are pale. She has failed to regain her birthweight. Her total bilirubin is 135 μmol/L (normal <100 μmol/L) with a conjugated fraction of 65 μmol/L (normal <20 μmol/L). Her full blood count and reticulocytes are normal. What is the most likely diagnosis?

A Physiological jaundice

B Biliary atresia

C Spherocytosis

D Glucose-6-phosphate deficiency

E Urinary tract infection

12. A 3-year-old girl of Irish parents presents with a history of diarrhoea since birth. The stool is pale and offensive smelling. She was born on the 25th centile but is now on the 0.4th centile for weight and height. She has been admitted on four occasions with pneumonia and has a chronic cough. Which investigation is most likely to yield her diagnosis?

A Coeliac antibodies

B Sweat test

C Stool reducing substances

D Stool culture

E Endoscopy and colonoscopy

13. A 4-year-old boy attends accident and emergency with a history of 3 days of nonbilious vomiting and diarrhoea; today he has had two vomits with streaks of blood in them. He has a low-grade fever but is well hydrated and tolerates a fluid challenge. What is the most likely diagnosis?

A Gastro-oesophageal reflux

B Oesophagitis

C Peptic ulcer disease

D Gastritis

E Mallory-Weiss tear

14. A 15-year-old girl attends clinic concerned about her episodic abdominal pain and loose stool over the last year. She describes crampy abdominal pain followed by the need to pass a stool which happens about twice a month. Her bowel habit is normal on the other days. There has never been any blood, and she has not lost any weight. She dates it back to when she changed schools the previous September, and symptoms usually occur on weekdays. Which of the following is most likely to be the underlying cause of her symptoms?

A Coeliac disease

B Ulcerative colitis

C Irritable bowel syndrome

D Overflow diarrhoea secondary to constipation

E Dysmenorrhoea

Chapter 6 Renal and genitourinary conditions

1. A 9-year-old girl is brought to her general practitioner with a several-day history of dark-coloured urine. She says her urine 'looks like Coca-Cola'. She has never experienced anything like this before. On examination, she is hypertensive, there is no fever and her abdomen is soft and nontender. A urine dipstick is positive for blood with a trace of protein. Blood tests show a normal full blood count, impaired renal function and normal electrolytes. What is the most likely additional symptom/sign she reports in the history?

A Puffy swelling of the arms, legs and around her eyes

B Blood-stained loose stools

C A recent sore throat with exudate on the tonsils

D A purple rash and joint pain

E Burning sensation on passing urine

2. An 11-year-old girl presents following 6 days of fever, abdominal pain and bloody diarrhoea. She has become increasingly irritable and lethargic. Blood tests reveal: Hb 7.5 g/dL, whole cell count 15×10^9/L, platelets 40×10^9/L, urea 9.0 mmol/L, creatinine 200 μmol/L and blood film shows red blood cell fragments. What is the most appropriate initial management?

A Rapid intravenous (IV) broad-spectrum antibiotics and IV fluid resuscitation

B   Oral penicillin and oral rehydration solution

C   Supportive treatment with IV fluids in a high-dependency setting

D   High-dose oral steroids with a reducing regimen

E   Urgent renal transplantation

3. A 4-month-old baby boy is brought to see the general practitioner due to swelling in the scrotum. His parents say he was born at term by a normal vaginal delivery and has been well since birth. He has not been distressed, has had no fever or vomiting. He is feeding well and growing along the 25th centile. On examination, the baby is well with a small, soft, painless swelling which you can get above and cannot be reduced. The swelling transilluminates with a pen torch. His parents are concerned that he will need an operation. What is the most appropriate management step?

    A   Urgent referral to a paediatric surgeon

    B   Reassure parents that no treatment is required at this point

    C   Ultrasound scan of the lump

    D   Fine-needle aspiration of the lump

    E   Referral to a paediatric surgeon if the lump is still present at 6 months of age

4. A 2-year-old girl is referred to paediatric outpatients after experiencing multiple complicated urinary tract infections. The last one occurred a month ago and she was very unwell with a high fever, rigors and vomiting. She required hospital admission and intravenous antibiotics and was discharged home with oral antibiotics. A recent blood test reveals that her renal function is reduced. The paediatrician is concerned that she may have developed renal scarring. What is the best first-line investigation to assess for this?

    A   Micturating cystourethrogram (MCUG)

    B   Magnetic resonance imaging (MRI) of the urinary tract

    C   Computed tomography (CT) of the kidneys, ureter and bladder

    D   Static radioisotope scan (dimercaptosuccinic acid (DMSA)]

    E   Abdominal ultrasound scan

5. An 8-year-old boy is brought into his general practitioner by his parents. He has recently been complaining that he feels very thirsty and drinking a lot more than usual. He has also been passing urine much more frequently than he normally does. He has no medical history of note, and there is no relevant family history. On examination, he is apyrexial with normal blood pressure for his age and sex. He has moist mucous membranes and a soft abdomen with no palpable masses. What is the key initial investigation?

A   Send urine for microscopy, culture and sensitivity

B   Test blood glucose level

C   Test renal function

D   Ultrasound scan of the kidneys

E   Send urine for osmolarity

6. A 24-month-old girl is brought into the emergency department by her mother with fever. At triage, her temperature is 38.7°C, other vital signs all within normal limits, and she is given antipyretics pending medical review. She is reviewed by the doctor 90 minutes later, and her temperature is now 37.7°C. Clinical examination reveals a well-hydrated and clinically well child with good social interaction. There are no localizing features and no apparent source for her fever. What is the most appropriate next stage in her care?

    A   Request a chest X-ray (CXR)

    B   Take bloods for inflammatory markers

    C   Take a blood culture

    D   Request a urine dipstick

    E   Discharge the child home

7. On routine newborn examination, a baby is noted to have bilaterally undescended testes. Genitalia appear to be male. Which is the most important initial investigation?

    A   Karyotype with fluorescent in situ hybridization (FISH) for sex-determining region of the Y chromosome

    B   Abdominal ultrasound scan

    C   Abdominal computed tomography scan

    D   17-Hydroxyprogesterone levels

    E   Urea and electrolytes (U&Es)

8. A 12-year-old boy presents to accident and emergency with a history of groin pain for the past 4 hours. He is complaining of nausea and has vomited twice. On examination there is tenderness and swelling of the scrotum and right testicle, with absence of the cremasteric reflex on the side. There is no fever or erythema. Routine blood tests are normal. He describes several previous episodes of pain which were short lived. What is the most likely diagnosis?

    A   Testicular torsion

    B   Torsion of the hydatid of Morgagni

    C   Inguinal hernia

    D   Renal stone

    E   Epididymo-orchitis

9. A 3-month-old baby girl presents with a fever of 38.6°C, crying and with vomiting. A dipstick demonstrates white cells and protein in her urine. Which of the following organisms is most likely to be responsible for her urinary tract infection?

A *Enterococcus* spp.
B *Pseudomonas*
C *Proteus*
D *Escherichia coli*
E *Klebsiella*

10. Many conditions that require surgery can be deferred until the risk of anaesthetic has lessened with age. However, some require surgery in early infancy. Which of the following would require surgery within the first 6 months of life?
A Hydrocele
B Umbilical hernia
C Posterior urethral valves
D Inguinal hernia
E Single undescended testis

Chapter 7 Endocrine system and growth

1. A 7-day-old male baby is brought into the emergency department with a 1-day history of poor feeding and vomiting. He was born at term by spontaneous vaginal delivery weighing 3200 g, and his initial postnatal period was uneventful. On arrival, he appears lethargic and has moderate dehydration. His weight is 2750 g. His blood glucose is 2.0 mmol/L, and his blood gas reveals a sodium of 124 mmol/L and a potassium of 6.8 mmol/L. Following resuscitation and stabilization, what is most likely to confirm the diagnosis?
A Abdominal ultrasound scan
B Adrenocorticotrophic hormone level
C Karyotype
D 17-Hydroxyprogesterone level
E Chloride level

2. A 5-year-old boy is referred to a paediatric specialist by his general practitioner with tall stature. On examination, he has testicular enlargement and fundoscopy reveals bilateral papilloedema. What is most likely to confirm the diagnosis?
A Magnetic resonance imaging brain scan
B Karyotype
C Adrenocorticotrophic hormone level
D 17-Hydroxyprogesterone level
E Bone age

3. A 2-day-old baby is admitted to the neonatal unit with respiratory distress and jaundice. A full septic screen is performed which yields gram-negative rods on blood culture. Ophthalmological assessment confirms the presence of cataracts. What is the most likely diagnosis?

A Galactosaemia
B von Gierke disease
C Phenylketonuria
D Medium-chain acyl-coenzyme A dehydrogenase deficiency
E Maple syrup urine disease

4. A 14-year-old boy is admitted with diabetic ketoacidosis. Intravenous insulin has been running at 0.1 U/kg/h for the last 12 hours alongside a 500-mL bag of 0.9% normal saline. His last blood sugar is 22 mmol/L, and he has a good urine output. Which of the following are most likely to be decreased?
A Serum sodium
B Serum potassium
C Serum lactate
D Serum chloride
E Serum calcium

5. An 11-year-old girl presents to the emergency department with a 4-day history of cough and fever. A working diagnosis of right middle lobe pneumonia is made, and she is commenced on intravenous antibiotics and admitted to the ward. Her blood tests reveal a plasma sodium of 127 mmol/L with normal renal function. Further investigations reveal a low plasma osmolality and a raised urinary sodium level. What is the most likely diagnosis?
A Syndrome of inappropriate secretion of antidiuretic hormone (SIADH)
B Cushing syndrome
C Diabetes insipidus
D Secondary adrenal insufficiency
E Adrenal hyperplasia

6. A 13-year-old boy attends his general practitioner as he is concerned that he is developing breast tissue. On examination he is tall with clear gynaecomastia. There is sparse pubic hair and small testes. He has been struggling with his schoolwork and is behind his peers. What is the likely diagnosis?
A Marfan syndrome
B Klinefelter syndrome
C Congenital tall stature
D Hyperthyroidism
E Growth hormone excess (gigantism)

7. A 5-year-old boy is referred by the school nurse as his weight and height are on the 99th centile at school entry weighing. He appears a healthy child with tall parents. He has no birthmarks, and his blood pressure is normal. Which of the following actions is appropriate?
A Thyroid function tests

B 9 a.m. Cortisol level
C Calculate mid-parental height
D Dietary assessment
E Genetic studies for Prader-Willi syndrome

8. Breastfeeding is the best for babies, and there are very few contraindications. Which of the following is an absolute contraindication to breastfeeding in the UK?
A Galactosaemia
B Phenylketonuria
C Neonatal jaundice
D Cleft palate
E ABO incompatibility

9. A 14-month-old baby girl is brought to the outpatient clinic as her parents are concerned about her size. She is on the second centile for weight and height and head circumference. She was born on the second centile. She is taking cow's milk and is fully weaned, her stool is normal and examination unremarkable. Her parents are concerned as they are both short and do not want her to be small when she is older. Which of the following is the most likely cause of her size?
A Constitutionally small
B Cow's milk protein enteropathy.
C Hypothyroidism
D Growth hormone deficiency
E Skeletal dysplasia

10. A 12-year-old girl is referred by her general practitioner to the paediatric endocrinology clinic for evaluation of delayed pubertal development. Following clinical assessment, constitutional delay of growth is diagnosed. What investigation is most likely to confirm this diagnosis?
A Magnetic resonance imaging brain
B Gonadotrophin hormone levels
C Growth hormone levels
D Bone age
E Karyotype

11. A newborn baby is noted to have coarse facies, a large fontanelle and hypotonia on routine examination. He also has jaundice. His blood sugar levels are normal. Which of the following investigations would be most likely to reveal the underlying diagnosis?
A Growth hormone
B Karyotype
C Thyroid function tests
D Blood group
E Creatine kinase (CK)

Chapter 8 Oncology

1. Brain tumours are the most common solid tumour of childhood, and presentation may be insidious leading to late diagnosis. Which of the following statements regarding brain tumours in childhood is true?
A They are usually supratentorial
B Signs of raised intracranial pressure are rare
C Astrocytomas carry poor prognosis
D Medulloblastoma is the most common type
E Metastasis is common

2. A 3-year-old boy is brought to his general practitioner with abdominal distension. He is otherwise well. There is no family history of note. On examination there is a large, smooth mass palpable in the left flank. There is no lymphadenopathy. Urinalysis shows 2+ blood; urinary catecholamines are not raised. What is the most likely diagnosis?
A Wilms tumour (nephroblastoma)
B Neuroblastoma
C Polycystic kidney disease
D Multicystic kidney disease
E Horseshoe kidney

3. A 2-year-old boy undergoes a computed tomography scan for abdominal mass. The scan demonstrates a large mass arising from the renal parenchyma. Following surgical resection, a histological diagnosis of nephroblastoma is made. Which of the following statements regarding nephroblastoma is true?
A It usually causes hypertension
B It is associated with Beckwith-Wiedemann syndrome
C A susceptibility gene is found on chromosome 22
D Metastasis at presentation is common
E Presentation is usually with abdominal pain and weight loss

4. A 2-month-old baby who was born at 36 weeks' gestation is brought to the general practitioner as a family photo shows a discrepancy in her eyes. On examination a red reflex is present in one eye only. She is otherwise healthy. Which of the following is the most likely diagnosis?
A Retinoblastoma
B Retinopathy of prematurity
C Congenital cataract
D CMV retinitis
E Glaucoma

5. A 15-year-old boy presents with a 6-week history of pain in his lower leg. On examination there is a painful swelling in

the proximal tibia. X-ray of the limb shows a sunburst appearance. What is the most likely diagnosis?

A Ewing sarcoma
B Rickets
C Osteosarcoma
D Osteomyelitis
E Chondrosarcoma

Chapter 9 Haematology

1. Haemoglobin production differs through foetal life and extrauterine life and the molecule itself changes with age. Which of the following statements regarding haemoglobin is correct?

A At birth, adult haemoglobin (HbA) is predominant
B Hb concentrations fall after birth until around 7 weeks
C Haematopoiesis mainly occurs in the liver and spleen at term
D The lifespan of a normal red blood cell is 10 days
E Foetal haemoglobin has a lower affinity for oxygen

2. An 11-month-old Caucasian boy attends his general practitioner as his mother has been struggling to wean him. He drinks cow's milk at regular intervals and eats some baby rice but refuses most other solids. On examination he appears very pale but otherwise well. There is no hepatosplenomegaly. A full blood count is arranged in view of the pallor which shows: haemoglobin (Hb) 7.8 g/dL, mean corpuscular volume 69 fL. What is the most likely cause of his anaemia?

A Sickle cell anaemia
B Thalassaemia
C Iron-deficiency anaemia
D Vitamin B12 deficiency
E Folate deficiency

3. A 4-year-old boy presents with pain in his abdomen and joints for the past 24 hours. He is afebrile. On examination he has diffuse abdominal tenderness but there are no masses, no lymphadenopathy and no hepatosplenomegaly. A widespread purpuric rash is present over the legs and buttocks. A urine dip shows 2+ blood. Routine bloods are normal. What is the most likely diagnosis?

A Idiopathic thrombocytopaenic purpura
B Meningococcal sepsis
C Acute lymphoblastic leukaemia (ALL)
D Vitamin C deficiency (scurvy)
E Henoch-Schönlein purpura (HSP)

4. A 3-year-old Afro-Caribbean girl presents with severe pain in her hands and abdomen. On examination there is mucosal pallor, yellow sclera and generalized abdominal tenderness with hepatosplenomegaly. Blood tests were taken including a full blood count: haemoglobin (Hb) 6.1 g/dL, mean corpuscular volume 78 fL, white cell count 6.0×10^9/L, platelets 300×10^9/L. What is the most likely cause of her anaemia?

A Thalassaemia
B Iron-deficiency anaemia
C Sickle cell disease
D Anaemia of chronic disease
E Glucose-6-phosphate dehydrogenase deficiency

5. An 8-month-old girl with Greek-Cypriot parents is brought to her general practitioner as her parents are worried that she is not growing well and is very pale. On examination there is pallor and mildly icteric sclera. She has a distended abdomen with hepatosplenomegaly, and there is mild frontal bossing. She was born on the 25th centile and her weight has fallen to below the 2nd centile. Blood tests show a microcytic hypochromic anaemia. What is the likely diagnosis?

A Sickle cell disease
B Hereditary spherocytosis
C β-Thalassaemia major
D Glucose-6-phosphate dehydrogenase deficiency
E Iron-deficiency anaemia

6. A 5-year-old boy attends accident and emergency with a nosebleed that his mother has been unable to stop for the past 45 minutes. He saw his general practitioner for a viral upper respiratory tract infection 1 week ago but is otherwise well. His nosebleed is stopped with pressure, but on examination, he is noted to have multiple petechiae on his chest, legs and abdomen. Blood tests reveal: haemoglobin (Hb) 10.4 g/dL, white cell count 13×10^9/L, platelet count 15×10^9/L, clotting screen normal. Which of the following is the most likely diagnosis?

A Henoch-Schönlein purpura
B Haemophilia B (Christmas disease)
C Immune (idiopathic) thrombocytopaenic purpura (ITP)
D Meningococcal septicaemia
E Haemolytic-uraemic syndrome

7. A 14-month-old boy is brought to accident and emergency by his mother with pain and swelling in his right knee. He is unable to weight bear, and on examination several large bruises are noted over the lower limbs and arms. He has blood tests, including a full blood count and clotting screen, which show: haemoglobin (Hb) 10.5 g/dL, white cell count 11×10^9/L, platelet count 340×10^9/L, prothrombin time 13.3 seconds, activated partial thromboplastin time >120 seconds. Which is the most likely diagnosis?

A   Vitamin K deficiency
B   Haemophilia A
C   von Willebrand disease
D   Immune (idiopathic) thrombocytopaenic purpura
E   Nonaccidental injury

8. A 7-year-old Ghanaian boy presented to accident and emergency, 3 days ago, on his return from holiday in West Africa, with high fever and rigors. A diagnosis of malaria was made, and he was started on primaquine. His mother is concerned that he has begun to look increasingly jaundiced. On examination there is deep jaundice, and he is looking pale and breathless. A full blood count and film are taken which show: haemoglobin (Hb) 5.5 g/dL, white cell count 15 × 10^9/L, platelet count 200 × 10^9/L, blood film shows red cell fragments and bite cells with Heinz bodies on staining. What is the most likely underlying diagnosis?
A   Glucose-6-phosphate dehydrogenase deficiency
B   Pyruvate kinase deficiency
C   Sickle cell disease
D   β-Thalassemia
E   Hereditary spherocytosis

9. A 4-year-old girl is undergoing chemotherapy for acute lymphoblastic leukaemia. She presents 8 days after her last treatment with a fever of 39°C. She has a portacath in situ. Her full blood count shows a white cell count 1.0 × 109/L, neutrophils 0.4 × 109/L, platelets 100 × 109/L, haemoglobin 10 g/dL. What is the most important step in her management?
A   Packed red blood cell transfusion
B   Platelet transfusion
C   Administration of G-CSF
D   Antipyretics
E   Intravenous antibiotics

10. A 14-year-old boy presents with a history of lethargy, constipation and shortness of breath on lying flat. On examination he has an enlarged, fixed lymph node in his left neck. He is investigated with blood tests and a CXR which demonstrate anaemia and a large mediastinal mass. A biopsy is taken from the mass in the neck which shows the presence of Reed-Sternberg cells. What is the likely diagnosis?
A   Tuberculosis
B   Non-Hodgkin lymphoma
C   Hodgkin lymphoma
D   Sarcoidosis
E   Epstein-Barr infection

Chapter 10   Fever, infectious diseases and immunodeficiency

1. A 14-month-old girl is brought into the emergency department with a 7-day history of fever and general malaise. On examination, she is very miserable, has bilateral conjunctivitis, cracked lips and bilateral cervical lymphadenopathy. A maculopapular rash is noted over her trunk. What is the most important investigation in this child's management?
A   Full blood count
B   Throat swab
C   Antistreptolysin O titre
D   Echocardiogram
E   Eye swab for microscopy, culture and sensitivities

2. A 9-year-old boy is brought into the emergency department by ambulance with an acute history of reduced consciousness. His mother described him complaining of headache and fever earlier in the day. On examination, he is pyrexial with a Glasgow Coma Scale score of 14/15 and is cardiovascularly stable. A few petechiae are noted on his legs. What is the single most effective immediate management for this child?
A   Arrange an urgent computed tomography brain scan and perform a lumbar puncture
B   Give a 20 mL/kg normal saline fluid bolus
C   Administer high-flow oxygen and call an anaesthetist for urgent intubation
D   Gain intravenous access, take blood cultures and administer broad-spectrum antibiotics
E   Administer vitamin K and refer to haematology

3. A 6-month-old female infant is admitted with a 3-day history of high fever >40°C with no focus. A full septic screen is performed which yields negative cultures and normal inflammatory markers. On day 4 of her illness, she develops a blanching morbilliform rash all over her body and her fever subsides. What is the most likely diagnosis?
A   Measles
B   Rubella
C   Roseola infantum
D   Scarlet fever
E   Chicken pox

4. A 4-month-old male infant has a history of failure to thrive, diarrhoea and has been admitted twice to hospital with pneumonia since birth. On examination, his abdomen is soft with no organomegaly or skin lesions to note. There is evidence of oral thrush. Lymphopaenia is noted on his full blood count. What is the most likely diagnosis?
A   Chronic granulomatous disease
B   Selective IgA deficiency

C Severe combined immunodeficiency (SCID)

D X-linked agammaglobulinaemia (Bruton disease)

E Human immunodeficiency virus infection

5. A 2-month-old male infant is brought into the emergency department by her father with fever. At triage, his temperature is 39.5°C but other vital signs are within normal limits. On examination, he has no respiratory distress, normal heart sounds, and good tone and activity. The infant is well perfused, and there are no localizing features to indicate a source for his fever. What is the most appropriate next step in this infant's management?

A A full septic screen followed by intravenous antibiotics

B A full blood count and C-reactive protein

C A clean catch urine sample

D Admission for observation

E Discharge with reassurance

6. A 10-year-old boy has a 2-week history of sore throat, fever and lethargy. Upon clinical examination there is pharyngitis, hepatosplenomegaly and bilateral shotty cervical lymph nodes are palpated. Blood tests reveal atypical lymphocytes and an alanine aminotransferase (ALT) of 190 U/L. What is the most likely causative pathogen?

A Coxsackievirus

B Hepatitis B

C Varicella zoster virus

D Epstein-Barr virus

E Cytomegalovirus

7. A 6-week-old female infant has been admitted with an acute febrile illness. A full septic screen is performed and intravenous antibiotics are commenced. The cerebrospinal fluid gram stain is reported as gram-positive cocci in chains. What is the most likely organism?

A *Neisseria meningitidis*

B *Haemophilus influenzae*

C Group B streptococcus

D *Staphylococcus aureus*

E *Listeria monocytogenes*

8. A 12-year-old boy returns from a holiday to Kenya with a febrile illness. It is associated with a headache and rigors. On examination he has hepatomegaly, is jaundiced and there are some lesions on his arms and legs that look like insect bites. Which of the following investigations is most likely to confirm the suspected diagnosis?

A Blood culture

B Full blood count

C Thick and thin blood films

D Hepatitis serology

E Liver function tests

Chapter 11 Allergy and anaphylaxis

1. An 8-year-old girl is brought to hospital following ingestion of a cereal bar containing peanuts. She is noted to have a widespread urticarial rash and swelling of the face and lips. She is finding it difficult to speak, and there is widespread wheeze on auscultation. The single most important step in her management is which of the following?

A Intramuscular 1 µg/kg adrenaline (epinephrine; 1:1000)

B Intravenous adrenaline (epinephrine), 1 µg/kg (1:10,000)

C Intramuscular 1 µg/kg adrenaline (epinephrine; 1:10,000)

D Oxygen

E Intravenous adrenaline (epinephrine), 1 µg/kg (1:1000)

2. A 1-year-old child is brought to the general practitioner by his mother. He has a history of severe egg allergy with previous confirmed anaphylactic reaction. Mum is concerned about him receiving his measles, mumps and rubella (MMR) vaccination as she has heard it contains egg. What is the most appropriate advice to give her?

A He can safely receive all vaccines

B He must not be given the MMR as it contains egg and he is at risk of severe allergic reaction

C He should avoid all live vaccines as they may precipitate a reaction

D He can safely receive the MMR, preferably in hospital, but should not receive the influenza or yellow fever vaccines

E He can be given the MMR but should receive antihistamine at the same time

3. A 4-year-old girl with a family history of atopy attends her general practitioner. Her older brother suffers from nut allergy and hay fever from grass and pollen. Her mother is very keen to have her tested before introducing her to nuts and requests skin-prick testing. Which of the following statements is true regarding skin-prick testing?

A The severity of an allergic reaction is accurately predicted by the size of skin-prick reaction

B It is suitable for identifying both immunoglobulin E (IgE)- and non-IgE-mediated allergy

C It is more accurate than blinded food challenge

D Positive (histamine) and negative (saline) controls should be injected, along with other allergens to confirm success of testing

E Tests for levels of specific IgE to allergens in the serum

4. A 6-month-old boy attends clinic with a history of bloody diarrhoea and failure to thrive. There is no vomiting and examination is normal. A diagnosis of cow's milk allergy is suspected. Which of the following statements regarding food allergy is true?

A It is commonly non-immunoglobulin E (IgE) mediated

B RAST will accurately identify all food allergies

C   A positive skin-prick test to soya means that the child is allergic

D   Elimination-reintroduction programme is unhelpful

E   It is rare for children to outgrow their allergies

5. A 5-year-old girl is being discharged after an admission for anaphylaxis. She is being referred to allergy clinic, is being discharged with an adrenaline autoinjector and her parents have been trained and they are being educated on signs of anaphylaxis to look out for. Which of the following is a red flag sign of life-threatening anaphylaxis?

A   A feeling of impending doom

B   A hoarse voice

C   A widespread urticarial rash

D   Abdominal pain and vomiting

E   Swelling around the eyes

Chapter 12   Dermatology

1. A previously healthy 7-year-old boy is brought in to see his general practitioner with a 3-day history of fever and coryzal symptoms. On assessment, the child is clinically well, and he has a rash composed of several distinctive erythematous lesions, both macular and papular and of differing sizes, distributed all over his body. The lesions have a central faded area. What is the most likely diagnosis?

A   Erythema nodosum

B   Erythema toxicum

C   Erythema marginatum

D   Erythema multiforme

E   Erythema chronicum migrans

2. A 3-month-old baby is seen in clinic with a severe nappy rash. The rash covers the perineal area including the skin folds and features satellite lesions. There is also a white coating to the baby's tongue. Otherwise, the baby is well and thriving. Which of the following is the most appropriate treatment?

A   Topical flucloxacillin preparation

B   1% Hydrocortisone ointment

C   Barrier cream (e.g., zinc and castor oil cream)

D   Antifungal preparation (e.g., miconazole)

E   Aim to keep the nappy off as much as possible

3. An 8-month-old develops an itchy rash which seems most distressing at night. His mother has started to develop similar symptoms. On examination the rash is affecting the whole body but worst on the soles of the feet, head and neck. The lesions are small fluid-filled vesicles and excoriations are visible. What is the most likely diagnosis?

A   Hand, foot and mouth disease

B   Scabies

C   Tinea capitis

D   *Molluscum contagiosum*

E   Impetigo

4. A 3-year-old boy has a crop of six small pedunculated lesions with a central punctum on his trunk. They are not itching and he is otherwise well and thriving. His older sister has similar lesions on her trunk. Which of the following is the most appropriate management?

A   Topical steroid therapy

B   Oral antibiotics

C   No treatment required

D   Investigation of immune function

E   Silver nitrate cautery of lesions

5. An 11-year-old girl presents to her general practitioner with a pink macular rash over her back and chest. It began 2 days ago with a scaly patch on her back. She is well in herself, but her mother is very concerned as she has never had a rash like this before. What is the best next step for the management of this child?

A   Refer to a paediatric dermatologist

B   Topical emollients with a soap substitute in the bath

C   Reassurance and discharge without treatment

D   Moderate-potency topical steroids

E   Antifungal treatment for the girl and her family

Chapter 13   Nervous system

1. A 6-week-old female infant has been admitted with an acute febrile illness. A full septic screen is performed and intravenous antibiotics are commenced. The cerebrospinal fluid Gram stain is reported as gram-positive cocci in chains. What is the most likely organism?

A   *Neisseria meningitidis*

B   *Haemophilus influenzae*

C   Group B streptococcus

D   *Staphylococcus aureus*

E   *Listeria monocytogenes*

2. A 14-month-old is seen in clinic as his mother is concerned that he may be having seizures. The episodes occur when he is angry or upset. He has colour change followed by collapse and occasional jerking movements. What is the most likely diagnosis?

A   Breath-holding spells

B   'Tet' spells

C   Myoclonic epilepsy

D   Nonepileptic seizure

E   Vasovagal syncope

3. A 6-year-old boy is falling behind at school. His mother is concerned he is inattentive. She describes him daydreaming frequently, during which time it is difficult to attract his attention. Routine blood tests are normal. An electroencephalogram (EEG) demonstrates spikes at 3 Hz. The likely diagnosis is which of the following?
   A Attention deficit hyperactivity disorder (ADHD)
   B Absence seizures
   C Juvenile myoclonic epilepsy
   D West syndrome
   E Nonepileptic seizures

4. A 5-month-old boy is brought in by his mother. She is concerned that he is frequently irritable. She is worried that he may be in pain as he tenses and describes him bending his head up and flailing his arms. An electroencephalogram (EEG) is performed which shows large-amplitude slow waves with spikes and sharp waves. What is the most likely diagnosis?
   A Absence seizures
   B Benign rolandic epilepsy
   C Gastro-oesophageal reflux
   D West syndrome (infantile spasms)
   E Breath-holding attacks

5. A 12-year-old girl with known epilepsy is brought in by ambulance. She has been fitting for 15 minutes. Her parents administered buccal midazolam after 5 minutes as part of her rescue regimen. On arrival, tonic-clonic movements are ongoing. The ambulance crew have inserted a cannula and are giving high-flow oxygen via facemask. What is the next step in management?
   A Intravenous lorazepam
   B Rectal diazepam
   C Rapid sequence induction
   D Loading dose phenytoin
   E Intravenous phenobarbital

6. A 12-year-old girl presents with a second generalized tonic-clonic seizure. She required lorazepam to terminate the seizure, and a decision is made to start antiepileptic treatment. Which of the following would be an appropriate first-line therapy?
   A Carbamazepine
   B Sodium valproate
   C Vigabatrin
   D Ethosuximide
   E Phenytoin

7. A 9-year-old girl is brought to her general practitioner with a 2-month history of headaches. Which of the following features of her headaches is a red flag symptom?
   A Unilateral pain
   B Eye watering
   C Morning headache
   D Associated with vomiting
   E Band-like in nature

8. A 2-year-old boy is referred to outpatients by his general practitioner as there is a family history of neurofibromatosis type 1 (NF1). Which of the following features would be diagnostic of this condition?
   A Presence of three café-au-lait spots
   B Acoustic neuroma
   C Ash-leaf macules
   D Lisch nodules
   E Adenoma sebaceum

9. Duchenne muscular dystrophy is the most common muscular dystrophy seen in children. Which of the following statements regarding Duchenne muscular dystrophy is true?
   A It is an autosomal dominant condition
   B The average age of onset is 14 years
   C Gower sign is an uncommon feature
   D Mutation is in the dystrophin gene
   E Calf pseudohypertrophy is rare

10. Cerebral palsy is a nonprogressive lesion of the central nervous system that can result in disordered movement and posture. Which of the following statements about cerebral palsy is correct?
   A Birth asphyxia is the most common cause
   B Infants with cerebral palsy are always hypertonic
   C Tendon reflexes are brisk
   D It is diagnosed based on magnetic resonance imaging (MRI) findings
   E Can occur past 1 year of age

Chapter 14 Musculoskeletal system

1. A 12-year-old Afro-Carribean girl has been referred by her general practitioner with a 2-month history of right-sided painful limp. There is no history of trauma, and she is previously fit and well. On examination, her weight is 65 Kg (98th-99.6th centile), she is pyrexial and there is painful restriction of external rotation of her right hip joint. She has normal inflammatory markers, and the X-ray is shown below. What is the likely diagnosis?

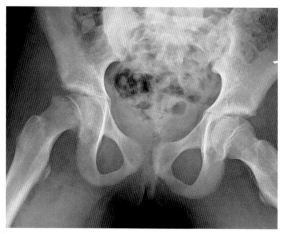

(Source: Churchill's Pocketbooks of Orthopaedics, Trauma and Rheumatology, Second Edition, 2017)

    A Transient synovitis
    B Osteomyelitis
    C Perthes disease
    D Juvenile idiopathic arthritis
    E Slipped upper femoral epiphysis (SUFE)

2. An 18-month-old female is presented to the emergency department with a 12-hour history of refusal to weight-bear on her left leg. There is no history of trauma and no other preceding symptoms. On examination, her temperature is 39.5°C, heart rate is 160 beats/min and she appears uncomfortable at rest. Her left knee is swollen, erythematous and held in flexion. What is most likely to confirm the diagnosis?
    A Left knee X-ray
    B Left hip X-ray
    C Left knee joint aspiration and fluid culture
    D Inflammatory markers
    E Blood culture

3. A 6-week-old baby girl, born by elective caesarean delivery for breech, is brought in to her general practitioner (GP) for routine check-up with her GP. Antenatal history reveals oligohydramnios during pregnancy. On inspection, the baby is noted to have bilateral talipes. For which condition is this baby at greatest risk?
    A Perthes disease
    B Scoliosis
    C Developmental dysplasia of the hip (DDH)
    D Torticollis
    E Arthrogryposis

4. A 7-year-old African-American boy with known sickle cell disease presents to the emergency department with a 3-day history of fever and an immobile left leg. On examination, he is pyrexial at 39.8°C, refusing to weight-bear on the left or for you to move his leg at all. You do not see any skin changes or deformity. What is the most likely diagnosis?
    A Perthes disease
    B Transient synovitis
    C Juvenile idiopathic arthritis
    D Slipped upper femoral epiphysis
    E Osteomyelitis

5. A 5-year-old girl is referred to a paediatrician by her general practitioner (GP). She has a 7-week history of intermittent left knee and elbow pain that has been becoming more frequent. More recently, she has also been complaining of pain in her right ankle. Her GP performed blood tests that revealed positive antinuclear antibodies. To which subspecialty should this child be referred as part of her management?
    A Paediatric cardiology
    B Paediatric ophthalmology
    C Paediatric respiratory
    D Paediatric gastroenterology
    E Paediatric nephrology

6. An 8-year-old boy attends the emergency department following a minor injury while playing football. An X-ray confirms a mid-shaft fracture of his tibia. His records show that he has sustained multiple fractures in the past and is under the paediatric ear, nose and throat team for conductive hearing loss. The emergency doctor thinks that his sclerae may have a blue tinge to them. What is the most likely diagnosis?
    A Osteogenesis imperfecta type I
    B Osteogenesis imperfecta type II
    C Osteogenesis imperfecta type III
    D Osteogenesis imperfecta type IV
    E Osteogenesis imperfecta type V

7. A 4-year-old boy is referred to the paediatricians by his general practitioner due to a purple rash over both his eyelids. On further examination he has red nodules on both elbows and a red rash over his metacarpal phalangeal joints. As he plays in the clinic room, you notice that he struggles to get up from sitting position and tires easily. What is the most likely diagnosis?
    A Childhood eczema
    B Juvenile dermatomyositis
    C Systemic lupus erythematous
    D Psoriasis
    E Juvenile idiopathic arthritis

8. You see a 5-year-old child with a limp. Which of the following features would rule out transient synovitis from your list of differential diagnosis?
   A Symptom duration 24 hours
   B Cough, cold and runny nose the week prior to onset
   C Fever of 39.2°C
   D Partially weight-bearing
   E C-reactive protein <2 mg/L

Chapter 15 The newborn

1. A baby is delivered by caesarean at 38 weeks following a prolonged and obstructed labour. He requires full resuscitation and his initial capillary blood gas shows a pH of 6.9 (normal range 7.35–7.45). At 10 minutes of age, his APGAR score was 5 and he is hypotonic. Which of the following management options is correct?
   A Encourage the baby to feed early
   B Keep warm in an incubator
   C Send the baby to the postnatal ward but review in 1 hour
   D Begin cooling therapy
   E Start continuous positive airway pressure (CPAP) and repeat a gas in 1 hour

2. A baby girl, born by elective caesarean section delivery for breech, is brought in to her general practitioner for her routine 6-week check. The history reveals oligohydramnios during pregnancy. On inspection the baby is noted to have bilateral talipes. For which condition is this baby at greatest risk?
   A Perthes disease
   B Scoliosis
   C Developmental dysplasia of the hip (DDH)
   D Torticollis
   E Arthrogryposis

3. A mother on the postnatal ward is concerned that her toddler has chicken pox. The rash developed 2 days ago, and she has not previously had chicken pox. Her baby boy is 1-day old and is well, with no rash. What is the most appropriate management of the baby?
   A Check maternal antibodies; if negative, give varicella immunoglobulin
   B Observe on postnatal ward for development of chicken pox
   C Discharge home, advise avoid contact with toddler until lesions crusted
   D No precautions necessary
   E Treat baby with acyclovir

4. A male infant born by normal delivery at 29 weeks is now 4 hours old. He has developed an oxygen requirement, there is tachypnoea and severe intercostal and subcostal recession. Chest X-ray (CXR) demonstrates ground glass appearance. The most likely diagnosis is which of the following?
   A Transient tachypnoea of the newborn
   B Respiratory distress syndrome (RDS)
   C Congenital pneumonia
   D Pneumothorax
   E Congenital heart disease

5. A female infant born at 28 weeks is now 10 days old. She had been doing very well and breast milk was started 2 days ago via nasogastric tube. She has become increasingly unwell over the past 12 hours with abdominal distension, temperature instability and bile-stained aspirates from the nasogastric tube. Some blood is noted in the stools. Abdominal X-ray shows air within the bowel walls. What is the most likely diagnosis?
   A Sepsis
   B Intestinal obstruction
   C Necrotizing enterocolitis
   D Malrotation
   E Duodenal atresia

6. A term female infant is seen on the postnatal ward. She is 18 hours old and has not been feeding well. Her mother was told she needed to have antibiotics prior to labour but delivered too quickly to receive them. She is admitted to the neonatal unit with suspected sepsis, and chest X-ray confirms congenital pneumonia. What is the most likely causative agent?
   A *Streptococcus pneumonia*
   B *Escherichia coli*
   C *Listeria monocytogenes*
   D Group B haemolytic streptococcus
   E *Chlamydia pneumoniae*

7. A term infant born by home delivery is brought to accident and emergency on day 4. His mother noticed a small amount of bleeding from the umbilical stump, which is still oozing some blood at present. His mother mentions that her other children received vitamin K in the hospital, but she cannot recall her newborn receiving this. Which of the following blood results is likely to be abnormal?
   A Platelets
   B Prothrombin time
   C Activated partial thromboplastin time
   D Haemoglobin
   E Antiplatelet antibodies

8. A 7-month-old infant presents with a 12-hour history of intermittent inconsolable crying; he is mottled, has cool peripheries and has vomited several times. Examination reveals a mass in the right upper quadrant of the abdomen. What is the most likely cause of his symptoms?
   A Colic
   B Incarcerated hernia
   C Gastroenteritis
   D Intussusception
   E Gastro-oesophageal reflux

9. A 6-day-old baby girl who is breastfeeding well and thriving is referred by the midwife because she appears jaundiced. She has pigmented stools and is passing urine normally. Examination is unremarkable. Her bilirubin is 68 µmol/L (normal <100 µmol/L) with a conjugated level of 8 µmol/L (normal <20 µmol/L). Which of the following would be your management plan for this infant?
   A Complete a prolonged jaundice screen
   B Commence phototherapy
   C Top-up feeds with formula milk
   D Repeat bilirubin level in 8 hours
   E No treatment required

10. A 6-week-old baby is referred by the health visitor as she has only just regained her birthweight. She is being fed with formula milk and her stools are normal. On examination she appears thin but otherwise normal. She is admitted to the ward and is fed by the nursing staff for a week as her mother is readmitted with an infection. She demonstrates excellent weight gain during this period. What is the most likely cause for her initial poor weight gain?
   A Cow's milk protein intolerance
   B Gastro-oesophageal reflux
   C Cystic fibrosis
   D Inadequate intake/neglect
   E Urinary tract infection

Chapter 16 Genetics

1. A 15-year-old girl is referred by her general practitioner to the paediatric endocrinology clinic for assessment of delayed puberty. On examination, her height plots on the 0.4th centile, she has an ejection systolic murmur. Her gonadotrophin levels are raised. What is the most likely diagnosis?
   A Turner syndrome
   B Klinefelter syndrome
   C McCune-Albright syndrome
   D Hypothyroidism
   E Silver-Russell syndrome

2. A pregnant mother is being counselled regarding screening for trisomies 13, 18 and 21, as she has previously had a baby with Edwards syndrome. She asks the consultant which test would best exclude these. Which of the following tests would be diagnostic?
   A Ultrasound scan
   B Pregnancy-associated plasma protein A levels (PAPP-A)
   C Amniocentesis
   D Foetal magnetic resonance imaging (MRI)
   E β-Human chorionic gonadotrophin level (β-HCG)

Chapter 17 Developmental assessment and developmental delay

1. A mother brings her 22-month-old girl to her general practitioner with concerns regarding development. She is able to sit unsupported and cruises around furniture. She can point to parts of her body, gives her name and puts words together. The mother reports that she takes off her shoes and uses a spoon. During the consultation, the girl is observed to build a tower of five cubes. What is the most appropriate next step in the care of this girl?
   A Reassure mother that her daughter's development is within normal limits
   B Arrange a review appointment in 4 weeks
   C Order a creatinine kinase (CK)
   D Refer to a general paediatrician for assessment
   E Refer to a community paediatrician for assessment

2. At a routine health visitor consultation, a 12-month-old boy is noticed to be cruising around furniture, responding to his name and says 'mama' and 'papa'. He is holding a crayon in his left hand with a pincer grip, and his father informs the health visitor that he only uses his left hand at home. Which of the statements is true regarding his development?
   A He is advanced in his gross motor skills
   B His speech is delayed
   C Left-hand dominance is common in under 5-year olds
   D He is displaying early hand preference
   E He should be using a tripod grasp

3. A 3-year-old boy is referred to a community paediatrician with concerns regarding development. At assessment, he is able to walk up and down stairs holding the railing and jumps with both feet. The doctor observes poor eye contact and limited speech. The child is also repeatedly opening and closing the drawers in the desk. What is the most likely finding here?

A Gross motor delay
B Fine motor delay
C Speech and language delay
D Play and social skills delay
E Global delay

4. You are observing a young boy in the waiting room of the paediatric outpatient clinic. He is running and jumping around the room but cannot quite hop like the bigger children. You notice that he has drawn a circle on a piece of paper and he shares his crayons. What developmental age is this child?
    A 4
    B 3
    C 5
    D 2
    E Unable to estimate

5. Which of the following are developmental 'red flags'?
    A 'Bottom shuffling'
    B Not walking by 15 months
    C Not walking by 18 months
    D Hand preference at 20 months
    E Not sitting by 4 months

Chapter 18 Child and adolescent mental health

1. A 15-year-old girl attends her general practitioner with lethargy and irregular menstruation. She has also been experiencing intermittent palpitations. She has previously had regular periods and has developed secondary sexual characteristics. On examination she is slim and has firm parotid swelling bilaterally. There is poor dental hygiene. Blood tests are arranged which show: sodium (Na) 134 mmol/L, potassium (K) 3.0 mmol/L, chloride 90 mmol/L. What is the most likely diagnosis?
    A Mumps
    B Polycystic ovarian syndrome
    C Anorexia nervosa
    D Bulimia nervosa
    E Hypothyroidism

2. A 14-year-old girl is brought to her general practitioner by her mother who is concerned that she has been losing weight. Her weight has dropped noticeably over the past year, and she has become increasingly withdrawn. She is very active and plays for her school netball team. She is quiet and tends to eat most of her meals in her room. On examination, she is bradycardic, her body mass index (BMI) is 13 kg/m^2 and fine lanugo hair is noted over her upper body. What is the best management of her condition?
    A Thyroid function tests and carbimazole
    B Admission for feeding and psychological treatment
    C A gluten-free diet

D Regular blood sugar monitoring and insulin
E Commence fluoxetine

3. An 8-year-old boy is referred by the educational psychologist with a suspected diagnosis of attention deficit hyperactivity disorder (ADHD). He has been struggling at school and finds it hard to concentrate on an activity. Teachers have been finding it hard to manage his behaviour as he is restless and constantly running around the classroom. Which of the following would suggest a diagnosis other than ADHD?
    A Easily distracted by other children
    B Difficulty waiting for his turn
    C Symptoms only present at school
    D Constantly talking, often interrupting others
    E Symptoms present at home and at school

4. A 4-year-old boy is referred to his general practitioner by his teacher at nursery. She has noticed that he has delayed speech and has only a handful of words. He struggles with imaginative play and usually plays alone. He becomes upset if there is a change to the daily routine. In the GP surgery, he is quiet with poor eye contact and does not approach the doctor. There are no dysmorphic features. What is the most likely diagnosis?
    A Selective mutism
    B Normal development
    C Autism
    D Speech delay
    E Fragile X

5. A 6-year-old boy is brought to the general practitioner with bed-wetting. His mother is concerned that he has never been dry at night and wants to know if this is normal. When counselling his mother which of the following statements regarding nocturnal enuresis is correct?
    A It is commonly due to urinary tract infection
    B Children are commonly dry at night by age 4
    C Primary nocturnal enuresis is commonly related to stressful events
    D Cutting down fluid in the evening is ineffective
    E Bell alarms may be helpful in children who sleep very deeply

6. Which of the following features suggests a diagnosis of conduct disorder rather than oppositional defiant disorder?
    A Getting into arguments with other children at school
    B Age 7 years
    C Not listening to teachers
    D Refusing to go to bed on time
    E Setting fire to a neighbour's shed

Chapter 19 Community paediatrics, public health and child protection

1. There are very few absolute contraindications to live vaccinations. Which of the following is a contraindication to vaccination with a live vaccine?
    A   Family history of adverse reaction to immunization
    B   High-dose steroid therapy
    C   Prematurity
    D   Previous malignancy
    E   Less than 2.5 kg

2. A 3-month-old baby is sadly found unresponsive in her cot. She was born in July at 41 weeks to a mother who smoked during the pregnancy and afterwards. Which of the following factors is the most likely to have influenced her sudden infant death?
    A   Maternal smoking
    B   Sleeping in her own cot rather than in bed with her parents where she could be supervised
    C   Supine sleeping position
    D   Born in summer months
    E   Postterm delivery

3. A 5-month-old baby with no previous attendances at hospital is brought to the hospital by his distraught parents with a swollen left upper arm. Both parents tell you separately that he was playing on the floor and fell to one side. They noticed he was crying so phoned an ambulance to come to hospital. A radiograph of the arm shows a spiral fracture of his left humerus. Which of the following features suggest nonaccidental injury?
    A   Immediate presentation at hospital
    B   History of incident does not fit with injury
    C   Parents appearing distraught
    D   No previous attendances at hospital
    E   Both accounts of the incident matching

4. A 13-year-old girl is made to stay at home to clean the house while her two younger sisters attend ballet lessons on Saturday mornings. Her mother tells her that she has to do it as she is too fat and clumsy to go to ballet. What category of abuse does this fit most closely?
    A   Physical abuse
    B   Neglect
    C   Emotional abuse
    D   Child maltreatment
    E   Fabricated and induced illness

5. A 16-year-old girl is admitted to hospital and diagnosed with appendicitis. She is due to undergo an appendicectomy. She is accompanied by her mother, her stepfather who she lives with and her birth father who she sees once a month. Which of the following are best placed to provide consent for the operation?
    A   The mother
    B   The stepfather
    C   The birth father
    D   The girl
    E   The doctor performing the procedure

Chapter 20 Accidents and emergencies

1. A 3-year-old girl is 'blue-lighted' into the local emergency department with reduced consciousness. Her mother informs the paramedic that her daughter has been unwell for the last 8 days with vomiting and profuse diarrhoea. On arrival, she is apyrexial, has a heart rate of 170 beats/min and respiratory rate of 20 breaths/min. Her systolic blood pressure is 75 mmHg, and she has a capillary refill time of 5 seconds. She is barely responsive to pain. Resuscitation begins and a blood gas reveals a pH 6.9, base excess −18 mmol/L and blood sugar of 2.2 mmol/L. What is the most likely clinical syndrome?
    A   Anaphylactic shock
    B   Septicaemic shock
    C   Cardiogenic shock
    D   Hypovolaemic shock
    E   Neurogenic shock

2. A mother brings her toddler son into the emergency department following a burn. She tells the triage nurse that she had just finished making a cup of tea and left it on the kitchen worktop to attend to her crying 4-month-old girl infant. She heard screams from the toddler who had pulled the cup of tea over his right hand. She gave immediate first aid and came to hospital immediately. Mother appears distressed and tearful. Analgesia and suitable dressings are applied. What is the most appropriate next step in the management of this toddler?
    A   Discharge home
    B   Take blood for routine investigations
    C   Get intravenous fluids
    D   Call the duty social worker to express your concerns
    E   Discuss the case with the regional burns centre

3. A known person with epilepsy is brought into the local emergency department in status epilepticus. The paramedic crew have given rectal diazepam 10 minutes ago, but the patient continues to have generalized tonic-clonic seizures. He now has intravenous access, and his blood sugar is 5.5 mmol/L. What is the most appropriate next drug treatment to be given?
    A   Intravenous lorazepam
    B   Intravenous phenytoin

C Intravenous thiopental
D Rectal paraldehyde
E Buccal midazolam

4. A 14-year-old girl self-presents to her local emergency department with a history of deliberate self-poisoning following an argument with her boyfriend. She agrees to blood tests which reveal high paracetamol blood levels at 4 hours postingestion, necessitating treatment. Which is the appropriate treatment for this teenager?
    A Intravenous desferrioxamine
    B Intravenous *N*-acetylcysteine
    C Active cooling
    D Alkalinization of urine with bicarbonate
    E Activated charcoal

5. A previously well 5-year-old boy is brought in by ambulance to the emergency department with an acute onset of breathing difficulty. On arrival, he appears unwell, pale with audible stridor and is sitting upright unable to speak. His temperature is 40°C and he is drooling. What is the first priority in this child's management?
    A Lie the child down
    B Take a throat swab
    C Obtain intravenous access
    D Give oral dexamethasone
    E Summon immediate anaesthetic help

6. A 14-year-old boy is admitted with diabetic ketoacidosis (DKA). Intravenous insulin has been running at 0.1 units/kg per hour alongside a 500-mL bag of 0.9% normal saline for the last 12 hours. His last blood sugar is 22 mmol/L, and he has a good urine output. Which of the following are most likely to be decreased?
    A Serum sodium
    B Serum potassium
    C Serum lactate
    D Serum chloride
    E Serum calcium

7. A 24-month-old boy is brought into the emergency department by ambulance in cardiac arrest following a near-drowning incident. Resuscitation is in progress. Which of the following will indicate a poor prognosis for outcome?
    A Submersion time of 3 minutes
    B Core temperature of 35°C on arrival
    C Arterial pH of <7.0 postresuscitation
    D Near-drowning in seawater
    E No respiratory effort within 90 seconds

8. A 9-year-old boy in asystole is brought in by ambulance to the emergency department. The various members of the cardiac arrest team arrive and resuscitation begins. Which is the most important drug of choice?
    A Adrenaline (epinephrine)
    B Sodium bicarbonate
    C Atropine
    D Amiodarone
    E Lidocaine

9. A 3-year-old girl is brought into the emergency department by ambulance with a 4-hour history of listlessness, high fever and reduced responsiveness. Her temperature is 40.0°C, she has a heart rate of 170 beats/min, a respiratory rate of 35 breaths/min and saturations of 100% in 15 L of high-flow oxygen. On examination, she is responsive to voice and maintaining her airway. Systemic examination is unremarkable; her capillary refill time is 4 seconds. What is the first priority in the management of this child?
    A Intubation and ventilation
    B 10 mL/kg bolus of normal saline
    C 20 mL/kg bolus of normal saline
    D 15 mL/kg packed red cells
    E 3 mL/kg bolus of dextrose

Chapter 21 Nutrition, fluids and prescribing

1. A 3-year-old boy of Asian origin presents to his general practitioner accompanied by his father. He has a 6-month history of bilateral leg pains and occasionally finds it difficult to walk and has to rest. On examination, he has bowing of his legs but otherwise appears developmentally normal with no other neurological or musculoskeletal findings. His father mentions that his son is also due to see the dentist for 'bad teeth'. What is the most appropriate initial blood test to aid in diagnosis?
    A Bone profile
    B Liver function
    C Full blood count
    D C-reactive protein
    E Renal function

2. An 11-year-old girl presents to the emergency department with a 4-day history of cough and fever. A working diagnosis of right middle lobe pneumonia is made, and she is commenced on intravenous antibiotics and admitted to the ward. Her blood tests reveal a plasma sodium of 127 mmol/L with normal renal function. Further investigations reveal a low plasma osmolality and a raised urinary sodium level. What is the most likely diagnosis?
    A Syndrome of inappropriate antidiuretic hormone secretion (SIADH)
    B Cushing syndrome
    C Diabetes insipidus
    D Secondary adrenal insufficiency
    E Adrenal hyperplasia

3. A 14-year-old girl is brought to her general practitioner by her mother who is concerned that she has been losing weight. Her weight has dropped noticeably over the past year, and she has become increasingly withdrawn. She is very active and plays for her school netball team. She makes her own meals at home, rather than eating with the family. She has not reached menarche. On examination her body mass index is 15 kg/m² and fine lanugo hair is noted over her upper body. The most likely cause for her weight loss is which of the following?

   A   Hyperthyroidism
   B   Anorexia nervosa
   C   Malabsorption
   D   Diabetes mellitus
   E   Depression

4. A 12-year-old boy comes into hospital with right lower quadrant pain and anorexia. He is diagnosed with suspected appendicitis and is made nil by mouth pending a laparotomy. His weight is 32 kg: what are his maintenance fluid requirements?

   A   2240 mL/d
   B   1600 mL/d
   C   1740 mL/d
   D   2100 mL/d
   E   2600 mL/d

5. A 6-year-old boy attends accident and emergency due to lethargy and vomiting for 24 hours. He is listless and tachycardic, with dry mucus membranes and sunken eyes. His blood sugar is 28 mmol, blood gas showed pH 7.01 kPa, partial pressure of carbon dioxide (pCO_2) 3.2, bicarbonate (HCO_3^-) 14 mmol/L, base excess −7 mmol/L and his urine dipstick showed glucose 3+, ketones 3+. You diagnose severe diabetic ketoacidosis (DKA). After giving one 10 mL/kg bolus of 0.9% saline for shock, what is the correct next step in his fluid management?

   A   Prescribe full maintenance intravenous fluids over 24 hours
   B   Prescribe full maintenance intravenous fluids over 48 hours, and subtract the fluid given in as boluses
   C   Prescribe double maintenance intravenous fluids over 24 hours due to signs of dehydration
   D   Prescribe full maintenance intravenous fluids over 48 hours, plus the fluid deficit and subtract the fluid bolus
   E   Prescribe full maintenance fluids over 48 hours, plus the fluid deficit, but do not subtract the fluid bolus

UKMLA SBA Answers

Chapter 3 Cardiovascular system

1. B. Transposition of the great arteries often presents suddenly in the first days of life following spontaneous closure of the ductus arteriosus. If there is not an associated septal defect (e.g., VSD/ASD) to allow mixing of oxygenated and deoxygenated blood, babies are often unwell with severe cyanosis not responsive to oxygen and a metabolic acidosis. This baby should be started on a prostin infusion to try to maintain ductal patency whilst waiting for an emergency balloon atrial septostomy.

2. D. Explain that this is most likely to be an innocent murmur and inform the GP to reevaluate the child once she has recovered from her hospital admission. This patient has an innocent murmur, which can be more pronounced in the presence of an intercurrent febrile illness. Typical features of innocent murmurs are soft, systolic, normal heart sounds; an asymptomatic child; no accompanying signs or symptoms suggestive of cardiac disease and no radiation and variation with posture. An ECHO would be indicated if the murmur persisted. If infective endocarditis is suspected, three blood cultures are necessary to guide management.

3. A. This baby has clinical features of trisomy 21, and hence an atrioventricular septal defect is the most likely lesion, accounting for 40% of heart lesions in trisomy 21. The next most common is a ventricular septal defect, which accounts for approximately 30%.

4. E. This baby has congenital cyanotic heart disease, most likely transposition of the great arteries until proven otherwise, and an infusion of prostaglandin is mandatory for patency of the ductus arteriosus to allow mixing of blood.

5. C. *S. viridans* accounts for approximately 90% of cases of infective endocarditis (IE). Management consists of a 4- to 6-week course of intravenous antibiotics. Peripheral stigmata of disease are less commonly encountered in children with IE but include splinter haemorrhages and Osler nodes.

6. E. This baby has features of congenital rubella, including the absent red reflexes (cataracts) and growth restriction. The commonest cardiac lesions in this case are a patent ductus arteriosus and pulmonary stenosis.

7. D. There should be no added sounds with innocent murmurs. Innocent murmurs follow the rule of 'S': soft, short, systolic, symptom-free, signs – none. A split-second heart sound is normal.

8. B. Tetralogy of Fallot comprises pulmonary stenosis, overriding aorta, ventricular septal defect and right ventricular hypertrophy. Other forms of cyanotic congenital heart disease include transposition of the great arteries, tricuspid atresia, total anomalous pulmonary drainage and hypoplastic left heart. Infants with cyanotic heart disease are often dependent on the ductus arteriosus and it is vital to keep this open with prostaglandin infusion until surgery can be performed. The other answers are all examples of congenital acyanotic heart disease.

9. D. These ECG signs are in keeping with supraventricular tachycardia; the rate is above 220 beats/min and regular, the QRS complexes are narrow and P waves are not visible. Adenosine would be the first-line treatment in this instance as patients are symptomatic. If the child showed signs of haemodynamic compromise, then DC cardioversion can be tried in an emergency. In a well child you could consider vagal manoeuvres, although if successful, this is often a transient fix and difficult in unhappy toddlers. A fluid bolus would be indicated in sinus tachycardia as a result of sepsis, for example.

10. D. A raised antistreptolysin O titre or a positive throat swab for streptococcus is a required diagnostic requirement. Pericarditis, polyarthritis, chorea, subcutaneous nodules and erythema marginatum are major criteria. Raised acute phase reactants (erythrocyte sedimentation rate/CRP/white cell count), prolonged PR interval, fever, arthralgia and previous rheumatic fever are minor criteria. At least two major or one major and two minor criteria are required for diagnosis. Chorea is a rare feature of rheumatic fever.

Chapter 4 Respiratory system

1. D. This history of sudden onset of cough, stridor and respiratory distress after playing alone is suggestive of inhalation of a foreign body. As the child is too young to give an accurate history and there were no witnesses, an urgent chest X-ray is indicated. In cases of acute stridor, ENT and anaesthetic help should be summoned if there

are airway concerns and investigations and treatments kept at a minimum so as not to distress the child further.

2. C. The isolated speech delay and poor behaviour in an otherwise well 5-year-old are suggestive of a hearing problem which will need assessment. The most common cause is chronic otitis media with effusion. The history is not suggestive of attention-deficit/hyperactivity disorder or an autistic spectrum disorder, and although this child may benefit from the input of community paediatrics, the most important next step is a hearing assessment.

3. A. Asthma cannot be diagnosed in this age group. Her age and lack of crackles on examination make bronchiolitis unlikely but still possible.

4. D. This child has deteriorated and is demonstrating features of life-threatening asthma. Urgent action is required and the next step is to proceed with IV magnesium sulphate. Other second-line management options include IV salbutamol and IV aminophylline.

5. The history of delayed passage of meconium and findings of finger clubbing raise suspicion for cystic fibrosis, which must be excluded. The gold standard for diagnosis is the sweat test and a cystic fibrosis genotype will also detect common mutations.

6. C. Parainfluenza viruses account for up to 80% of cases of croup. Other viruses that cause croup are adenovirus and RSV. The characteristic symptoms of cough and stridor of croup typically follow symptoms of an upper respiratory tract infection and it has its peak incidence in the second year of life in the winter.

7. E. Summon immediate anaesthetic help. Acute epiglottis is now rare in children following the introduction of the *Haemophilus influenzae* vaccine (Hib) as part of the routine immunizations schedule. It is a life-threatening emergency and securing the airway is of paramount importance prior to intravenous antibiotics.

8. C. Admit and give nasogastric feeds. Her saturations are acceptable, and hence supplemental oxygen is not needed. However, as a general rule, less than 50% of oral intake warrants admission for feeding support and given the minimal recession, nasogastric feeds would be more physiological than intravenous fluids.

9. E. Add a long-acting β agonist. This child needs escalation of her asthma treatment. She should be reviewed to see if the long-acting β agonist has been beneficial. The stepwise approach to asthma is available on the British Thoracic Society website within the asthma guidelines.

10. A. In pneumonia, age is a good predictor of the likely pathogens. Viruses alone are found as a cause in younger children in up to 50%. In older children, when a bacterial cause is found, it is most commonly *S. pneumoniae* followed by *Mycoplasma* and *Chlamydia* (chlamydial pneumonia).

11. C. This infant may be entering the peak stage of her bronchiolitis where typically things can get worse before they get better. In view of her respiratory status and metabolic acidosis, high flow is the next most effective step. Stopping NG feeds and proning may also be of benefit.

12. A. The clinical findings of worsening respiratory distress and 'stony dull' percussion note suggest an empyema. This is not an uncommon complication of pneumonia and a chest X-ray is needed followed by an ultrasound scan to assess the extent of the empyema. In some hospitals, an ultrasound may be advised as first-line imaging.

Chapter 5 Gastrointestinal and hepatobiliary systems

1. C. This infant is likely to have pyloric stenosis, which is supported by the history and clinical findings. The typical findings on blood gas are of a hypokalaemic, hypochloraemic metabolic alkalosis caused by repeated vomiting. E is a respiratory alkalosis.

2. B. This is usually associated with diarrhoea, particularly *Escherichia coli* 0157 (Shiga toxin producing). Onset is around 5–10 days after development of diarrhoea. There is a triad of microangiopathic haemolytic anaemia, thrombocytopenia and acute kidney injury. Clinical features can mimic inflammatory bowel disease and dehydration may produce acute kidney injury in gastroenteritis; however, these would not cause haemolysis.

3. D. Bulimia nervosa is characterized by binge eating and purging (often through vomiting and excessive exercise). There is abnormal body image and obsession with food and bodyweight, although BMI may be normal. Vomiting can lead to electrolyte imbalances as seen in this case, particularly hypokalaemia, hypochloraemia and metabolic alkalosis. The parotid swelling is a consequence of recurrent vomiting; there may also be erosion of dental enamel.

4. E. The most likely diagnosis is Hirschsprung disease where there is an aganglionic segment of bowel which may be small or involve most or all of the colon. The delayed passage of meconium and infrequent passage of stool are classical. Histology of a biopsy of the rectum will show an absence of ganglionic cells. Treatment involves surgical resection of the aganglionic segment.

5. C. This is a classic description of coeliac disease where there is an autoimmune reaction caused by dietary gluten. The damage to the small intestine in coeliac disease leads to loss of the absorptive surface which can lead to an iron-deficiency anaemia, as described here. As well as diarrhoea and weight loss, there can be abdominal bloating and discomfort. Treatment involves complete exclusion of gluten from the diet.

6. A. The symptoms described may be common to Crohn disease and ulcerative colitis; however, the findings at endoscopy and colonoscopy point to Crohn disease as it can affect any part of the intestinal tract and tends to occur in skip lesions. Ulcerative colitis causes continuous inflammation, starting in the rectum and extending proximally.

7. D. This presentation is typical of intussusception where a part of the bowel telescopes inside itself. Peak age of onset is 6 to 9 months. Symptoms include episodic severe abdominal pain with inconsolable crying, pallor, vomiting, 'red currant jelly' stool and eventually shock. Abdominal ultrasound may reveal the 'doughnut sign' of bowel within bowel. Treatment is by air reduction enema or surgery if this is not effective.

8. D. Reassurance and no further investigation. Functional abdominal pain is the most likely diagnosis and no further investigation is required. Reassuring features in the history include the fact that the pain is short-lived and responds to simple analgesia and that she is thriving. It is of note that it does not occur at weekends. The nearer the pain is to the umbilicus the less likely it is to be significant. Often, after a thorough assessment, simple reassurance is all that is required.

9. E. The symptoms described are of an infective colitis. *Campylobacter* typically causes a bloody diarrhoea and is transmitted by infected chicken amongst other foods. The fact that other members of the family are affected and the timing of onset in symptoms after the takeaway are classical. No treatment is usually required but the Health Protection Agency should be informed.

10. A. This history is suggestive of appendicitis: classically there is abdominal pain which starts periumbilically and then localizes the right iliac fossa. Tenderness on examination warrants prompt surgical review to evaluate if an appendicectomy is required. The surgical team may ask for further investigations to be done but these should not delay their review.

11. B. This infant has prolonged jaundice which is conjugated and associated with pale stools and faltering growth which is caused by biliary atresia until proven otherwise. This is a serious condition which requires surgical correction via the Kasai procedure as soon as possible for the best outcome. If it is not diagnosed early, the Kasai procedure may not be successful and then liver transplantation is required.

12. B. The most likely diagnosis is cystic fibrosis due to the combination of respiratory symptoms and faltering growth and diarrhoea. Many cases are now diagnosed via the newborn screening programme. However, a sweat test is the test of choice at this age. Cystic fibrosis is more common in Celtic populations.

13. E. A Mallory-Weiss tear is a small tear in the oesophageal mucosa after prolonged forceful vomiting. It can lead to blood in the vomit and is a complication of gastroenteritis. It is a self-limiting condition that requires no treatment. Other causes of haematemesis are rare in children.

14. C. Irritable bowel syndrome can cause symptoms in response to stressful situations. The fact that she gets pain and diarrhoea infrequently, and most often on school days, makes a more serious diagnosis unlikely. In addition, she is growing well, which is reassuring.

Chapter 6 Renal and genitourinary conditions

1. C. The description here is of acute nephritis (haematuria, hypertension, reduced renal function). The most common childhood cause is poststreptococcal glomerulonephritis which classically presents with 'cola'-coloured urine 10 to 14 days after a throat or skin infection. You would expect a purpuric rash and joint pain in Henoch-Schönlein purpura and bloody diarrhoea in haemolytic-uraemic syndrome, two less common causes of acute nephritis. Peripheral and periorbital are common in nephrotic syndrome which is not described here, and dysuria in a urinary tract infection is not expected to cause hypertension or affect renal function.

2. C. This description is of haemolytic-uraemic syndrome, the most common cause of an acute kidney injury in a previously healthy child. Management is supportive, but antibiotics are contraindicated as they can induce expression and release of the Shiga toxin and therefore exacerbate the patient's condition. High-dose oral steroids are the treatment for nephrotic syndrome and renal transplantation would not be considered initially as 90% of children recover full renal function.

3. B. The description here is of a hydrocele, a fluid-filled scrotal swelling caused by a small opening of the processus vaginalis. The majority will resolve spontaneously by 12 months and treatment is only needed in the first 2 years if very large. No imaging or intervention is required.

4. D. The description here is of multiple complicated urinary tract infections requiring further investigation, which should be done according to National Institute for Health and Care Excellence (NICE) guidelines (see Tables 6.3–6.4). Renal scarring is best seen on nuclear medicine radioisotope scans, the first line of which is a static scan, DMSA. An MCUG allows visualization of the urinary tract and detects reflux, an underlying cause of multiple infections. An abdominal ultrasound scan is a useful initial investigation but does not have high sensitivity for the detection of scarring. Neither CT nor MRI would be indicated in this patient, due to the risks of irradiation with CT and the need for sedation for both CT and MRI in a patient of this age.

5. B. In a patient with polyuria and polydipsia, the key investigation is to test the blood glucose (and also to dipstick the urine for glucose and ketones) to rule out a new diagnosis of diabetes mellitus.

6. D. This is a well child presenting with fever without apparent focus. The examination findings do not suggest any 'red' or 'amber' features and hence, in accordance with the National Institute for Health and Care Excellence (NICE) 'traffic light' guidance of fever management, the next step is to request a urine dipstick and CXR only if there are signs of pneumonia (not in this case). If the urine is clear of infection, then the child could be discharged home with advice.

7. E. In an infant with bilaterally undescended testes it is important to consider complex genital anomaly. The most common cause for this is congenital adrenal hyperplasia (CAH). A number of investigations are warranted including rapid FISH for sex determination, ultrasound of the abdomen to determine placement of the testes (or identify female internal genitalia) and 17-hydroxyprogesterone (raised in the most common form of CAH). However, the immediate risk to the infant is a CAH salt-wasting crisis, therefore U&Es should be done as soon as possible.

8. A. Testicular torsion occurs when the testis turns on the remnant of the processus vaginalis and blood supply is restricted. It presents most commonly with testicular pain of less than 12 hours duration, although lower abdominal or inguinal pain can also occur. There may be swelling of the testis and overlying erythema. Epididymo-orchitis is often associated with urinary symptoms. Doppler of the testes may help differentiate these (blood flow reduced in torsion and increased in epididymitis) but shouldn't delay surgery. Torsion of the hydatid of Morgagni presents similarly to testicular torsion but is much less common.

9. D. E. coli is the most common cause of urinary tract infection in the structurally normal kidney.

10. C. Failure to treat posterior urethral valves (by temporary urinary drainage followed by definitive surgical management) leads to irreversible renal damage. Hydroceles and umbilical hernias usually resolve spontaneously. A unilaterally undescended testicle warrants surgical referral if undescended at the age of 1 year. Inguinal hernias frequently require repair but there is no definite urgency to do this within the first 6 months of life.

Chapter 7 Endocrine system and growth

1. D. 17-Hydroxyprogesterone level. This baby has presented with a 'salt-losing' adrenal crisis as reflected by the hyponatraemia and hypoglycaemia. Clinical presentation of congenital adrenal hypertrophy can either be classic or nonclassic and symptoms are due to androgen excess and cortisol deficiency.

2. A. Precocious puberty in boys is always pathological and requires investigation. The finding of papilloedema suggests an intracranial cause and therefore a brain tumour must be excluded.

3. A. This autosomal recessive condition is associated with cataracts, liver failure and Escherichia coli sepsis. It is diagnosed by decreased or absent galactose-1-phosphate uridylyltransferase in red blood cells. Treatment is by a lactose-free diet and no breastfeeding.

4. B. Insulin drives potassium into cells and therefore serum potassium falls. Intravenous fluids should be given with potassium (i.e., 0.9% sodium chloride and 20 mmol KCl/500 mL) when treating diabetic ketoacidosis (DKA). Patients with DKA require 6- to 8-hour monitoring of urea and electrolytes and blood gases.

5. A. The laboratory findings here all point to SIADH. This is a common stress response and in this case is secondary to pneumonia. Other causes of SIADH include central nervous system disease and treatment is by treating the underlying cause and fluid restriction.

6. B. Boys with Klinefelter syndrome (47, XXY) are tall (particularly long legs). They often have small testes and gynaecomastia; learning and attention difficulties are common. Hyperthyroidism would explain the height and gynaecomastia but not the small testes or learning difficulties.

7. C. It is reassuring that his height and weight are both on the 99th centile. Most endocrine causes of obesity are associated with short stature. As his parents are tall, it is likely that he has the appropriate weight and height for his age but calculation of the mid-parental height would confirm this.

8. A. Galactosaemia is a disorder of the metabolism of galactose which can result in liver dysfunction, coagulopathy and cataracts. Treatment is by removing any source of galactose from the diet including breast milk.

9. A. This baby is following the centile she was born on and has small parents. There is no suggestion of any organic illness and she is healthy. Some parents request treatment to increase height, but the use of growth hormone is restricted to a few very specific indications.

10. D. In constitutional delay of growth, bone age will reveal delayed skeletal maturity. By contrast, normal skeletal maturation is seen in familial short stature.

11. C. The combination of features suggests congenital hypothyroidism. In the developed world this is most commonly due to agenesis or failure of migration. Thyroxine should be started as soon as possible to preserve neurological function. Karyotype could be indicated if there were features of trisomy 21 which can be

associated with hypothyroidism. A blood group would be part of your workup of jaundice but is not a diagnostic test. CK is used to diagnose muscular dystrophies and growth hormone is used to assess pituitary function.

Chapter 8 Oncology

1. C. Brain tumours are mainly infratentorial. Diagnosis is often late, with signs of raised intracranial pressure. Metastasis of CNS tumours is rare. Astrocytomas are the most common form and continue to have poor prognosis despite treatment.
2. A. The most common renal tumour, nephroblastoma, presents mainly in the under 5 year olds with painless, smooth abdominal mass. Children are usually well at diagnosis. It is associated with syndromes including Beckwith-Wiedemann, hemihypertrophy, WAGR and Denys-Drash. Metastasis at diagnosis is uncommon. Mutations have been found on chromosome 11.
3. B. It is associated with Beckwith-Wiedemann syndrome. Beckwith-Wiedemann is a genetic overgrowth condition caused by deregulation of genes on chromosome 11. There is gigantism (i.e., hemihypertrophy) and macroglossia. It is associated with exomphalos and predisposes to tumours, particularly nephroblastoma (Wilms tumour).
4. A. Retinoblastoma can occur unilaterally but 40% of cases are bilateral. Checking for a red reflex is one of the most important parts of the newborn and 6- to 8-week checks. Although this baby was born prematurely, babies who are considered at risk of retinopathy of prematurity are those born at <34 weeks' gestation or weighing <1.5 kg at birth.
5. C. Primary malignancies of the bone are rare. They occur most frequently in adolescent boys. The sunburst appearance on X-ray is suggestive of osteosarcoma. Ewing sarcoma is associated with onion-skin appearance on X-ray. There are no features suggestive of rickets or osteomyelitis. Chondrosarcomas are rare and found mainly in the axial skeleton.

Chapter 9 Haematology

1. B. Early foetal haematopoiesis begins in the liver, spleen and lymph nodes; however, bone marrow begins production around the fourth month of gestation and is the main source by term. Most haemoglobin is foetal haemoglobin (HbF) at term – this has a higher affinity for oxygen to facilitate gas exchange at the placenta. A gradual changeover occurs after delivery. Hb concentration is high at birth and falls until around 7 weeks to a nadir of about 9 g/dL.
2. C. Iron deficiency is extremely common in childhood, affecting around 3% of toddlers. It is usually dietary and there is often a history of fussy eating. Under 1 year olds consuming unmodified cow's milk are particularly at risk. It

is a microcytic, hypochromic anaemia and is usually asymptomatic. If severe, it can lead to lethargy, breathlessness and even cardiomyopathy. There is increasing evidence that iron deficiency impacts neurodevelopmental outcomes in childhood.

3. E. HSP is characterized by palpable purpura in the absence of thrombocytopaenia or coagulopathy, abdominal pain, arthralgia and renal involvement. Immune thrombocytopaenic purpura would have low platelets. A raised white cell count with or without lymphadenopathy would be expected with ALL. Scurvy can cause purpura but there is no indication of this here.
4. D. Sickle cell disease (HbSS) causes an anaemia, often normocytic, which may be quite profound. It is characterized by intermittent 'crises' where the abnormal haemoglobin precipitates, leading to 'sickling' of red blood cells which clump together. This produces a variety of clinical manifestations in addition to acute haemolysis. The most common presentation is with painful vasoocclusive crisis (bone pain). Splenomegaly is present in young children but autosplenectomy secondary to recurrent splenic infarctions occurs in older children.
5. C. β-Thalassaemia is a quantitative defect in haemoglobin production. Homozygous mutation produces thalassaemia major which presents as foetal haemoglobin (HbF) levels decline in infancy. There is a microcytic hypochromic anaemia and children are transfusion dependent. Frontal bossing is produced by extramedullary haematopoiesis.
6. C. ITP most commonly presents with bruising or petechiae in an otherwise well child. The platelet count is low (production of platelets is normal, but they are rapidly consumed). Around 60% of cases are preceded by a viral infection. Management is usually supportive as it tends to self-resolve.
7. B. Haemophilia A (factor VIII deficiency) is an X-linked recessive condition resulting in abnormal clotting. Infants usually get through birth and the initial neonatal period without significant problems, although intracranial bleeding is a risk. Presentation is usual during early childhood, often with excessive bleeding (e.g., following circumcision), or, as in this case, with haemarthrosis and easy bruising as the child begins to mobilise.
8. A. This is an X-linked disorder of red cell enzyme. It reduces the ability of the red blood cells to respond to oxidative stress. It is characterized by haemolysis in response to infection, drugs (including primaquine), acidosis (e.g., diabetic ketoacidosis) and fava beans. It is common in Afro-Caribbean groups.
9. E. Febrile neutropenia is a common side effect of chemotherapy. It occurs most frequently 8 to 10 days postchemotherapy. Prompt management is vital and would include peripheral and central blood cultures, and

rapid initiation of intravenous antibiotics according to local protocol. G-CSF injections can be used to stimulate a rise in the neutrophil count but only under guidance of a haematologist. Supportive treatment with platelet/red blood cell transfusions is often required in patients with ALL but these are not indicated here.

10. C. The differential diagnosis of lymphadenopathy is vast. In this case, the histology is diagnostic with Reed-Sternberg cells being pathognomonic for Hodgkin lymphoma. The shortness of breath is due to superior vena caval obstruction from the mediastinal mass on lying flat.

Chapter 10   Fever, infectious diseases and immunodeficiency

1. D. This child's clinical features satisfy the diagnostic criteria for Kawasaki disease. It is an autoimmune disease in which the medium-sized blood vessels throughout the body become inflamed and is largely seen in children under 5 years. The most important complication is coronary artery aneurysms which can occur in 20% to 25% of untreated cases. Aneurysms have a peak frequency at around 4 weeks of onset of illness.

2. D. Meningococcal sepsis is a catastrophic diagnosis if missed with serious potential long-term complications. The management, as with any emergency, is paying attention to airway, breathing and circulation followed by definitive treatment with broad-spectrum intravenous antibiotics (e.g., ceftriaxone). In this scenario, the child is maintaining his own airway with a Glasgow Coma Scale score 14/15 and is cardiovascularly stable.

3. C. This is a typical presentation of human herpesvirus (HHV)-6 or HHV-7 infection and is a well-recognized cause of febrile convulsions in 10% to 15% of cases due to high fevers.

4. C. This infant gives a classic presentation for SCID which must be considered. SCID is an X-linked disorder and cure may be possible with bone marrow transplantation.

5. A. This infant warrants a full septic screen as indicated by the age group of <3 months and high fever. The infant is not unwell and not displaying any signs of shock or compromise. In this type of scenario, inflammatory marker results should be looked at retrospectively to not delay investigations and treatment.

6. D. Both clinical and biochemical findings point to Epstein-Barr virus causing glandular fever. Hepatomegaly occurs in approximately 10% of cases and splenomegaly in about 50% of cases. Treatment is symptomatic and supportive.

7. C. *Neisseria* and *Haemophilus* are gram-negative organisms. *S. aureus* is also gram-positive but occurs in clusters. *Listeria* is a gram-positive rod.

8. C. Thick and thin blood films for malaria parasites. The history of travel to a malarial area in conjunction with a febrile illness, hepatomegaly and jaundice means that malaria must be excluded.

Chapter 11   Allergy and anaphylaxis

1. A. Anaphylaxis is a medical emergency and rapid treatment can be life-saving. Treatment is with the airway, breathing, circulation (ABC) approach. If possible, the allergen should be removed (e.g., drug infusion). Intramuscular adrenaline (epinephrine) is the most important pharmacological treatment and may be given by adrenaline (epinephrine) autoinjector if available. Oxygen will be needed but will not stop the reaction. Intravenous steroids (e.g., hydrocortisone) and antihistamine (e.g., chlorphenamine) should also be given but do not take immediate effect and are not the most important step in treatment here.

2. D. The MMR does not contain egg, although it is produced on chick fibroblasts. If there is a history of severe anaphylaxis to egg, advice should be sought about location of vaccination. Yellow fever and influenza vaccines contain egg and must not be given to egg-allergic children.

3. D. Size of reaction does not correlate with clinical symptoms. Skin-prick testing is only suitable for diagnosis of IgE-mediated allergy. Radioallergosorbent testing (RAST) measures serum-specific IgE levels.

4. A. For this reason, RAST (which identifies specific IgE) may not identify food allergies. A positive skin test does not necessarily correlate with clinical allergy (there may be cross-reactivity) and should be taken in context. Children frequently outgrow their allergies (especially cow's milk allergy). An elimination–reintroduction test may be extremely helpful in diagnosing allergy.

5. B. Although all of these signs can be seen in anaphylaxis, it is the hoarse voice which is the most worrying as it suggests laryngeal oedema and impending airway obstruction.

Chapter 12   Dermatology

1. D. The description is highly suggestive of erythema multiforme. It is usually idiopathic and self-limiting, but in this scenario, it may be secondary to streptococcal or mycoplasma infection.

2. D. The most likely diagnosis is candidiasis. The hallmarks of this rash are satellite lesions and the fact it is affecting the tongue and nappy area. Treatment using an antifungal preparation is indicated and can be given orally and to the nappy area to ensure eradication.

3. B. *Sarcoptes scabiei* is a mite that can be transmitted from person to person by skin-to-skin contact. It causes intense itching and can affect the whole body in infants. The classical hallmarks are burrows visible on the wrists or between the fingers. It may affect other members of the family.

4. C. The lesions are suggestive of *Molluscum contagiosum* which is caused by a pox virus. If they are all over the body, then an immune workup may be indicated but small crops are common in childhood. They resolve spontaneously and no treatment is required.

5. C. This description is typical of pityriasis rosea, a benign condition thought to be caused by an underlying viral infection. The typical pattern is of a 'herald patch' as described here, with the rash spreading over the trunk in a 'Christmas tree' pattern after 1 to 3 days. This rash resolves usually in 6 to 8 weeks and no treatment is required.

Chapter 13 Nervous system

1. C. *Neisseria* and *Haemophilus* are gram-negative organisms. *S. aureus* is also gram-positive but occurs in clusters. *Listeria* is a gram-positive rod. Group B *Streptococcus* is the most common causative agent in neonatal sepsis and it can occur early (i.e., symptomatic at birth) or late (up to 3 months).

2. A. These occur in children between 6 months and 2 years and are triggered by high emotion (tantrums, etc.). The child holds their breath, becomes pale or cyanotic, loses consciousness and falls to the floor. There may be tonic-clonic movements. History is vital in distinguishing this from other forms of syncope. 'Tet' spells are episodes of cyanosis occurring in tetralogy of Fallot due to a temporary increase in right ventricular outflow obstruction. Myoclonic epilepsy is characterized by jerking movements of the muscles, particularly on wakening. Vasovagal syncope is uncommon in this age group.

3. B. Absences can occur very frequently during the day and may be mistaken for poor concentration or daydreaming. This history is typical and the EEG is characteristic. First-line treatment is with sodium valproate or ethosuximide. The EEG would be normal in ADHD and nonepileptic seizures. West syndrome is associated with infantile spasms, and myoclonic epilepsy is muscle jerks typically occurring on wakening.

4. D. This seizure disorder presents in infancy, often with the salaam seizures described here, and has a characteristic EEG (hypsarrhythmia). It is treated with vigabatrin or adrenocorticotrophic hormone. The EEG would be normal in reflux and breath-holding attacks. Benign rolandic epilepsy affects older children and typically causes focal seizures.

5. A. The protocol for status epilepticus is described in Chapter 20. First-line treatment is with benzodiazepines. The first dose has been given in the community as buccal midazolam. A second dose is indicated if the seizures continue 10 minutes after administration of the first dose. This could be given as rectal diazepam but intravenous access has already been obtained and thus lorazepam is the drug of choice.

6. A. First-line therapy for generalized tonic-clonic seizures includes carbamazepine, sodium valproate and lamotrigine. Sodium valproate should be avoided in girls who have reached puberty due to its teratogenic effects, providing that their seizures can be controlled by another drug. Phenytoin is generally avoided in view of its side-effect profile. Ethosuximide is useful in absence of seizures and vigabatrin is first-line therapy for infantile spasms.

7. C. This suggests raised intracranial pressure. Most headaches are benign; however, there are some sinister causes. About 70% of brain tumours present as headache. Red flag symptoms are those of raised intracranial pressure, any focal neurology, weight loss, sudden onset or progressive in nature. Migraine is typically unilateral and associated with vomiting and band-like pain suggests tension headache. Eye watering is nonspecific but can occur with cluster headaches, which are uncommon in children.

8. D. Diagnostic criteria for NF1 include at least two of the following: six or more café-au-lait patches, two or more neurofibromas (or one plexiform neurofibroma), axillary freckling, Lisch nodules, optic glioma or first-degree relative with NF1. Acoustic neuromas are a feature of neurofibromatosis type 2; ash-leaf macules and adenoma sebaceum are features of tuberous sclerosis.

9. D. Duchenne muscular dystrophy is X-linked. It is associated with calf pseudohypertrophy, proximal muscle weakness (with positive Gower sign) and cardiomyopathy. Onset is generally early with most patients requiring a wheelchair by 12 years of age.

10. C. Tendon reflexes are brisk, as cerebral palsy is an upper motor neuron lesion. The commonest group of causes is antenatal causes, which include cerebral dysgenesis and congenital infections. Intrapartum causes such as birth asphyxia result in 10% of cases. Cerebral palsy is a clinical diagnosis and MRI is often not required. Infants are initially hypotonic and can have feeding difficulties. Tone increases with age making the diagnosis more apparent.

Chapter 14 Musculoskeletal system

1. E. This is a child with 'risk factors' for SUFE. He is black, overweight and in the correct age group for children with SUFE to present. The lack of fever does not suggest an infective cause. The X-ray shows SUFE of the left hip – the femoral head has slipped off the metaphyseal neck.

2. C. This is septic arthritis until proven otherwise. This can be difficult to distinguish from osteomyelitis as both present with limp in children who are unwell and febrile. The key differences are that osteomyelitis is more insidious, may not have skin changes/swelling and there is typically pain on

movement and weight-bearing, not at rest. Inflammatory markers may be normal at this stage and X-rays may also be nonconclusive. It is vital that joint aspiration be performed as soon as possible followed by broad-spectrum antibiotics to prevent joint destruction.

3. C. Risk factors for DDH include first born, female, oligohydramnios, breech delivery, family history of DDH, congenital muscular pathology and congenital foot abnormalities (e.g., talipes and clubfoot). This child should have had a screening ultrasound of her hips organized based on her risk factors, regardless of examination findings.

4. E. Children with sickle cell disease have increased susceptibility to osteomyelitis, specifically due to encapsulated organisms like *Salmonella*. Other examination findings may include erythema of the affected limb with warmth, but not always. Acute-phase reactants are likely to be elevated. Any child with fever and limp has osteomyelitis until proven otherwise.

5. B. This girl has oligoarticular juvenile idiopathic arthritis as suggested by the duration of symptoms (>6 weeks), number of joints involved (four or fewer) and the asymmetrical pattern of joint involvement. These patients are at high risk for developing anterior uveitis and hence ophthalmological screening is very important.

6. A. There are eight types of osteogenesis imperfecta but type I is the commonest and accounts for 50% of all people with osteogenesis imperfecta. Blue sclerae are often present but not always. Diagnosis is by culturing skin fibroblasts that show a reduced amount of type 1 collagen.

7. B. The rash described on the eyelids is a heliotrope rash and the rash on the metacarpophalangeal joints is the Gottron papule, typical of this condition. He also has symptoms of proximal muscle weakness. Raised muscle enzymes (e.g., creatinine kinase), an electromyography and muscle biopsy would confirm the diagnosis.

8. C. The other symptoms described are typical features of a child with transient synovitis. The natural course would be for this to resolve within 7 days from the onset of symptoms. The treatment of transient synovitis is regular nonsteroidal antiinflammatories and careful safety netting, with a clinical review in 7 days. The presence of fever warrants further investigation for suspected osteomyelitis or septic arthritis.

Chapter 15 The newborn

1. D. This baby is at risk of hypoxic-ischaemic encephalopathy and meets criteria A and B (outlined by the TOBY trial) for cooling therapy. You would therefore not want to warm the baby and he is too sick to be sent to the postnatal ward. Low tone has implications for his swallow and he could be at risk of aspiration if fed. You are not given information about respiratory status here and it

is more likely that this is a metabolic acidosis, meaning CPAP would not be indicated.

2. C. Risk factors for DDH include first born, female sex, oligohydramnios, breech delivery, family history of DDH, congenital muscular pathology and congenital foot anomalies (e.g., talipes). Scoliosis is not associated with oligohydramnios. Perthes is idiopathic osteonecrosis of the femoral head occurring in older children, typically boys. Arthrogryposis would present as contractures in multiple joints, and torticollis is a neck deformity which although it can be congenital is not associated with oligohydramnios.

3. A. This baby does not have congenital varicella syndrome and we are told he is well. The neonate is at risk if a mother is exposed 5 days before and 2 days after birth due to transmission of the virus without time for the mother to develop antibodies. Therefore, the neonate should be given varicella immunoglobulin if the mother tests negative for varicella zoster virus antibodies. Acyclovir is given if lesions develop in the newborn.

4. B. RDS is associated with prematurity due to surfactant deficiency and a ground glass appearance on CXR is characteristic. Transient tachypnoea of the newborn is more common in caesarean deliveries and usually resolves by 4 hours. A pneumothorax should be detected on CXR and there may be focal consolidation in pneumonia. Although patent ductus arteriosus is common in preterm babies, it is unlikely to be the cause of such severe respiratory distress.

5. C. This baby is at risk of necrotizing enterocolitis (NEC) due to prematurity and this is a typical presentation. Other risk factors include low birthweight and formula feeding. Pneumatosis (air within the bowel wall) is highly suggestive of NEC. Intestinal obstruction, malrotation and duodenal atresia are important differentials but abdominal X-ray would normally distinguish these. The abdominal signs make sepsis less likely, although she would be treated with antibiotics.

6. D. Approximately 30% of women are colonized with group B haemolytic streptococcus and in some countries, it is routinely screened for in pregnancy (not the UK). All the organisms listed are causes of neonatal sepsis, but group B *Streptococcus* is the most likely causative agent.

7. B. The bleeding is caused by vitamin K deficiency – also called 'haemorrhagic disease of the newborn'. Low vitamin K results in a prolonged prothrombin time and so a raised international normalized ratio.

8. D. All of the above are causes of vomiting; however, this is an acute presentation with an unwell child and so this rules out colic and reflux. Diarrhoea and fever would make gastroenteritis more likely. Common sites for hernias in babies are inguinal and umbilical – a mass in the right upper quadrant would not fit. Intussusception occurs when

part of the bowel telescopes inside itself, which is the palpable mass. It is thought that an initial infection may lead to an increase in size of lymphoid tissue in the bowel which can act as the lead point. Peak onset is 6 to 9 months. Symptoms include episodic severe abdominal pain, pallor and eventually shock and red currant jelly stool. Treatment is by air reduction enema or surgery if this is not effective.

9. E. This baby has physiological jaundice of a low level that does not require any treatment. It may be exacerbated by breastfeeding but this does not mean breastfeeding should not be encouraged. Breast milk may delay the maturation of the liver enzymes involved in the metabolism of bilirubin but should be continued. The bilirubin would not be above the phototherapy threshold and prolonged jaundice occurs at >14 days old.

10. D. There is no suggestion of an organic illness in the history. The fact that the infant gained weight quickly when adequate intake was offered makes previous inadequate intake likely. This may have been due to lack of understanding of the needs of the baby or neglect, but it needs thorough assessment before discharge.

Chapter 16 Genetics

1. Causes of delayed puberty can be classified into central causes (low gonadotrophins) and gonadal failure (high gonadotrophins). The ejection systolic murmur suggests coarctation of the aorta which is the commonest heart lesion in Turner syndrome.

2. C. Amniocentesis allows for karyotyping to be performed which will give a definitive diagnosis. An ultrasound scan is used to measure nuchal translucency (skin neck fold thickness) which if increased could be a sign of trisomy 21. It can also be increased in other chromosomal anomalies and congenital heart defects, so it is not a specific test. You can also see false positives. Whilst PAPP-A and β-HCG levels are sensitive markers, they are never used in isolation. Foetal MRI would not be indicated in this scenario.

Chapter 17 Developmental assessment and developmental day

1. E. This toddler has specific gross motor delay as she is not walking by 18 months, which warrants developmental assessment by a community paediatrician. Always regard concerns raised by parents over their child's development as serious. Investigations are likely to be needed in this case.

2. D. This is a worrying sign at 12 months of age. This may signify hemiplegia, for example, in cerebral palsy and warrants further assessment. His speech is appropriate as children have one or two words at 12 months.

3. D. This child is showing strong signs of a social communication disorder (e.g., autistic spectrum disorder). Autism has a prevalence rate of approximately 1 in 100 people and boys are four times more likely to develop it than girls. The average age at diagnosis is 3 years although speech concerns occur from about 2 years onwards. The gross motor skills described are age appropriate.

4. B. Whilst you may not know the chronological age of the child, observing their behaviour and play can be helpful in estimating their developmental age. Children can jump at 2 years, but hopping is usually mastered at age 4. Children can draw a line at age 2, a circle at age 3, a square at age 4 and a person with a body at age 5. Sharing toys typically happens around 3 years.

5. C. Bottom shuffling can be a normal variant, but these children are often late walkers. Children are expected to be walking by 12 to 15 months and should be referred if not walking by 18 months. Hand preference is expected to develop from 18 to 24 months but earlier than this is a red flag. The ability to sit unsupported requires head support and is not expected until 6 months.

Chapter 18 Child and adolescent mental health

1. D. Bulimia nervosa is characterized by binge eating and purging (often through vomiting and excessive exercise). There is abnormal body image and obsession with food and bodyweight, although body mass index may be normal. Vomiting can lead to electrolyte imbalances as seen in this case, particularly hypokalaemia, hypochloraemia and metabolic alkalosis. The parotid swelling and enamel erosion are also sequelae of recurrent vomiting.

2. B. This is anorexia nervosa, characterized by low bodyweight and a fear of weight gain. There is distorted body image and pubertal delay or amenorrhea may be a feature. With a BMI of 13 kg/m^2 and bradycardia, she is likely to need inpatient admission for refeeding. The other answers describe treatments for other causes of weight loss; however, the fixation with food, social withdrawal and excessive exercise make anorexia the most likely cause.

3. C. The core features of ADHD are inattention, hyperactivity and impulsiveness. Features of these must be present in more than one setting (e.g., at school and at home) for a period of more than 6 months. The term has become increasingly popular with parents and the diagnosis should only be made following careful evaluation, including exclusion of other conditions, for example, autism or developmental delay, and consideration of psychosocial factors.

4. C. Autism is a pervasive developmental disorder characterized by speech delay and impairment of social communication skills. Autistic children may struggle to

interpret nonverbal communication and to form relationships with peers. Autistic behaviours are associated with a number of syndromes including fragile X, untreated phenylketonuria and Williams syndrome; however, in this scenario, there are no dysmorphic features.

5. E. Primary nocturnal enuresis (where a child has never been dry) is usually secondary to deep sleep and failure to wake to a full bladder or inadequate antidiuretic hormone secretion. Secondary enuresis is more commonly associated with emotional stress. Conditions such as urinary tract infection, neuropathic bladder and constipation may lead to enuresis but are uncommon.

6. E. Most of these behaviours are common to oppositional defiant disorder and conduct disorder, but oppositional defiant disorder is typical in younger children (<8 years) and does not feature the severely antisocial behaviour such as destruction of property that defines a conduct disorder.

Chapter 19 Community paediatrics, public health and child protection

1. B. High-dose steroid therapy means that the appropriate immune response to the vaccination will not occur. Other contraindications are immunosuppression due to medications or an inherited condition such as severe combined immunodeficiency. Premature and low-birth-weight babies can receive live vaccines, as can those with previous malignancy who are not currently immunosuppressed. A family history of adverse reaction is not a contraindication.

2. A. Maternal smoking during pregnancy and after pregnancy has been shown to increase the rates of sudden infant deaths. Parents should be counselled about this prior to conception. The infant should be placed supine in a cot or Moses basket to sleep and not in the parental bed. Neonates born very early or late have higher rates of sudden infant death, but this is less of a factor than smoking.

3. B. A spiral fracture suggests a twisting force has been applied to the arm. This is unlikely from falling from a sitting position. A spiral fracture at this age is unusual and raises the suspicion of nonaccidental injury. No previous attendances, immediate presentation at hospital, accounts which match and the attitude of the parents are all reassuring here.

4. C. Emotional abuse can be manifested as persistent and malicious criticism. In this case the girl is made to feel that she is not worthy of ballet lessons like her siblings as she is clumsy and fat. This can lead to behaviour problems and self-esteem and confidence issues in later life.

5. D. At the age of 16, a young person has the same rights to consent as an adult. Therefore she can consent to the treatment irrespective of her parents' wishes; however, it is

good practice for them to be aware of her decision if she agrees. The only difference is that she cannot choose to refuse life-saving treatment until she is 18 years old.

Chapter 20 Accidents and emergencies

1. D. This girl has hypovolaemic shock likely secondary to gastroenteritis. Her observations, clinical status and blood gas analysis imply decompensated shock and urgent intervention is required to prevent irreversible shock and death. An intraosseous needle is likely to be needed due to poor perfusion with aggressive fluid resuscitation (after stabilization of airway and breathing).

2. E. There are no concerns in this case to arouse suspicion for child abuse. Burns involving the face, hands or perineum are an indication for discussion with the regional burns centre and it is very likely they would want to review the child as soon as possible.

3. A. This is the next step in the status epilepticus protocol once intravenous access has been gained. No more than two doses of benzodiazepines should be given to avoid the risk of respiratory depression. The next step on the advanced paediatric life support algorithm is rectal paraldehyde if easily available, otherwise intravenous phenytoin.

4. B. Liver function tests and clotting studies must also be checked as liver failure may occur. Psychiatric evaluation is needed for all children presenting with deliberate poisoning.

5. E. Acute epiglottis is now rare in children following the introduction of the *Haemophilus influenzae* vaccine (*H. influenzae* type b (Hib)) as part of the routine immunizations schedule. It is a life-threatening emergency and securing the airway is of paramount importance prior to intravenous antibiotics. Options A, B and C would risk upsetting the child which can lead to complete airway obstruction. Steroids are of uncertain benefit in epiglottitis and are not routinely used. Following intubation, antibiotic administration is the next priority.

6. B. Insulin drives potassium into cells and therefore serum potassium falls. Intravenous fluids should be given with potassium (i.e., 0.9% sodium chloride and 20 mmol KCl in 500 mL) when treating DKA. Patients with DKA require 6- to 8-hour monitoring of urea and electrolytes and blood gases.

7. C. See Table 20.10 for a summary of other poor prognostic indicators in near drowning.

8. A. Asystole is the commonest cardiac arrest rhythm in children. It is the only drug used in management of nonshockable rhythms, in addition to ongoing cardiopulmonary resuscitation and providing adequate oxygenation. Amiodarone is used after the third and fifth shock in the management of shockable rhythms.

9. B. This girl has clinical features of shock (likely septic shock in view of the high fever). As with any emergency, attention

must be paid towards airway, breathing, circulation, disability, exposure (ABCDE). Her airway is patent and is receiving oxygen. She does, however, have circulatory compromise with tachycardia and delayed capillary refill time (CRT), and therefore requires a fluid bolus, which should be given in 10 mL/kg aliquots up to 40 m/kg prior to asking for PICU assistance. Antibiotics should be given within the first hour.

Chapter 21 Nutrition, fluids and prescribing

1. A. This boy has rickets (vitamin D deficiency) as suggested by the bowing of legs and dental problems. Bone profile will reveal a raised alkaline phosphatase and the serum calcium may or may not be low. The vitamin D level should also be checked.
2. A. The laboratory findings here all point to SIADH. This is a common stress response and in this case is secondary to pneumonia. Other causes of SIADH include central nervous system disease and treatment is by treating the underlying cause and fluid restriction. Diabetes insipidus results in hypernatraemia.
3. A 14-year-old girl is brought to her general practitioner by her mother who is concerned that she has been losing weight. Her weight has dropped noticeably over the past year and she has become increasingly withdrawn. She is very active and plays for her school netball team. She makes her own meals at home, rather than eating with the family. She has not reached menarche. On examination her body mass index is 15 kg/m^2 and fine lanugo hair is noted over her upper body. Which of the following is most likely to be the cause of her weight loss?
   A. Hyperthyroidism
   B. Anorexia nervosa
   C. Malabsorption
   D. Diabetes mellitus
   E. Depression
4. C. This is calculated by: 100 mL/kg for the first 10 kg, 50 mL/kg for the second 10 kg and 20 mL/kg for the remaining kilogram. Therefore, the answer is reached by (100 × 10) + (50 × 10) + (20 × 12) = 1740 mL.
5. E. This is severe DKA as indicated by a pH of <7.1. He has signs of dehydration and likely shock, hence the fluid bolus. The correct management of a child in DKA is to replace the maintenance fluid over 48 hours and to correct any fluid deficit (in this case a severe DKA is estimated to be 10% dehydrated). Fluid given as boluses is not subtracted from the total unless replaced but only anything above 20 mL/kg.

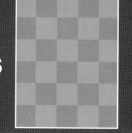

OSCEs and Short Clinical Cases

STATION 1 – HISTORY TAKING

Student instructions

Please take a history from Greg, a 14-year-old boy presenting with abdominal pain and loose stools. You have 8 minutes to complete this. You will be asked for a diagnosis and to answer some follow-up questions.

Patient instructions

You are a 14-year-old boy with a 6-week history of abdominal pain and diarrhoea. It started gradually and is worsening. You are having up to six watery, mucousy stools per day. The stools are brown in colour and flush easily. Previously, you opened your bowels once or twice a day with a formed stool. There is no blood in your stool.

You have intermittent abdominal pain; this is crampy in nature in the lower part of your abdomen, it doesn't radiate. Nothing makes it better or worse.

You're not hungry and you feel exhausted all the time.

You think you've lost weight because you need a belt to hold up your trousers.

Only volunteer if asked:

- You've been having mouth ulcers over the past few weeks making eating painful.
- You've also noted a red skin rash on your shins these past 2 days.

If asked, you have no upper GI symptoms/abdominal distension/arthralgia/visual disturbance/chest pain/reflux/SOB. You also have no perianal symptoms.

Past medical history: You're usually fit and well, you've not been unwell like this before and have never been to hospital.

Drug history: You have no allergies. You take no medications. You take paracetamol but this doesn't really help the pain.

Social History

You're in Year 10 and have started your GCSEs. You want to study engineering. You're worried about the impact of missing school on your GCSEs. You don't drink alcohol or smoke.

Family history: Your maternal half-uncle has ulcerative colitis.

ICE

You have no idea what's wrong. You're worried it's something serious; could it be cancer? You want to get good grades to go to university and missing school due to pain is preoccupying your thoughts. You're also missing going out with your friends in the evenings and at weekends.

Examiner instructions

The student has 8 minutes from the bell to take a history from the patient. At 8 minutes you should stop the student and use the next 3 minutes to ask the questions below. Please use the following mark scheme to assess the student.

Mark scheme

	Inadequate	Attempted	Performed adequately
Introduction	0	0	1
Establishes details of abdominal pain + diarrhoea	0	1 or 2	3
Enquires about associated symptoms	0	1 or 2	3
Enquires about mouth ulcers	0	0	1
Enquires about rash	0	0	1
Takes a Past Medical History	0	0	1
Takes a drug history	0	0	1
Enquires about foreign travel	0	0	1
Enquires about impact on schooling and life	0	0	1
Takes a relevant FH	0	0	1
Communication skills: rapport, active listening, responding to cues, signposting	0	1	2
Enquires about ICE	0	1	2
Patient's marks	0	1	2

Examiner's questions: 1, 2, 3, 4, 5
Total marks: /25

Questions

1. What do you think the diagnosis is?

   Inflammatory bowel disease – specifically Crohn disease
   1 mark

   (Mouth ulcers and perianal disease are highly indicative of Crohn disease, PR bleeding tends to be more indicative of ulcerative colitis).

2. Name two features that differentiate Crohn disease from ulcerative colitis macroscopically and histologically.

   Crohn's: Transmural inflammation, cobblestone mucosa (clustering of ulcers that resembles a cobblestone street), skip lesions, 'Rose-thorn' ulcers, fistulae
   1 mark (0.5 for each)

3. Name two extraintestinal features of inflammatory bowel disease.

   Ankylosing spondylitis, enterohepatic arthritis, skin – erythema nodosum/pyoderma gangrenosum, visual disturbance – uveitis/scleritis.
   1 mark (0.5 for each)

4. What is the initial first-line treatment for inducing remission in Crohn disease?

   Either exclusive enteral nutrition with an elemental or polymeric diet or steroids.
   1 mark

5. Can you explain why a patient with IBD may be anaemic?

   Normocytic anaemia of chronic disease.

   If they've had bowel resected, they may have malabsorption depending on the location, potentially iron, vitamin B12 and folate deficiency. This can result in either a microcytic or macrocytic anaemia
   1 mark for either

STATION 2 – COMMUNICATION

Student instructions

Maria is a 15-year-old girl who has recently been diagnosed with epilepsy. She has had three tonic-clonic seizures over the past 3 months. An ECG, blood tests and CT Head scan are all normal. She will be starting an antiepileptic medication tomorrow.

You have 10 minutes to talk to Maria and explain the diagnosis, the need to start medication and anything important you feel she should be aware of.

Patient instructions

You are a 15-year-old girl. In the past 2 months you have had three generalized tonic-clonic seizures. All of your investigations have so far come back normal and the doctor has diagnosed you with epilepsy.

You don't really understand what epilepsy is, you just know it causes you to have seizures. You'd like it to be explained so that you understand properly. You know you need to take medication but haven't been told anything more. Your main concerns are the impact it'll have on your life as you are a county swimmer. Will it stop you swimming? You're also embarrassed to tell your friends and are worried if you have a seizure in front of them.

You'd be very shocked to hear about needing contraception, you don't have a boyfriend and feel quite embarrassed/offended, but you're pleased that you're now aware.

Questions you'd like to ask:

- Can you drive?
- How long do you need to take the medication for?

Examiner instructions

The student has 10 minutes from the bell to speak to the patient. At 10 minutes you should stop the student and use the next 3 minutes to ask the questions below. Please use the following mark scheme to assess the student.

Introduction	0	1	
Takes a brief history	0	1	
Elicits current understanding through open questions	0	1	2
Elicits worries and concerns regarding the diagnosis	0	1	2
Explains what epilepsy and seizures are	0	1	2
Explain triggers	0	1	
Explain complications of epilepsy	0	1	2
Explain need to start treatment + duration	0	1	
Side effects of treatment	0	1	
Teratogenicity of medication and the need for both barrier and hormonal contraception if sexually active	0	1	
Lifestyle recommendations, e.g., showers not baths, don't lock doors, use of helmets, informing friends	0	1	2
Communication skills: rapport, active listening, responding to cues, signposting	0	1	2
Patient marks	0	1	2

Total: /20

Summary

There are many ways to explain seizures. Here is an example below:

'The brain is constantly sending electrical signals along the nerves in the body containing instructions for your body to move and undertake normal activities. A seizure happens when the electrical signals in the brain misfire causing a temporary disruption to the signals; this is what causes seizures. Epilepsy is diagnosed when a person continues to have seizures with no clear cause. There are different types of seizures involving different parts of the body, they may look frightening to others but usually, they are short-lasting and not painful. Triggers can include bright or flashing lights, sleep deprivation, stress, fever and certain foods'.

There are multiple different types of antiepileptic medications each with their own side effect profile. Generally speaking, most are teratogenic – they have the potential to cause severe birth defects if taken by a woman during pregnancy. Therefore, if a teenager is sexually active, then they should use a hormonal form of contraception and a barrier form (e.g., condoms). If taking a combined oral contraceptive, then often a higher dose may be required. Often, most patients take medications for two years and then reassess, particularly if they have been seizure free but it varies in each individual. Patients should be prepared for medications to be used in the medium to longer term.

It is usually helpful to explain that it is important for friends and family to be aware of their epilepsy and know how to help. Carrying buccal midazolam to terminate a seizure lasting more than 5 minutes is very important. Some family members should have training to use this, and they should know to call 999 if the seizure doesn't stop after this.

From a lifestyle perspective, it's important to not lock doors and to opt for showers rather than baths. The use of helmets is encouraged if riding a bike. If swimming, it is usually advised that there is another adult around who can supervise and knows about the epilepsy.

Patients with epilepsy should notify the DVLA if they want to drive. It may affect someone's ability to drive legally if they have not been seizure free for a certain length of time. It is helpful to look at the latest DVLA advice on their website.

STATION 3 – EXAMINATION

Student instructions

Theo, a 5-year-old boy, is having difficulty climbing the stairs. Please perform a lower limb neurological examination. Please summarize your findings at the end of the examination and give an appropriate differential diagnosis. The examiner will ask you follow-up questions.

Examiner instructions

The student has 8 minutes from the bell to examine the patient. At 8 minutes you should stop the student and use the next 3 minutes to ask the questions below. Please use the following mark scheme to assess the student.

Introduction/consent	0	1	
Ensures the patient is not in pain	0	1	
Assess gait	0	1	
Perform Romberg's test	0	1	
Inspect the lower limbs	0	1	
Assess tone	0	1	2
Assess for clonus	0	1	
Assess power throughout the lower limbs	0	1 or 2	3
Assess lower limb reflexes	0	1	2
Perform heel-shin test	0	1	
Assess light touch sensation	0	1	2
Assess proprioception	0	1	
Assess vibration	0	1	
States would not assess pain or temperature in a child	0	1	
States would plot height and weight on a growth chart	0	1	
Examines opportunistically and professionally	0	1	
Communication – builds rapport, cooperation, explanation	0	1	2
Summarizes key findings	0	1	
Provides the correct diagnosis	0	1	

Examiner's questions: 1, 2, 3, 4, 5

Total: /30

Findings for case and questions:

Theo is a 5-year-old boy with calf hypertrophy on inspection. He walks with a 'waddling' gait indicative of proximal myopathy. He has reduced thigh muscle bulk. His tone is normal but hip flexors are weak with a 4/5 MRC power grading. Knee reflexes are absent. He has normal sensation and coordination. In summary, these findings are consistent with a diagnosis of Duchenne muscular dystrophy.

Questions:

1. What classical sign can be demonstrated when asking the child to stand from sitting position on the floor?

   Gower's sign.

   1 mark

2. How is this condition inherited?

In an X-linked recessive manner with mutations in the dystrophin gene.

1 mark

3. What investigations can help confirm the diagnosis?

Creatine kinase will be raised. Diagnosis can be confirmed by genetic studies of the dystrophin gene.

1 mark

(Previously, muscle biopsy and EMG were used diagnostically prior to the widespread use of genetic testing.)

4. Name two complications that may arise.

Complications include scoliosis, dilated cardiomyopathy, recurrent respiratory infections and restrictive lung disease.

1 mark (0.5 mark each)

5. What is the prognosis for children?

Survival rates have increased over time, but median survival is around 20 years of age. Children lose the ability to walk by their teenage years, using a powered wheelchair for mobility.

1 mark

STATION 4 – HISTORY

Student instructions

You have 7 minutes to take a history from Sarah, who is concerned about her 3-year-old son, Arthur. You will be asked for a diagnosis, and to answer follow-up questions.

Patient instructions

Your son is 3 years old and you've noticed over the past few weeks that he has some bruises and nonblanching spots. You're unsure whether he has fallen over at nursery or how he's got them. He can't remember where they're from. They are distributed across his limbs and back.

Over the past few weeks, he's been tired, looks pale and not interested in running around with his friends at nursery. You've also noticed he seems short of breath. He has told you that his legs hurt. You've not noticed a fever and you're not sure if he's lost weight. He has had two infections in the past 6 weeks – a urine infection and a viral URTI. There has been no active bleeding.

If specifically asked, there are no current headaches, sore throats, cough, coryza, neck lumps, visual disturbance, vomiting, abdominal pain or meningism. You have not noted any abdominal distension or masses.

He is drinking and passing urine but has a reduced appetite.

Past medical History: 37+0 NVD. No NICU, fit and well, growing along the 25th centile for height and weight. No developmental concerns.

Drug history: No allergies and no regular meds. Fully up to date with immunizations.

Social history: You're separated from your husband, though he is fully involved in the children's lives. Arthur has an older sister, Violet who is 5 years old. She is fit and well.

Family history: Nil.

ICE

You hope it's nothing serious, children are often clumsy and it's common to get lots of bugs at this time of year. Hopefully, the doctor can reassure you that this is just simple bruising. You would be shocked and devastated if it was anything significant.

Examiner instructions

The student has 8 minutes from the bell to take a history from the patient. At 8 minutes you should stop the student and use the next 3 minutes to ask the questions below. Please use the following mark scheme to assess the student.

	Inadequate	Attempted	Performed adequately
Introduction	0	0	1
Establishes details of bruising	0	1 or 2	3
Enquires about symptoms of marrow suppression (anaemia/infections/bleeding)	0	1 or 2	3
Enquires about chest and abdominal symptoms	0	1	2
Enquires about recent fever + meningism	0	0	1
Takes a past medical history	0	0	1
Takes a drug history	0	0	1
Enquires about impact on life and nursery	0	0	1
Take a relevant FH, e.g., bleeding disorders	0	0	1
Communication skills: rapport, active listening, responding to cues, signposting, etc.	0	1	2
Enquires about ICE	0	1	2
Patient's marks	0	1	2

Examiners questions: 1, 2, 3, 4, 5
Total marks: /25

Questions:

1. What do you think the diagnosis is?

    Acute lymphoblastic leukaemia.

    1 mark

2. Name two differentials for bruising in a child.

    Immune thrombocytopenic purpura (ITP), platelet function disorders (e.g., Glanzmann thrombasthenia), clotting disorders such as Von Willebrand disease, collagen disorders such as Ehler-Danlos syndrome.

    1 mark (0.5 marks each)

3. What complications are children at risk of when they start induction therapy?

    Tumour lysis syndrome.

    1 mark

4. Which chromosome is associated with a poorer prognosis?

    The Philadelphia chromosome t(9;22).

    1 mark

5. Which classical cells might be visible on a blood film?

    Blast cells.

    1 mark

STATION 5 – COMMUNICATION

Student instructions

Steve's son, Max, was admitted to paediatrics following an anaphylactic reaction to hazelnuts at a friend's house. He required a dose of adrenaline before the symptoms started to improve. He has been observed in hospital for 24 hours and is ready for discharge with an adrenaline autoinjector (EpiPen, Jext or Emrade).

You have 10 minutes to talk to Steve and explain the diagnosis and how to use the adrenaline autoinjector.

Patient instructions

Max is your 4-year-old son who developed wheezing, difficulty breathing, lip and facial swelling and a rash after eating scrambled eggs at a friend's house. 999 were called and they administered adrenaline. The symptoms began to improve in the ambulance on the way to the hospital. He received some more medication in the hospital and was admitted for observation overnight.

No one in your family has allergies so you found it very scary to hear he had gone to hospital with breathing problems. You don't really understand how he had such severe symptoms or really understand how allergies work. Max is usually fit and well.

Your main concern is that it will happen again and it may be worse this time and he could even die. You've never used an 'EpiPen' but are very keen to learn how.

Examiner instructions

The student has 10 minutes from the bell to speak to the patient. At 10 minutes you should stop the student and use the next 3 minutes to ask the questions below. Please use the following mark scheme to assess the student.

Introduction	0	1	
Takes a brief history	0	1	
Elicits current understanding through open questions	0	1	2
Elicits worries and concerns regarding the diagnosis	0	1	2
Explains allergies and anaphylaxis	0	1	2
Explain triggers	0	1	
Explain symptoms and complications	0	1	2
Explain why an EpiPen is needed	0	1	
Explain how to use it	0	1	2
Mention the importance of having 2 pens (one for home and one for nursery)	0	1	
Other recommendations including follow up and avoiding triggers	0	1	2
Communication skills: rapport, active listening, responding to cues, signposting	0	1	2
Patient Marks	0	1	2

Total marks: /21

Summary

Here is an example of how to explain anaphylaxis:

'An allergy is a response by the body's immune system to a substance that is not necessarily harmful in itself. However, some children are sensitive to it and have a reaction when exposed to it. The word anaphylaxis is used to describe a very serious form of allergic reaction which can be life-threatening. Certain foods, insect venoms, medications and latex are common triggers for this reaction. Food is the most common trigger in children.

During anaphylaxis, the immune system goes into overdrive by responding to a trigger, this causes the normal body functions to be completely disrupted.

Symptoms include swelling of the lips, tongue and throat. Breathing problems including wheeze, hoarseness and shortness of breath. Swelling can completely block your airway, meaning oxygen cannot be breathed into the lungs. Some children also develop a red, raised itchy rash'.

It is important to train parents and the child how to use the adrenaline autoinjector – there are three main devices – EpiPen, Jext or Emerade. Children should have two devices (of the same type) – one for use at home and for use at school or nursery. It is important that school staff know how to use these as well. If a parent needs to use the device, this should trigger a 999 call as the child is in anaphylaxis.

To use an adrenaline autoinjector you should:

- Remove the safety cap
- Hold the pen firmly, and move it from about 10 cm away and push strongly into the upper outer thigh (it can be used through cotton clothing in emergencies)
- There will be automatic release of adrenaline into the muscle
- Hold the pen in position for 10 seconds and then release
- Massage the area for 10 seconds

If a child has had an anaphylactic reaction, they should be followed up in an allergy clinic in 6 to 8 weeks. Sometimes, when a child is older, food challenges are considered but in the interim, avoidance of the triggering food is recommended. Antihistamines can be used in the case of more mild reactions. Sometimes reactions can become more severe over time.

STATION 6 – EXAMINATION

Diagnosis: Cystic fibrosis

Student instructions

Albie, a 12-year-old boy, suffers from shortness of breath. Please perform an examination of his respiratory system.

Examiner instructions

The student has 8 minutes from the bell to examine the patient. At 8 minutes you should stop the student and use the next 3 minutes to ask the questions below. Please use the following mark scheme to assess the student.

Introduction and consent	0	1	
General inspection and observation around the bedside	0	1	
Inspects the hands	0	1	2
Examines for a fine and coarse tremor	0	1	2
Checks radial pulse	0	1	2
Inspects the face and mouth	0	1	2

Assess for cervical lymphadenopathy	0	1	2
Examines JVP	0	1	2
Inspects the chest	0	1	
Examines for tracheal deviation	0	1	2
Locates the apex beat	0	1	2
Assess chest expansion correctly (upper and lower lobes anterior and posterior)	0	1	2
Percusses the chest anteriorly and posteriorly	0	1	2
Auscultates the chest anteriorly and posteriorly	0	1	2
Performs vocal resonance	0	1	
Assess for ankles/sacral oedema	0	1	2
States would plot height and weight on a growth chart	0	1	
End pieces – states that they would request oxygen saturations, peak flow, sputum sample	0	1	2
Examines opportunistically and professionally	0	1	
Communication – builds rapport, cooperation, explanation	0	1	2
Summarizes key findings	0	1	
Provides the correct diagnosis	0	1	2

Examiner's questions: 1, 2, 3, 4, 5
Total marks: /42
Findings for case and questions:

Albie is a thin, underweight boy who appears pink. His respiratory rate is 24 and he is noted to be using his accessory muscles. On inspection, clubbing of the fingers and chest hyperexpansion are evident. Occasional, scattered crepitations are heard on auscultation bilaterally. A pot with yellow sputum and vitamin supplements can be seen next to the bed. In summary, these findings are in keeping with a diagnosis of cystic fibrosis and likely infective exacerbation.

Questions:

1. With which respiratory conditions is clubbing associated?

   Cystic fibrosis, bronchiectasis, fibrosing alveolitis, chronic empyema, primary ciliary dyskinesia.

   1 mark

2. Name one nonrespiratory cause of clubbing.

   Atrial myxoma, infective endocarditis, congenital cardiac disease, inflammatory bowel disease.

   1 mark

3. How is this condition inherited?

CF is inherited in an autosomal recessive pattern, defects are in the CF gene on chromosome 7. 1 in 25 people in the UK are carriers.

1 mark

4. How is CF diagnosed?

If asymptomatic (as follows newborn screening; with genetic testing and sweat test); if symptomatic then either sweat test or genetic studies diagnose CF (rarely it can be diagnosed by symptoms alone if these tests are negative).

1 mark

5. Name two nonrespiratory complications of CF.

Pancreatic insufficiency, meconium ileus, nasal polyps, infertility in most males, reduced fertility in females, diabetes mellitus, rectal prolapse, delayed puberty, growth faltering/being underweight, liver disease – portal hypertension, biliary cirrhosis, reduced bone mineral density.

1 mark (0.5 for each)

SAQS

SAQ 1 – The oedematous child

A 3-year-old boy is seen with his mother in the children's assessment unit. He was born at term and is up to date with his vaccinations. She reports that he has had puffy eyes and swollen ankles for one week. He seems more tired than usual but has not had a fever or any other symptoms. The only medical history of note is recurrent tonsillitis. The last episode was around one month ago.

O/E: he is alert and appropriate. He has generalized oedema. Heart sounds are normal and his chest is clear. His abdomen is soft but mildly distended. HR 100, BP 84/40, RR 20, temperature 36.7°C, SpO_2 97%.

a) From the history, what is the most likely diagnosis? (2 marks)
b) What simple investigations could be performed to confirm the diagnosis? (2 marks)
c) What two initial treatments should be commenced and why? (4 marks)
d) Name three complications of this presentation. (3 marks)
e) Give two indications for more invasive investigations. (2 marks)
f) Before discharge, her mother informs you that his sister has had chickenpox for 3 days and that Joseph has never had this himself. Varicella serology confirms this. Does Joseph require any treatment? (5 marks)

SAQ 2 – Child with polydipsia

Sophie is a 6-year-old girl being seen in the Emergency Department with her mother. Her mother has brought her to hospital because she was unable to get a GP appointment. She is worried because Sophie has been extremely thirsty and has been seen drinking from the tap and dog bowl. She also has been passing urine up to 12 times a day which is not normal for her.

a) What are your differentials for this presentation? (3 marks)
b) How would you urgently make a working diagnosis in the Emergency Department? (2 marks)
c) What is the urgency of making a working diagnosis in this presentation? Why is this and what further tests would you need to diagnose it? (5 marks)
d) Can you name three long-term complications of this diagnosis that Sophie will be monitored for all her life? (3 marks)

SAQ 3 – Murmur in a child

Albert is a 6-week-old baby who was born via normal vaginal delivery at term. He has no antenatal concerns nor any postnatal concerns aside from a murmur heard on his newborn examination. Mum was reassured that this can be normal and he will receive a follow-up in 6 to 8 weeks. Albert's mum has brought him to the GP as she is concerned as he has started feeding poorly and hasn't been gaining much weight. His mum notes she can't feed him his full bottle anymore as he needs multiple breaks compared to a few weeks ago.

On examination he is warm, well perfused and alert. He has a notable increased work of breathing that is equal on both sides and no added sounds are heard (saturations 98% in air). On examination of his heart a loud systolic murmur 4/6 is heard over the left lower sternal edge, capillary refill is less than 2 seconds. His abdomen is soft and nontender, but distended and a 3 cm hepatomegaly is felt.

a) What are your differentials for the presentation? What is the most probable diagnosis and why? (2 marks)
b) What bedside investigation will give you the diagnosis of what is happening? (1 mark)
c) What do the symptoms Albert's mum has described indicate? What medications would be used to address this? Will any further treatments be required? (4 marks)
d) Which nonmedical professional would it be appropriate to have early support from when considering his weight loss? (1 mark)

SAQ 4 – The breathless child

Gemma is an 8-year-old girl who was diagnosed with asthma when she was 5 years old. She has been brought into A&E by her parents as her breathing has not been right for the past day or two. Her parents have been helping her use the blue inhaler (Gemma does not have any other coloured inhalers) around 15 times yesterday, but overnight her breathing has gotten worse and they feel she is struggling to breathe.

On examination Gemma is not able to speak in full sentences, she requires supplementary oxygen to keep her saturations around 91% and has both subcostal and intercostal recession with tracheal tug. Her respiratory rate is 50 breaths per minute. Her peak flow is 70 L/min (her best is 225 L/min when well).

a) What is your diagnosis? (2 marks)
b) The attending FY2 performs a capillary blood gas and the following results come back:
    -   pH 7.30, pO$_2$ 11, pCO$_2$ 6, BE -3, lactate 1.9, glucose 6.9.
    Does this change your diagnosis from the above one? Which results do you base this decision upon? (3 marks)
c) What level of severity for this presentation do all of these results indicate? What is the next best step in her management? Who should you inform? (3 marks)
d) At discharge what treatments and advice are important for this presentation? (5 marks)

SAQ 5 – Nonblanching rash

Fiona, an 18-month-old girl has been brought in by her parents to the A&E as they are concerned that their child isn't well. Her parents report she's been under the weather over the past 2 days, and that they feel something has been going around at nursery. She has been off her food and drink, has a fever and her parents have noted today that she has been quieter today. Over the past 3 to 4 hours they have noticed a new rash come out on her legs, which isn't fading with pressure.

Her observations are: HR 165, RR 42, saturations 98% in air, capillary refill time 4 s, BP 90/50, temperature 38.9°C.

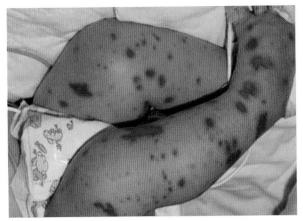

(Source: Srinivas Murthy, Peter N. Cox, Infectious Syndromes in the Pediatric Intensive Care Unit, in Zimmermann, J. Pediatric Critical Care, Fifth Edition, 2017.)

a) From the above – do you think this child is sick? (1 mark)
b) What is your number 1 diagnosis in this child? (2 mark)

c) What are your key management steps – to complete in the first 5 minutes of presenting to the Emergency Department? (6 marks)
d) Give four key investigations. (6 marks)

SAQ 6 – Jaundice in a 4-day-old baby

Jack, a 4-day-old baby, has been referred to the Children's Assessment Unit by the community midwives due to poor feeding and being a bit yellow. Jack was born at 40+1 weeks via normal vaginal delivery. He had no antenatal or postnatal concerns and his newborn exam was normal. Of note his mum's blood group is O+ve.

His observations are normal aside from a mildly raised heart rate. His ability to feed is quite poor as his mum notes he is a bit more tired than previously.

On examination you note he is active and alert, has icteric sclera, the abdomen is soft, nontender, with no organomegaly, no murmurs are auscultated, the work of breathing is normal, the anterior fontanelle is level and the capillary refill is less than 2 seconds.

a) What are the differentials? (2 marks)
b) What investigations would you like to perform and why? Are there any resources you would need for these results, and why? (12 marks)

SAQ 7 – The child with abdominal pain

Sarah is a 4-year-old girl who has been brought to the GP by her parents due to her being picky with her food and complaining of tummy pain on and off. Her mum states she has always been a good eater but over the past 3 months her appetite and fussiness have increased and has been having bouts of loose stools. She is concerned that since Sarah isn't eating enough, she won't be putting on weight and growing.

On further questioning you find out that Sarah's maternal aunt has type 1 diabetes and her paternal grandma has rheumatoid arthritis.

On examination you note Sarah is slim but with a distended abdomen, her abdomen is soft and nontender, her chest and heart sounds are both normal, she appears to have wasting of her buttocks on further inspection.

a) What are the differentials for this presentation and why? (4 marks)
b) What investigations would you use to evaluate the presentation against your differentials? What is your investigation strategy and why? (10 marks)
c) Beyond achieving the diagnosis, what further investigations should be performed to check her general health? (4 marks)
d) What dietary management might be used for the differential diagnoses considered? (4 marks)

SAQ 8 – The child with growing pains

Tom is an 8-year-old boy who has been brought to A&E by his parents because of the pains in his legs. They have seen the GP multiple times and were told these were normal growing pains. The pain often occurs at night and doesn't hurt as much during the day. Tom's appetite of late has been poor and his parents think he has lost some weight. Over the past 2 months, his parents think he has been unlucky as he's had lots of viral infections and some requiring antibiotics.

On examination you see a slim boy who is pale in colour compared to his parents. His chest and heart sounds are normal, his abdomen is soft and nontender but full and distended. There is no bruising or reduced range of motion with either leg, but on general inspection you note a fine petechial rash over his body.

a) What are your differential diagnoses, in what order of probability would you place these? (6 marks)
b) It is difficult getting the blood tests, you have obtained 0.5 mL; Tom's mother asks for a brief period to let Tom calm down. What investigations would you prioritize? (4 marks)

c) Tom's observations are done and it is noted Tom has a temperature of 38.5°C. What result in the investigation you prioritized are you most interested in, and why? (3 marks)

SAQ 9 – The dysmorphic child

Baby Wright is a 1-day-old baby that the midwives have asked you to see on the postnatal ward due to poor feeding and being rather floppy when being held. She was born at 38+1 weeks via normal vaginal delivery. There were no antenatal concerns and her 20-week scan was normal.

Below is a picture of her on examination.

a) State what dysmorphic features are seen above. (5 marks)
b) What is your main differential diagnosis? (1 mark)
c) What else would you like to check for on history and examination? (2 mark)
d) What investigations should be performed in this clinical scenario before discharge? (4 marks)
e) Which specialist would be best placed to manage and coordinate the care of this child? (1 mark)

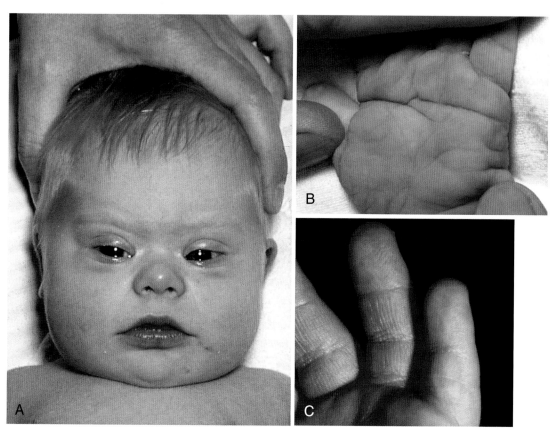

A

B

C

(Source: Zitelli, B. L., & Davis, H. W. [2012]. Atlas of pediatric physical diagnosis [6th ed.]. St. Louis: Mosby)

SAQ 10 – The fitting child

Frank, a 3-year-old child, is brought into the Emergency Department by ambulance having had a 2-minute self-terminating seizure at home witnessed by his mum. He is otherwise fit and well. His aunt has epilepsy which is under control. Developmentally, he is normal and his immunizations are up to date.

His examination is largely normal aside from an erythematous pharynx and palpable lymph nodes on the anterior cervical chain.

His observations show that he is mildly tachycardic and has a mild temperature of 37.9°C.

a) What are your top two differential diagnoses? What extra questions would you ask in the history to help distinguish these? (5 marks)

b) Frank has repeated observations which show he has a temperature of 38.5°C, a nurse contacts informs you asking if you could prescribe an antipyretic (paracetamol) as Frank is miserable with the fever. You prescribe this but are urgently called because Frank is having a further seizure. As you attend Frank with the nurse, the nurse is very upset and asks if the seizure is because the antipyretic hadn't been given – what would you answer? (1 mark)

c) Frank continues to seize, the nurse has applied oxygen to Frank and asks what the next management will be – what single investigation will you ask for and what treatment will you request? (3 marks)

SAQ answers

1.

   a. Nephrotic syndrome; would also consider angioedema – either allergic or hereditary angioedema.

      i. See Chapters 6 and 11.

   b. Urinalysis – demonstrating heavy proteinuria and blood albumin – demonstrating hypoalbuminaemia (nephrotic syndrome think HOP; hypoalbuminaemia, oedema, proteinuria).

   c. Prednisolone (to induce remission – or to establish that is not responsive, and not consistent with minimal change disease, prompting consideration of renal biopsy and use of other agents – cyclophosphamide, tacrolimus, ciclosporin or levamisole) and penicillin V (to reduce the risk of secondary bacterial infection – notably with *Streptococcus pneumoniae*).

   d. Hypovolaemia (oliguria, peripheral vasoconstriction, raised packed cell volume and hypotension), infection (typically *Streptococcus pneumoniae*), thrombosis. (Nephrotic syndrome – HOP, see above – complications = HIT hypovolaemia, infection, thrombosis).

   e. Renal biopsy should be considered in children presenting with nephrotic syndrome who: are aged <1 or >12; fail to

respond to steroid therapy, develop renal failure, present with hypertension, a low C3, or frank haematuria.

   f. Yes; the concern will be of Joseph developing chickenpox – this is an indication of using varicella zoster immunoglobulin (VZIG); were Joseph to present with chickenpox, one should consider the use of aciclovir. VZIG use is authorized by a virologist. It would be prudent to discuss the case and results with a virologist.

      i. Whilst varicella vaccines exist, current guidance advocates their use either for nonimmune healthcare workers or healthy susceptible contacts of immunocompromised individuals (e.g., nonimmune siblings of a child being treated for leukaemia, or nonimmune children of a parent undergoing chemotherapy).

      ii. See Chapter 10.

2.

   a. Diabetes mellitus; this would be the most likely diagnosis in a child presenting at this age; 95% of childhood diabetes mellitus is type 1. Type 2 diabetes mellitus is more common in children with certain risk factors (obesity, family history, south Asian or Afro-Caribbean heritage and female sex). On closer questioning one would expect a history of weight loss and tiredness.

      i. Diabetes insipidus. Nephrogenic diabetes insipidus is rare and most cases in childhood are hereditary and would be unlikely in a presentation at this age; Central diabetes insipidus is most commonly idiopathic, but if confirmed would require neuroimaging to exclude intracranial disease, including infiltrating pituitary disease.

      ii. Psychogenic polydipsia; increased intake of fluids.

      iii. A urinary tract infection might cause polyuria but not polydipsia to the extent in this presentation – it should be considered as infection that can coexist in presentations of diabetes mellitus.

      iv. See Chapter 7.

   b. The most important diagnosis not to miss in this presentation is diabetes mellitus; this can be recognized by either:

      i. Urinalysis; in diabetes mellitus, one would expect this to show glycosuria +/–ketonuria, equally; urinalysis could exclude the possibility of a urinary tract infection.

      ii. Capillary glucose test >11.1 mmol/L (or >7 mmol/L if fasted).

      iii. And if confirmed diagnostic investigations can be collected and treatment commenced.

   c. Diabetic ketoacidosis (DKA) is a life-threatening complication of diabetes mellitus, ~40% of children presenting with a new diagnosis of diabetes mellitus are in DKA. DKA diagnosed by hyperglycaemia (to diagnose diabetes mellitus; >11.1 or >7.1 if fasted), metabolic acidosis (pH <7.3 or HCO_3 <15) and ketonaemia (blood ketones)>3 mmol/L

    i. See Chapter 20.

  d. Cardiovascular disease, retinopathy, nephropathy, neuropathy, risk of DKA and hypoglycaemia.

3.

  a. The presentation is of respiratory distress – intriguingly with an unremarkable chest examination and normal saturations; in the context of previously recognized murmur becoming more apparent.

    i. Congenital heart disease; is going to be the lead differential; with either pressure or volume overload causing cardiac failure. In this case, the child is not cyanosed and is 6 weeks old – this would argue against pressure overload causes (obstructive lesions – coarctation of the aorta, tend to present in neonates). Volume overload (left-right shunts) present at this age is commonly a manifestation of either a ventricular septal defect or a persistent ductus arteriosus.

    ii. Respiratory disease; whilst respiratory conditions such as bronchiolitis are common, one would expect the presentation to demonstrate chest signs (wheeze and crackles) and reduced oxygen saturations. Importantly, the presence of chest signs would not exclude congenital heart disease – children presenting at this age with respiratory distress and a murmur always require careful consideration as to whether a cardiac cause may be responsible and is a not uncommon reason for requiring an inpatient echocardiogram.

  b. Echocardiogram

    i. Other investigations – ECG and chest X-ray may well be normal in cases of VSD.

  c. The presentations are suggestive of cardiac failure, with hepatomegaly and respiratory distress. Early presentations can be the result of a respiratory infection, and one should consider this carefully.

    i. Diuretics; furosemide, spironolactone and in some cases, ACE inhibitors are used to control these symptoms.

    ii. Many ventricular septal defects close spontaneously; close oversight and medical management allow safe determination of the need for closure of the VSD.

  d. Dietician

    i. See Chapter 3.

4.

  a. Asthma – life-threatening asthma.

  b. No, the result is consistent with asthma. The raised carbon dioxide in the context of tachypnoea (one would

expect this to be blown off' and low; it is not) implies tiring and is a grave sign – urgent treatment is required, with close observation to manage ongoing deterioration despite treatment.

    i. A differential of respiratory distress will be diabetic ketoacidosis (DKA) with Kussmaul breathing – this would cause hyperglycaemia, with a raised blood sugar level (however, salbutamol and steroids can also cause hyperglycaemia, blood ketones can be helpful in distinguishing between this iatrogenic hyperglycaemia and DKA).

  c. The peak flow rate is <33% of predicted; the oxygen saturations are <92% in supplemental oxygen indicating life-threatening asthma.

    i. There are further markers of this severity on the presentation; poor respiratory effort and fatigue are suggested from the history and inability to complete sentences; the blood gas result supports this interpretation, with hypercarbia – raised carbon dioxide in the context of tachypnoea.

    ii. Initial treatment should be with 'back:back', typically 3, nebulized bronchodilators – failing to improve is an indication of a very severe presentation; intravenous bronchodilators and steroids are likely to be required (IV magnesium sulphate, IV hydrocortisone; further IV bronchodilators – aminophylline or salbutamol may well be required).

    iii. This presentation mandates a discussion with your senior and consultant – the presentation is life-threatening, and despite optimum treatment may well continue to deteriorate needing critical care support.

  d. The presentation has been of life-threatening asthma.

    i. No preventers are in use – they should be commenced – inhaled corticosteroids (brown inhalers).

    ii. It is important to explain that the inhaled corticosteroids (brown inhalers) take some weeks before they take effect – they need to be taken every day and will have no effect if only used acutely when the child is unwell.

    iii. The presentation with life-threatening asthma implies a lack of understanding of severity (at best, if this were a recurrent occurrence, then it is evidence of life-threatening neglect – child abuse). It is important to provide, explain and document a written asthma plan – including management of exacerbations – using six puffs of the blue inhaler when required; if needing this more frequently than every 4 hours – the child should be taken to the Emergency Department and can be given ten puffs before leaving the house to the Emergency Department.

    iv. See Chapters 3 and 20

5.

a. Yes; critically ill.

b. Sepsis – meningococcal sepsis is perhaps the most likely cause. The incidence of this has fallen since routine immunization has been introduced, but vaccine failure still occurs (even if the vaccine has been administered).

c. Apply oxygen and call for help – ask for a medical emergency 'Crash call' to be placed – this is a prearrest presentation.

   i. Assess the airway and breathing, immediate support is not required; it is very likely that the child will require rapid sequence intubation and ventilation as a result of the illness and urgent treatments that are required.

   ii. Circulation: insert two wide bore cannulae, take investigations, give a fluid bolus 10 mL/kg, give broad-spectrum antibiotics (IV ceftriaxone or cefotaxime) and glucose if hypoglycaemic on blood gas.

   iii. (A helpful mnemonic is ABC, Don't Ever Forget the Glucose, no LP, PIC.)

d. Blood culture, blood gas, clotting, U&E, calcium, FBC, LFT, CRP, meningococcal PCR, throat swab.

   i. A blood culture is essential to aid diagnosis and tailor treatment, before antibiotics are given – if at all possible. If antibiotics have been given, the meningococcal PCR and throat swab (if taken shortly after antibiotics have been given) can still be diagnostic. Diagnosis has public health implications. (Score 3 marks)

   ii. Score 1 mark for any of the other investigations, up to a maximum total of 4:

   iii. The blood gas result is available in minutes, and contains a glucose level – this is often deranged – low, requiring urgent treatment. The blood gas also provides a baseline to appraise response to treatment.

   iv. Clotting is frequently deranged, and requires treatment with vitamin K.

   v. Potassium and calcium homeostasis are often deranged – requiring urgent treatment (both of these should be available on the blood gas result).

   vi. The white blood count may be normal or low – implying a poor response to the infection, and a graver prognosis.

   vii. LFT and CRP provide a baseline to evaluate response to treatment over the following days.

   viii. See Chapter 20.

6.

a. Neonatal jaundice (ABO incompatibility haemolytic jaundice should be considered, if excluded then physiological jaundice).

   i. Sepsis – this is less likely by the infant being alert and active with an examination (other than jaundice) being unremarkable – but should always be considered.

b. Bilirubin (total): to determine the need and nature of treatment (no treatment required, phototherapy, intravenous immunoglobulin – depending upon other tests and exchange transfusion). Often a result is available on a blood gas sample – more quickly than a formal laboratory sample.

   i. Glucose: infants who are jaundiced often feed poorly and may need further oversight or support.

   ii. Direct antigen test: if this is positive, then, depending upon the bilirubin level, one might consider intravenous immunoglobulin (IVIG) in addition to other treatments.

   iii. FBC: evaluate for possible (haemolytic) anaemia.

   iv. The bilirubin result needs to be interpreted against the treatment threshold graphs (which are different for infants of different gestations); hosted on the NICE guidance 'Jaundice in newborn babies under 28 days', many departments will have this as a 'bilirubin chart'.

   v. The first threshold line is for phototherapy; having exceeded this threshold, phototherapy should be commenced; depending upon the direct antigen test, and response to phototherapy, IVIG may also be indicated.

   vi. The second threshold is for exchange transfusion.

   vii. See Chapter 15.

7.

a. Coeliac disease. Growth faltering, with buttock wasting; in the context of a family history of autoimmune disease is a classical presentation of coeliac disease. (2 marks)

   i. Growth faltering with frequent loose stools would also suggest consideration of inflammatory bowel disease as a differential. (1 mark)

   ii. Infection; infective colitis is possible, but perhaps less likely to cause growth faltering; following gastroenteritis, transient lactose intolerance can occur, but tends to last for 6 to 8 weeks. (1 mark)

b. A coeliac screen; Ig A tissue transglutamase; if this is positive (more than 10 × above upper reference) and endomyseal antibodies are present – a biopsy (endoscopy) is not required for diagnosis.

   i. If the tissue transglutamase is positive, but not to this level, or endomyseal antibodies are not detected, a biopsy (OGD endoscopy) is required.

   ii. If the coeliac screen is negative, then inflammatory bowel disease or infection is more possible – in the context of frequent loose stools and growth faltering.

   iii. Faecal calprotectin, stool culture CRP, LFT, FBC. If these suggest inflammation and no infective cause, then one needs to resolve the possibility of inflammatory bowel disease, ultimately with endoscopy.

c. FBC (possible anaemia), LFT (can show elevated transaminases), B12 + folate (possible deficiencies), ferritin, bone profile (possible deficiencies).
d. Coeliac disease; gluten-free diet. (2 marks)
    i. Inflammatory bowel disease; elemental diet.
    ii. Growth faltering or identified deficiencies not as a consequence of either, dietetic nutritional support, possible lactose-free diet, iron or folate supplementation.

8.
a. Acute leukaemia; as a cause for nocturnal limb pains, petechial rash (thrombocytopaenia), weight loss and frequent infections.
    i. Idiopathic thrombocytopaenic purpura (ITP) is possible – but the limb pains, weight loss and frequent infections make this less likely.
    ii. Sepsis; a generalized petechial rash, particularly if spreading, or in the context of temperature, should make one consider the possibility of sepsis.
    iii. Growing pains; whilst possible, this must be a diagnosis of exclusion in this case, with the petechial rash (suggesting thrombocytopaenia) and weight loss.
b. FBC and film; is there evidence of pancytopaenia and blasts – suggesting leukaemia, is there only a reduced platelet count (thrombocytopaenia) suggesting ITP, are the results – reassuringly normal. This would be the priority investigation. (4 marks)
    i. Alternate answers: If any non blanching rash has a normal platelets, a clotting would be suggested. With the history of a petechial rash and frequent infections, a CRP would be an acceptable request, especially if there is any suspicion of fever.
    ii. A blood culture would be important, but since there is no plan to commence antibiotics, and the result will not be available for over 36 hours, this can be deferred. (1/2 mark)
    iii. CRP might be helpful when considering sepsis – but the urgency of treatment for sepsis should be based upon the clinical assessment; CRP does not resolve the other differentials. (1/2 mark)
c. Neutrophil count; if neutropaenic, should consider the possibility of neutropaenic sepsis; obtain blood cultures and commence treatment with broad-spectrum antibiotics – this most probable in the presentation. (3 marks)
    i. Or, CRP; if elevated consider sepsis – however, the antibiotics used in febrile neutropaenia tend to be different to those used for possible sepsis – one is potentially undertreating an infection. (1/2 mark)

9.
a. Upward slant of canthal folds of the eye; possibly tongue protrusion, short neck.
    i. straight simian crease
    ii. short little finger, not extending beyond the distal joint of the ring finger
b. Down syndrome.
c. Cardiac examination; clinical evidence for congenital heart disease (murmurs).
    i. vomiting; need to consider duodenal atresia
d. Confirmatory tests of the clinical Down syndrome diagnosis; rapid chromosomal analysis by follicular in situ hybridization (FISH) and karyotype to confirm the result. (3 marks)
    i. Echocardiogram and cardiac review. (1 mark)
e. Community paediatrician and multidisciplinary team.

10.
a. Febrile convulsion (simple febrile convulsion); seizure in the context of fever with normal development. However, would wish to know if there are risk factors for epilepsy (see below). (1 mark)
    i. Epilepsy – unmasked by fever. (1 mark)
    ii. Are there risk factors for epilepsy – which has been unmasked by the temperature; is there a history of premature birth or admission to the neonatal unit, have there been any significant head injuries (requiring neuroimaging or admission), is there a history of meningitis (might there be an epileptogenic focus as a result). (3 marks)
b. Antipyretics do not prevent febrile convulsions, they are used in children who have fever and distress.
c. Investigation: a child who is fitting, having attended to the ABCs – Don't Ever Forget Glucose; a blood sugar level should be obtained – either by capillary blood test, or when an IV cannula has been inserted. (1 mark)
d. Treatment – benzodiazepine (midazolam by buccal administration, or IV lorazepam) should be given if a seizure continues for more than 5 minutes. (2 marks)

Acute epiglottitis Life-threatening emergency; caused by infection with *Haemophilus influenzae* leading to inflammation of the epiglottis and upper air way obstruction.

Acute glomerulonephritis Acute inflammation of the glomeruli leading to fluid retention, hypertension, haematuria and proteinuria.

Acute otitis media An acute inflammation of the middle ear due to a viral or bacterial infection.

Apnoea of prematurity Episodes of apnoea seen in preterm infants due to immaturity of the respiratory centre.

Attention deficit hyperactivity disorder A condition characterized by lack of attention beyond normal for the child's age, hyperactivity and impulsiveness.

Autistic spectrum disorder A range of conditions usually with onset earlier than 3 years, characterized by impaired social interaction, impaired communication and a restricted pattern of behaviour.

Breath-holding attacks Episodes characterized by a screaming infant or toddler holding his/her breath in expiration, goes blue and limp for a few seconds followed by rapid recovery.

Bronchiolitis Acute inflammation leading to narrowing of the bronchioles and lower airways, most commonly caused by respiratory syncytial virus.

Caput succedaneum Diffuse swelling of the scalp in a neonate that crosses the suture lines, caused by oedema.

Cephalohematoma Subperiosteal haemorrhage into the scalp bones in a neonate, usually associated with birth trauma.

Cerebral palsy A disorder of motor function due to a nonprogressive lesion of the developing brain; the manifestations may evolve as the child grows, although the lesion itself remains the same.

Chronic lung disease of prematurity Preterm infant needing oxygen beyond 36 weeks' corrected gestation or beyond 28 days of age.

Congenital adrenal hyperplasia A group of disorders caused by a defect in the pathway that synthesizes cortisol from cholesterol, often presenting with female virilization, salt wasting and cortisol deficiency.

Craniosynostosis premature fusion of the cranial sutures.

Croup Acute inflammation of the upper airways (larynx, trachea and bronchi) most commonly caused by parainfluenza virus.

Cushing syndrome Syndrome caused by glucocorticoid excess either due to exogenous replacement or endogenous overproduction, characterized by short stature, truncal obesity, skin striae and hypertension.

Developmental dysplasia of the hip Progressive malformation of the hip joint leading to varying degrees of acetabular dysplasia and dislocation of the femoral head; previously known as 'congenital dislocation of the hip'.

Exomphalos Abdominal contents herniate through the umbilical ring, covered in a sac formed by the peritoneum and amniotic membrane.

Febrile convulsions Seizure episode associated with fever in a child between 6 months and 6 years of age in the absence of intracranial infection or any other neurological disorder.

Gastroschisis A developmental defect of the abdomen where whole or part of the bowel and viscera, without a covering sac, protrude through a defect in the abdomen adjacent to the umbilicus.

Gillick competence A child under 16 years of age can be deemed 'Gillick competent' if they have sufficient maturity and understanding to be able to give informed consent for a particular investigation or treatment.

Global developmental delay A significant delay in two or more developmental domains.

Guillain-Barré syndrome Acute demyelinating polyneuropathy, often following a viral or bacterial infection, typically characterized by hyporeflexia and an ascending paralysis.

Haemolytic-uraemic syndrome Clinical syndrome caused by verocytotoxin-producing *Escherichia coli* O157:H7, resulting in microangiopathic haemolytic anaemia, thrombocytopaenia and renal failure.

Haemophilia A X-linked recessive coagulation disorder due to reduced or absent factor VIII.

Haemophilia B X-linked recessive disorder of coagulation caused by deficiency of factor IX.

Henoch-Schönlein purpura A multisystem vasculitis of small blood vessels, affecting skin, kidneys, joints and the gastrointestinal tract.

Idiopathic thrombocytopenic purpura Immune-mediated destruction of platelets leading to thrombocytopaenia, for which no other cause is evident.

Inborn errors of metabolism Any inherited disorder that results from a defect in the normal biochemical pathways.

Infantile colic Recurrent episodes of inconsolable crying of unknown aetiology, often accompanied by drawing up of the legs, seen in the first few months of life.

Infantile spasms (West syndrome) A rare kind of epilepsy that has its onset in late infancy and is characterized by myoclonic spasms and a typical electroencephalogram (hypsarrhythmia).

Irritable hip Transient inflammation of the lining of the hip joint (transient synovitis), usually following a viral infection.

Juvenile idiopathic arthritis Arthritis involving one or more joints in a child, persisting for more than 6 weeks after excluding other causes; previously known as juvenile chronic arthritis/juvenile rheumatoid arthritis.

Kawasaki disease A systemic vasculitis causing fever, redness of eyes, lymphadenopathy, mucosal involvement and rash with a potential for late coronary aneurysms.

Legg-Calve-Perthes disease Idiopathic avascular osteonecrosis of the femoral head seen in children between 3 and 12 years of age.

Low birthweight Weight less than 2500 g.

Muscular dystrophies Group of disorders characterized by progressive degeneration of muscle in the absence of any storage material.

Necrotizing enterocolitis Inflammation and necrosis of the intestine, commonly seen in preterm infants and often predisposed by early and rapid introduction of formula feeds.

Neonatal encephalopathy A combination of abnormal consciousness, tone and reflexes, respirations, feeding and seizures in the early neonatal period due to various reasons, not necessarily from intrapartum asphyxia.

Neonatal screening This is done by the neonatal spot blood test, screening for phenylketonuria, hypothyroidism, cystic fibrosis, medium-chain acyl-coenzyme A dehydrogenase deficiency and certain haemolytic anaemias.

Nephrotic syndrome Clinical condition characterized by proteinuria, hypoalbuminaemia and oedema.

Neural tube defect Range of conditions caused by a failure of fusion of the neural plate, resulting in defects of the vertebra and/or the spinal cord.

Neurodegenerative disease Disorders of the central nervous system characterized by delayed development and a loss of acquired skills (developmental regression).

Nocturnal enuresis Involuntary voiding of urine during sleep beyond 5 years of age.

Otitis media with effusion Persistent fluid in the middle ear due to recurrent middle ear infections or poor eustachian tube ventilation.

Patent ductus arteriosus A vessel connecting the aorta to the left pulmonary vein that usually closes a few hours after birth.

Persistent fetal circulation High pulmonary vascular resistance leading to right to left shunt across the duct and at the atrial level, in the absence of any other congenital heart defect.

Physiological jaundice of the newborn Jaundice occurring between 2 and 14 days of life, in a term infant characterized by predominantly unconjugated hyperbilirubinaemia and a total bilirubin less than 350 μmol/L, in the absence of other causes.

Preterm Less than 37 completed weeks' gestation.

Pyelonephritis Infection of the upper urinary tract involving the renal pelvis.

Pyrexia of unknown origin Documented protracted fever for more than 7 days without a diagnosis despite initial investigations.

Reflex anoxic seizures Episodes, usually provoked by pain, where an infant or toddler turns pale and loses consciousness, sometimes associated with a few jerky movements followed by rapid recovery.

Respiratory distress syndrome Respiratory distress, usually in a preterm infant, due to surfactant deficiency.

Retinopathy of prematurity Abnormal vascular proliferation of the retina occurring in preterm infants in response to various injuries, especially hyperoxia.

School refusal An unwillingness to attend school, usually due to separation anxiety, stressors like bullying or adverse life events; these children usually tend to be good academically, but oppositional at home.

Short stature A height below 0.4th centile for age.

Slipped upper femoral epiphysis Uncommon condition characterized by progressive slippage of the femoral head from the neck at the epiphysis, most commonly seen in obese teenagers.

Small for gestational age Birth weight less than 10th centile for gestational age.

Still disease A systemic variant of juvenile rheumatoid arthritis characterized by high fever, typical rash, lymphadenopathy, hepatosplenomegaly and serositis.

Stridor Predominantly inspiratory noise due to narrowing of the extrathoracic airways.

Tetralogy of Fallot Cyanotic congenital heart disease characterized by a large ventricular septal defect, pulmonary stenosis, overriding of the aorta and right ventricular hypertrophy.

Thalassaemia A group of haemolytic anaemias characterized by defective globin chain synthesis.

Transient tachypnoea of the newborn A transient condition characterized by tachypnoea and respiratory distress due to delayed reabsorption of lung fluid.

Transposition of great arteries Cyanotic congenital heart disease where the aorta arises from the right ventricle and the pulmonary artery arises from the left ventricle, usually associated with an atrial septal defect, ventricular septal defect or a patent ductus arteriosus.

Wheeze Predominantly expiratory noise due to obstruction of the intrathoracic airways.

Note: Page numbers followed by *f* indicate figures, *t* indicate tables, and *b* indicate boxes.